Psychology in Counselling and Therapeutic Practice

Psychology in Counselling and Therapeutic Practice

Jill D. Wilkinson

and

Elizabeth A. Campbell

with contributions by

Adrian Coyle
Alyson Davis

JOHN WILEY & SONS
Chichester · New York · Weinheim · Brisbane · Singapore · Toronto

Other Wiley Editorial Offices

John Wiley & Sons, Inc., 605 Third Avenue,
New York, NY 10158-0012, USA

VCH Verlagsgesellschaft mbH
Pappelallee 3, 0-69469 Weinheim, Germany

Jacaranda Wiley Ltd, 33 Park Road, Milton,
Queensland 4064, Australia

John Wiley & Sons (Asia) Pte Ltd, 2 Clementi Loop #02-01,
Jin Xing Distripark, Singapore 129809

John Wiley & Sons (Canada) Ltd, 22 Worcester Road,
Rexdale, Ontario M9W 1L1, Canada

Library of Congress Cataloging-in-Publication Data

Wilkinson, Jill.
    Psychology in counselling and therapeutic practice / Jill D.
  Wilkinson and Elizabeth Campbell ; with contributions by Adrian
  Coyle, Alyson Davis.
        p.   cm.
    Includes bibliographical references (p.   ) and index.
    ISBN 0-471-95562-0 (pbk. : alk. paper)
    1. Counseling.   2. Psychotherapy.   I. Campbell, Elizabeth.
II. Coyle, Adrian.   III. Davis, Alyson.   IV. Title.
BF637.C6W55   1997
150—dc20   96-32463
                                                                        CIP

British Library Cataloguing in Publication Data

A catalogue record for this book is available from the British Library

ISBN 0-471-95562-0

Typeset in 10/12pt Times by Saxon Graphics Ltd, Derby
Printed and bound in Great Britain by Bookcraft (Bath) Ltd
This book is printed on acid-free paper responsibly manufactured from sustainable forestation, for which at least two trees are planted for each one used in paper production.

Contents

For Florence, Isla and Keith

About the Authors

Jill Wilkinson is a practising Chartered Counselling Psychologist and Lecturer in the Department of Psychology at the University of Surrey,. where she is Director of the three year post-graduate Practitioner Doctorate course in Psychotherapeutic and Counselling Psychology. She divides her time equally between her university work and her own independent therapy practice and holds an Honorary NHS appointment. She has been active in the development of Counselling Psychology in Britain and has served on the Executive Committee of the Division of Counselling Psychology of the British Psychological Society and as Chief Examiner for the BPS Diploma in Counselling Psychology.

Elizabeth Campbell is a Senior Lecturer in Clinical Psychology in the Department of Psychological Medicine, University of Glasgow. She has been very involved with post-graduate professional training in therapeutic and clinical psychology. She is an Honorary Consultant Clinical Psychologist with a Glasgow NHS Trust and also a member of the Board of Examiners of the Division of Counselling Psychology of the BPS. Her clinical and research interests include post-traumatic reactions and stress in the emergency services. She has recently co-authored (with Jennifer Brown) *Stress and Policing* (Wiley).

Adrian Coyle is a lecturer in the Department of Psychology at the University of Surrey and Research Tutor for the Practitioner Doctorate in Psychotherapeutic and Counselling Psychology. His research interests include coping with transition, identity, mental health issues and psychosocial aspects of HIV/AIDS. He has worked in the NHS as an HIV counsellor and has also fulfilled counselling roles within various voluntary organizations.

Alyson Davis is a lecturer in psychology in the Department of Psychology at the University of Surrey and Course Director of the BSc Honours Degree course in Psychology. Her research interests include: areas of children's social cognition, such as the assessment of children's imagination and childhood fears and children's understanding of hospitalization and medical procedures; children's representations (drawing, writing and number); and the relationship between early mathematical thinking and education.

The book was conceived and written by Jill Wilkinson and Elizabeth Campbell, with Alyson Davis and Adrian Coyle contributing to Chapters 8 and 9 respectively, and Adrian Coyle contributing to Chapter 7.

Preface

As counsellors, therapists and psychologists we derive our understandings of our clients, their problems and their presenting concerns from a variety of sources: from literature and philosophy, from our own personal experiences and, of course, from formal psychological theory. Most counsellors will be familiar with the major group of theories which traditionally inform therapeutic practice: humanistic theory, psychodynamic theory and cognitive behavioural theory. But there is also a much broader body of psychological knowledge which can contribute an important additional dimension to our understanding. It is this literature which forms the substance of this volume. We have selected the core topics in psychological theory and research and presented them in such a way as to be of particular relevance to the counsellor, therapist or trainee in the field. It is hoped that this literature will facilitate the counsellors' understanding of their clients, of themselves as counsellors and of the therapeutic process.

Throughout, we have used illustrative case history material to demonstrate how theory and research might inform practice. In so doing, we are, of necessity, offering one particular perspective on the examples in question. This is not to say that this is the best or the only way to understand the material. Indeed, there are usually a multitude of explanations or interpretations that could be made for any one example and those presented in this book are intended to be neither exhaustive nor prescriptive. We do however hope that the particular perspectives offered will shed a new or different light on the way in which such case history material can be conceptualized and possibly lead to new insights and understandings.

Where we have drawn from real-life case material, details have been changed to protect the anonymity of the clients. In such instances, clients have given their explicit consent to the use of the material.

Throughout this volume we will be referring to counsellors and to therapists, to counselling and to therapy. We have done this for purely pragmatic reasons. At the time of writing, the whole area of counselling and therapy is going through a period of growth and change. Some confusion is inevitable. We do not intend to add to this confusion but consider that there are some central tasks and concerns that are common to both of these two professional groups and activities.

This book is intended for all those involved in the practice of counselling and therapy. This will include counsellors and therapists accredited or recognized by bodies such as the British Association for Counselling (BAC) and the United Kingdom Council of Psychotherapists (UKCP), counsellors, therapists and counselling

psychologists in training and also those engaged in counselling as part of their professional activities. Such people might include occupational therapists, general practitioners,
teachers, psychiatric and community psychiatric nurses as well as counsellors working
in voluntary settings.

We would like to thank all those who have contributed to this book: Jonathan Chase
for his work on Chapters 5 and 7; Ian Davies and Lynne Milward for their helpful comments on Chapters 4 and 5 respectively; our families, friends and animals for their support, and, most importantly, our clients who have given their permission for the use of
the case material.

1

Psychology and Counselling

CONTENTS

1.1 INTRODUCTION

This chapter introduces the reader to the discipline of psychology; how it relates to common-sense understandings of human nature, and how the processes of formulating, testing and evolving our own implicit theories which we adopt in our everyday lives have been developed and refined into the methods employed in psychological research.

As counsellors and therapists, we use psychological theory both implicitly and explicitly in our work with clients. Our 'intuitive' understandings are usually derived from our own implicit theories and our more systematic formulations from explicit psychological theory.

This theme of the relationship between implicit and formal theory continues as we go on to look at the main theoretical perspectives in psychology: psychodynamic, behavioural, cognitive, humanistic and biological.

In order to present the reader with a comprehensive overview of the discipline in which to locate the contents of this volume, we will then outline the major research areas in psychology and the main fields of applied and professional psychology. The chapter ends with a brief summary of the book as a whole.

1.2 THE RELATIONSHIP BETWEEN IMPLICIT AND FORMAL THEORY

During the course of our everyday lives we are constantly looking for explanations and striving to understand the thoughts, feelings, actions and motives of ourselves and others. Everybody does this to a greater or lesser degree. It is not just the preserve of the counsellor or psychologist. We all have our own 'theories' about human nature and human functioning. These are sometimes called **implicit theories**. Many people will not have given much thought to the matter nor will have ever tried to articulate their own particular theoretical perspective, but it is evident from our everyday conversation that such theories exist.

Take the following scene; four or so people in an office or changing room at a sports club are talking about a rather shy person (John R) whom they all know and whom they have **observed** as having some difficulty.

A   *It always seems to me that he's really unsure of himself—somehow frightened of committing himself. I think it's got something to do with the fact that his father died when he was a baby. His mother must have had a really bad time of it—dealing with losing a husband and coping with a new baby at the same time. Although he probably doesn't remember it, I'm sure it must have affected him.*

B   *I think it's more likely to do with the fact that he's never learned to stand up for himself—It's as if he always has to say the 'right' thing or we won't like him. Have you met his mother? They seem very fond of each other but she's terribly overbearing—always has to be right.*

C   *I'm sure he's never really felt accepted or allowed to be himself—that must have affected him.*

D   *Well I think it's just the way he is. He was probably born that way. I bet his father was exactly the same.*

Here we have four different **explanations** of how this particular person has come to be as he is. Implicit in each of the statements made by the four people are different assumptions about the development of the personality.

A   *explains it in terms of a disruption in his early family relationships brought about by his father's untimely death. This view is based on the assumption that early experiences and relationships are important, even if the person has no recollection of them.*

B   *gives an explanation in terms of John never having 'learned' particular behaviours he considers necessary to function effectively. He also believes that John's evaluation of the possible consequences of behaving otherwise (that others' will not like him if he does not say what they expect to hear) has relevance. 'B' clearly believes in the importance of learning in the development of the person and also in the effect of perceived consequences on behaviour.*

C   *also sees environmental influences as significant, but this time the emphasis is on the importance of acceptance to the development of the person.*

D   *explains things in terms of genetic inheritance, taking the view that environmental influences have little or no effect and that it is all down to biology; nature rather than nurture which determines how people are and why they act as they do.*

These, as we might anticipate, are the views represented by the major theoretical approaches to the development of the **personality** in psychology. (Which will be discussed in detail in Chapter 2.) Stated rather more formally, these are:

- **Psychodynamic theories**—which stress the crucial role of both early experiences and of the unconscious in determining thoughts, feelings and behaviour.
- **Cognitive–behavioural theories**—which view many behaviours, including those which fall within the realm of personality, as being acquired through learning. They also emphasize the effect that mental processes, such as beliefs, thoughts and perceptions, have on behaviour.
- **Humanistic approaches**—which emphasize the individual's inborn striving for personal growth and, given the right environment, the ability to achieve his or her creative potential.
- **Biological theories**—which are primarily concerned with determining the extent to which genetic and other biological factors affect personality

    A's views, it can be seen, are consistent with psychodynamic theory, **B**'s with a cognitive–behavioural, **C**'s with humanistic and **D**'s with biological.

    Psychological theory therefore helps us to **explain** the relationship between specific behavioural patterns and mental processes and their causes. One of the difficulties with the explanations of the four individuals above, however, is that they are 'after the fact'. Any one of them sounds reasonable. If any theory is going to be put to the test, it needs not only to explain, but to **predict** future events.

    If this hypothetical conversation were to be taken a stage further we might overhear a discussion amongst the group about what might help this seemingly unfortunate man. This might take the form of predictions about the circumstances or conditions under which change may (or may not) occur. It could go something like this:

A   *I wish there was something we could do to help him but he's so insecure. Although he'd never admit it, he probably resents his mother deep down and feels really bad about what happened to him. He'd have to come to terms with such a lot.*

B   *No—what he needs is to learn to stand up for himself. To take a risk and speak his mind and find out that if he did we wouldn't hold it against him. And even if we did it wouldn't be the end of the world.*

C   *If you'd all stop wanting to change him and just accept and appreciate him for what he is, I'm sure that would help him to be more confident and do his own thing.*

D   *It's just the way he is. Nothing is going to change that, short of a head-transplant! Although, on second thoughts, maybe this new wonder drug Prozac might help him. I've even thought of getting some myself!*

Each member of the group has formulated his or her own **hypothesis**, or educated guess, derived from their respective theoretical approaches to personality, about what would be necessary to bring about change.

These suggested ways of helping do, of course, reflect the four main theoretical approaches to therapeutic intervention; the first three psychological, the fourth medical:

- **the psychodynamic approach (A)**, which seeks to help clients gain insight by recognizing, understanding and dealing with unconscious thoughts and feelings;
- **the cognitive/behavioural approach (B)**, which is aimed at helping clients to change the way in which they think as well as the way they behave;
- **the humanistic approach (C)**, which aims to create the conditions of trust to facilitate the client's personal growth and the achievement of their potential;
- **the biological approach (D)**, directed at changing the body's biochemistry.

There is, therefore, a direct relationship between the approach people take to personality, either implicitly or explicitly, in terms of formal theory, and the approach they take to helping.

A   believes the difficulty stems from early childhood experiences and has the idea that there is some possible area of early distress or conflict which must be resolved.

B   thinks the problem has arisen partly because the person had never learned the behaviours necessary to stand up for himself (possibly because attempts at assertive behaviour were not adequately reinforced by his dominant mother) and believes that he needs to learn to be assertive now.

C   regards feeling accepted is important and in using the phrase 'be himself' makes an important philosophical point about the nature of the person. C accordingly sees acceptance and appreciation at this stage of the person's life as being the most effective way helping him to 'grow' in a way that is meaningful to him.

D   feels that any difficulties are the result of his genetic biological make-up and considers the possibility that medication directed at biochemical change may help.

The terms used in this example of course would never be used in everyday conversation but nevertheless the psychological concepts which are implicit in the three statements made by the first three individuals are explicit in psychodynamic, cognitive–behaviourial and humanistic theories of personality and in psychological therapy and counselling.

People on the whole, however, do not develop or adopt one particular theoretical perspective and stick to it. They may have an overall orientation but **they may change or modify their theories** in the light of **evidence** from the external world.

Supposing, for example, the man in question became very much more confident and assertive over the following three or four months. D's (biological) hypothesis that nothing would change the way he is, except possibly medication, would not have been confirmed if she found that this had not been the case. So D's biological perspective might be revised to accommodate this new piece of evidence and include the conditions under which change could occur. The revised theory might state that in general people's genetic inheritance determines their personality, unless they have suffered a major trauma in childhood.

If however 'B', who has taken more of a learning theory approach, also notices a change, and subsequently discovers that John has been attending assertiveness classes, she would not be at all surprised. Her hypothesis would have been confirmed and as a result, her theory strengthened.

People therefore, in their everyday lives, develop and use implicit theory, psychological theory, to understand their interpersonal world and to make predictions about future events. From these theories they formulate hypotheses which are sometimes put to the test and provide evidence which may support or refute their original position and lead to a refinement of their theory.

If people in their everyday lives use implicit theory so, of course, do clients in counselling. The degree to which clients are able to conceptualize their difficulties before, during and, indeed, after counselling varies considerably. Some people are more accustomed to thinking 'psychologically' and may be fairly sophisticated in this respect. Others may never have developed a sufficiently coherent theoretical framework in which to understand their current difficulties. As counsellors and therapists, we need to recognize and respect our clients' implicit or explicit theoretical orientations, and particularly to be aware of discrepancies between the views held by our clients and those we, ourselves, adhere to.

Although counsellors and therapists are generally trained in a particular theoretical approach, they too are likely to use implicit theory in their counselling work. This is understandable. No one theory or theoretical approach has been developed which, on its own, addresses all the issues relating to the vast wealth and depth of human experience. Sometimes, however, there can be a conflict between the counsellor's implicit theory and the formal theory adopted, and integrating implicit theory into counselling practice can be problematic. If the counsellor is not aware of this, and the conflict is not resolved, it can cause difficulties for the client, as the following case demonstrates.

A relatively recently qualified General Practitioner, Dr C, in his late twenties, has been aware for some time of the importance of psychological factors in relation to physical health and, for this reason, has been attending quite an intensive humanistically orientated counselling course. He has been asked by a colleague to see one of her patients, a thirty-five-year-old woman who, when she brought her eight-month-old baby in for a check-up, told her that she was experiencing frequent headaches and having considerable difficulty in coping with the situation at home.

The patient, Mrs D, has given up a very good job in the City in order to be at home with her young son. She now finds that the new baby, although planned, has completely disrupted her life: her relationship with her husband has deteriorated, she feels worthless, she cannot see the way out of the mess and no—she doesn't want any antidepressants! Her GP immediately sees this as a good opportunity for Dr C to practise his newly acquired counselling skills. Mrs D. has no history of psychological disorder. Indeed she has always seemed to be remarkably well adjusted. It seems to Dr C to be fairly straightforward. He suggests that he sees her for five half-hour 'counselling' sessions to help her to sort out some of the difficulties she is facing as a result of the considerable changes in her life brought about by the birth of her son. This sounds like a good idea to her although she has no idea what to expect. Will he, like everyone else, tell her to go back to work? Of course she has thought about that but she really does not want her son to grow up with a working mother as she herself did. Will he want to know about her potty training?! She goes to their first session with some trepidation.

At the end of her first session she is really surprised. The time went so quickly. She didn't realize she had so much to say. But what did she say? She can't really remember but she feels almost elated. What did he say? Not much, it seems to her. He certainly didn't tell her to go back to work—nor to do anything else for that matter. And he never even mentioned the word 'potty' once. So why does she feel as she does. Of course it won't last; and it doesn't. Nothing has changed at home. Her husband still arrives home at the same time wanting his dinner. They used to do it together, or get a takeaway on the way home. The house still always seems a tip. And when it doesn't who cares anyway. You don't get 'brownie points' for dusting. Nobody comes in and says, 'My goodness! Haven't you dusted that table well'. But somehow, in spite of the fact that nothing has changed, she looks forward to her next session with Dr C.

The second session seems much like the first but this time she talks much more about her life in general. She remembers things she'd long since forgotten. They don't seem to be of any great significance—but you never know. She notices that she does not feel under any pressure to get it 'right' for him. She leaves the second session feeling thoughtful.

By the end of the third session Mrs D has begun to realize that she is thinking about things she's never thought about before. For example she realizes she has always done what has been expected of her. Everything has been planned for. She has never really worked out for herself what she wants, what she needs to do. Nobody until now, she feels, has really listened to her. She feels that Dr C is really 'on her side', that he won't somehow impose things on her. She still doesn't know what the answer is. Things at home are much the same but somehow she feels better within herself, more confident that things will be OK and she only had one headache last week. She still does not really understand what Dr C is doing or why she feels better but she knows she feels 'safe' with him; that she can talk to him about anything and it will be OK.

Meanwhile Dr C has been doing quite a lot of thinking himself. His own marriage has been under some strain recently with all the extra administration of the practice he has taken on. However he has always prided himself on confronting problems 'head on', on taking responsibility and on being a good problem-solver. He is attempting to reorganize things at work and has set out a plan for improving things at home, allowing time each day for the children and, perhaps more importantly, time for his wife—'quality time'. This has begun to work well and his efforts have been rewarded and home life is now much more satisfactory for him.

Dr C has also been thinking about his sessions with Mrs D and he is not at all sure where they are going. There are only two more sessions left and he feels he really hasn't achieved very much so far. He realizes of course that he is not supposed to solve her problems. His counselling training tells him that, but nevertheless he does feel a bit frustrated, even a little impotent in the situation.

The fourth session arrives at the end of a long surgery for Dr C. Mrs D has been doing quite a lot of thinking between the sessions and is keen to share her thoughts with her counsellor/doctor. Dr C opens the session, which is quite unusual for him, by sharing his ideas about how she might improve things at home for everybody. He has listened to her and although he thinks otherwise, has accepted that she doesn't want to go back to work. However if she could put a little more into her relationship with her husband he is sure it would pay off; get a baby-sitter and go out for a meal once a fortnight, make sure she puts aside some time especially for him etc. He says all this in a friendly and helpful way. He even shares with her the fact that this approach is working well for him and his family.

Mrs D can't believe it. Not what he is saying, but her response to it. Shock. Disbelief. Anger. Turmoil. Why? What he has said is perfectly reasonable. He has said nothing one of her friends might not have said. Yet she feels, in some quite fundamental way, betrayed. She feels herself 'closing down', 'shutting off'. They talk about the practicalities of motherhood and the difficulty of combining work and family life. The session seems to go on interminably. Finally the half-hour is up and Mrs D tells Dr C how helpful the sessions have been and she does not feel she needs the final one.

Dr C is also thrown by Mrs D's response. He cannot understand what has happened, and does not know what to make of it. After all, he was only trying to be helpful. Maybe she has some more fundamental problems after all. But he is worried. He noticed that after talking about what she could do they never regained the quality he can only describe as 'intimacy' that they had before. Something had gone. Something was lost.

Fortunately for Dr C's subsequent clients, he took this problem to supervision. That is, he discussed it with a senior counselling colleague in a meeting set up for that purpose. As a result of this meeting he began to understand what had happened and why Mrs D had responded as she had. Some weeks later Mrs D sought the help of an experienced counsellor and worked through some of her feelings which resulted from her earlier experiences in counselling and also addressed some of the issues which were beginning to emerge in those sessions.

To the more experienced counsellor, this may seem like a rather obvious example. Yet it can, and indeed did, happen. For the first three sessions Dr C followed the approach of his training; a non-directive approach derived from humanistic theory. This approach assumes that every individual, given the right circumstances, has the motivation and the ability to change, and suggests that the person themselves is the best qualified to decide on the direction such change should take. The goal of the humanistic counsellor, therefore, is to facilitate the exploration of the individual's own thoughts and feelings and to assist them in arriving at their own solutions. The counsellor strives to create the conditions of trust and 'empathetic understanding' which allows this process to take place.

In the first three sessions, Dr C provided these conditions. He created a situation of sufficient trust for Mrs D to risk exploring areas of her experience at quite an important and fundamental level. She felt safe. She also began to trust herself. So when Dr C switched tack at the beginning of the fourth session by taking a practical problem-solving approach derived from his own implicit theory of human nature, she experienced a sense of loss, both of the possibility of moving forward in her life and of the relationship which had enabled this process. This is not to say that a problem-solving approach would not have been appropriate in the situation, but because this way of working is based on a theoretical model which makes very different assumptions about the person and about ways of helping from humanistic theory, the two approaches are, in this context, incompatible. The GP did not have sufficient knowledge of the theoretical underpinnings of different approaches, nor an awareness of his own implicit approach, to understand what had gone wrong and his patient could not have been expected to know.

The problem with implicit theory is that it is implicit. Whilst such theory plays a fundamental role in people's understanding of their everyday world, when it is introduced arbitrarily into the counselling context, with no attempt to integrate it into the formal approach taken, it can lead to confusion.

Another difficulty with the use of implicit theory in a therapeutic or counselling context is that the process by which it is developed is, of necessity, fairly haphazard and often applied 'after the fact'. Real life does not always present us with the opportunities to test out our hypotheses and even if it does, we may ignore any evidence which does not 'fit'. Our theories, as a result, can be inconsistent and contradictory. This may not really matter in our everyday lives. It can, however, as we have seen, have a considerable impact on the counselling process.

1.3 METHODS OF PSYCHOLOGICAL RESEARCH

One of the major tasks of psychology is the development of theory in a formal and consistent way. Psychology uses methods similar to those used by people in their everyday lives in the development of their implicit theories: observation, explanation, proposing and testing hypotheses and formulating and developing theories which in turn can be used to generate new hypotheses. One important difference between an informal approach and the 'scientific' approach adopted in psychology is that the psychologist, having formulated a hypothesis, then sets up a programme of research using **empirical** methods of investigation to provide the evidence (Figure 1.1), rather than letting life take its course, as it did in the case of John in the first example. Facts, in scientific disciplines, must be established in this way rather than by logical argument. By the use of 'scientific' methods, psychology is constantly developing and refining theories in attempting to discover general laws or principles that govern human behaviour and mental processes which are intended to be generalizable to groups or populations, and not just applicable to John or whoever.

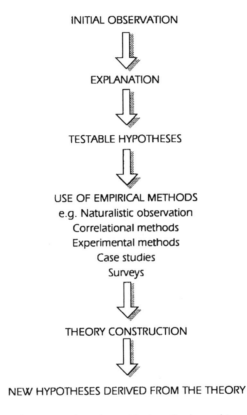

INITIAL OBSERVATION

EXPLANATION

TESTABLE HYPOTHESES

USE OF EMPIRICAL METHODS
e.g. Naturalistic observation
Correlational methods
Experimental methods
Case studies
Surveys

THEORY CONSTRUCTION

NEW HYPOTHESES DERIVED FROM THE THEORY

Figure 1.1   The scientific approach and empirical methods used in psychology

In testing hypotheses and developing theories, psychologists use a number of empirical methods in their research, the main ones being naturalistic observation, correlational methods, experimental methods, surveys and case studies.

1.3.1 Naturalistic Observation

This method involves observing behaviour in natural settings to gather useful information about behaviour as it occurs. Naturalistic observation only provides **descriptions** of behaviour and information about *possible* causal relationships.

Although some psychologists use descriptive methods, naturalistic observation is more frequently used as a starting point in research.

1.3.2 Correlational Methods

Correlational methods involve making measurements to discover relationships between naturally occurring events that, as with naturalistic observation, are not controlled by the researcher. This may also allow us to make predictions, but again, it does not tell us anything about causality.

For example, if a correlation, or association, was found between sleep and irritability, that is, that people who suffer from disturbed nights report being more irritable the next day than those who sleep well, we could not infer from this that poor sleep *causes* irritability, or vice versa. Indeed, both of the variables (sleep and irritability) may be caused by a third variable, for example, stress. We may, if the correlation is strong, predict that those whose sleep is disturbed are more likely to be irritable and that those who are anxious are more likely to get disturbed nights, but in order to infer causality, we need to employ experimental methods.

1.3.3 The Experimental Method

Here, techniques of controlled experimentation are used in order to draw conclusions about cause and effect. This involves changing in some way the conditions which are thought to be the cause, and recording whether this has any effect on the behaviour in question.

So if it was thought that disturbed sleep caused irritability, then sleep would be the condition which would be changed or **manipulated** in the experiment. The experiment would be conducted in the laboratory with one group, the **control group** allowed to go to sleep normally and the other group, the **experimental group**, say, woken up several times and kept awake for a part of the night in order to produce conditions of disturbed sleep.

Measures of irritability would then be taken so that the effects of lack of sleep could be ascertained. If we find that those whose sleep has been disturbed suffer from **significantly** higher levels of irritability than those whose sleep was not disturbed (that is, the difference is greater than could have occurred by chance), then we can say that disturbed sleep can be a causal factor in irritability. In order for that claim to be made, however, a number of other considerations relating to the research design would have to be met.

Thus experimental design at its very simplest involves:

1. creating two or more groups of subjects which should be alike in all ways except the condition you are varying;
2. directly varying a condition thought to cause changes in behaviour;
3. recording whether varying the condition has any effect on the behaviour.

Most psychological research is far more complex and often involves examining how several independent variables interact to produce an effect on one or even several dependent variables. These are known as **multivariate experiments.**

1.3.4 Case Studies

The goal of most case studies is to identify or illustrate certain principles of individual behaviour that are assumed to apply in a general case. Case studies are in-depth records of individual subjects and are used mainly in clinical settings. Most case studies are based on remembered events and records. This clearly requires a certain amount of reconstruction because it is usually only when the individual develops a problem that knowledge of the past becomes a matter of interest and importance in understanding the present behaviour. A case-study approach can also be used to study groups or whole organizations.

1.3.5 Survey Methods

Surveys provide information on attitudes and psychological functioning of large groups of people. An adequate survey requires a carefully constructed questionnaire and a sample of people selected to ensure that they are representative of the population to be studied.

1.3.6 Sampling

There are many variations on the methods briefly described above and often psychological research involves the use of more than one method. There are also a number of important considerations to be taken into account, including sampling. Because it is not usually possible to study every member of a particular group, research is usually restricted to a segment or **sample** drawn from a larger population. If the conclusions drawn from the research are going to apply to the larger population, then the sample must be **representative** of that group.

The nature of the sample must always be taken into account when interpreting research results. Findings of research on stress derived from a sample of male middle managers may well not apply to other populations, such as lone parents.

Conducting psychological research is clearly a complex process fraught with methodological problems. It also raises a number of important philosophical questions. Experimental approaches in particular have come in for considerable criticism for being reductionist and mechanistic (see Popper, 1959). At the other end of the spectrum, case studies have been considered to be subjective and less than scientific. One important consideration is that different methods are used for different purposes. Experimental methods are generally employed in the study of the various 'processes' (such as perception and memory) involved in human functioning, whereas case studies are more concerned with the lives of real individuals. Both approaches can provide us with useful information but the methods by which that information are obtained should not be accepted uncritically or without question.

1.4 THEORETICAL PERSPECTIVES IN PSYCHOLOGY

Because psychology has its roots in very varied disciplines, it is not surprising that it has developed a number of different ways of viewing the same topic, as we saw from the example of John R. in Section 1.2 above. There are usually considered to be five different perspectives, the psychodynamic, the cognitive, the behavioural, the humanistic and the biological. Sometimes the cognitive and behavioural are combined. Each perspective focuses on different aspects of functioning and on different causes of human behaviour. Although we have outlined above some of the characteristics of the different perspectives in relation to the development of personality, the topic warrants rather more attention than provided above.

1.4.1 Psychodynamic Perspective

The psychodynamic perspective is based on the work of Sigmund Freud. He created both a theory to explain personality and mental disorders, and the form of therapy known as psychoanalysis. The psychodynamic approach assumes that all behaviour and mental processes reflect constant and often unconscious struggles within the person. These usually involve conflicts between our need to satisfy basic biological instincts, for example for food, sex or aggression, and the restrictions imposed by society. Not all of those who take a psychodynamic approach accept all of Freud's original ideas, but most would view abnormal or problematic behaviour as the result of a failure to resolve conflicts adequately.

1.4.2 Behavioural Perspective

Whereas the psychodynamic perspective focuses mainly on the role of the unconscious and innate biological forces within us, the behavioural perspective stresses the role of the external environment, particularly the pattern of rewards and punishments, in shaping and governing our actions. Although few psychologists today would regard themselves as strict behaviourists, behaviourism has been very influential in the development of psychology as a scientific discipline.

1.4.3 Cognitive Perspective

The cognitive perspective brings the emphasis back to the person. But in contrast to the psychodynamic approach which focuses on the unconscious and non-rational mental forces, the cognitive approach views humans as rational problem-solvers whose actions are governed by conscious thought and planning. The emphasis with this approach is on the ways in which people perceive and mentally process incoming information, evaluate it and decide how to respond to it.

1.4.4 Humanistic Perspective

The humanistic perspective similarly rejects the notion that we are controlled by unconscious conflicts or by rewards and punishments and, in common with the cognitive approach, sees people as having the capacity to choose how to think and act and to control their own destiny. According to humanistic theories, all human beings are motivated by a tendency towards growth, the development of their potential and 'self-actualization' but need a supportive environment for this to occur. The humanistic viewpoint tends to be more of a philosophical position than a formal scientific theory and humanistic psychologists tend to be more interested in describing the inner life and experiences of individuals than in developing theories or in predicting behaviour. It is not therefore surprising that this approach is the one most favoured by many counsellors.

1.4.5 Biological Perspective

The biological perspective attempts to understand human thought, emotion, behaviour and motivation in terms of the physical processes which take place in the body. It emphasizes the biochemical processes that are involved in these activities, the role of the human brain, and the part played by genetic factors in our individual development.

Sometimes these psychological perspectives on a particular topic are contradictory and mutually exclusive. This tends to be the case when the different perspectives put forward different explanations for the same phenomenon as in the example of John R above. However, if the perspectives focus on different aspects of the same phenomenon, then each perspective can contribute to our overall understanding of a particular area.

If we take the example of obesity, there may be a number of different reasons why people overeat. Some of these reasons might be psychodynamic, for example, as a means of trying to cope with an anxiety-producing situation in a way which has always provided comfort; some may be cognitive, such as the breakdown of a systematic plan of eating and the ensuing feelings of loss of control; some of the reasons may be behavioural, for example, in response to specific stimuli such as eating in a restaurant or at a party; and from a humanistic perspective, the situation may not be conducive to the achievement of potential. There may also be biological reasons, possibly a genetic predisposition to obesity.

Although some research areas in psychology, such as that concerned with the biological basis of behaviour, clearly correspond to a particular perspective, other areas, e.g. motivation, can be viewed from some, or all of the perspectives discussed above.

1.5 RESEARCH AREAS IN PSYCHOLOGY

The range of psychological phenomena that are the focus of research is almost limitless. In the first section of this chapter psychological theory was discussed mainly in relation to personality, but this is only one of an enormous variety of topics which comprise the discipline of psychology.

Psychology is usually defined as the scientific study of behaviour and its causes. The term 'behaviour' is used in its broadest sense to include both **overt behaviours**, which are the actions which we can actually observe, and **covert behaviours**, such as thoughts, feelings, images and biological processes which are not available to direct observation. Psychology is concerned with body, mind and behaviour and relates to virtually every aspect of our lives. It is hardly therefore surprising that there appears an often bewildering array of topics, sections, subsections, speciality areas and perspectives relating to the discipline of psychology.

Psychologists have attempted to deal with the complexity of the subject by dividing up areas of human functioning into the separate research areas or subdivisions which are reviewed below. Most of the areas, however, are not discrete categories but are often interrelated and interdependent, so the divisions are somewhat artificial and to some extent arbitrary. This is why different basic texts on psychology will sometimes appear to cover different areas. The discipline of psychology is also constantly developing with different areas achieving prominence at different points in time.

Broadly speaking, these research areas can be divided into **process-based approaches**, which tend to look at the mechanisms that underlie various aspects of behaviour and **person-based approaches**, which are more immediately concerned with people as a whole. Process-based research areas would include the biological basis of behaviour, cognitive psychology (sensory processes, perception, memory, thinking and language), learning and conditioning, motivation, emotion and states of consciousness. Individual differences (intelligence and personality), social Psychology, lifespan psychology, stress and coping and abnormal psychology would come roughly under the heading of person-based approaches.

The person-based approaches appear, on the face of it, to be of more direct relevance to the therapeutic context. However, there is much that is intriguing and of value to the counsellor to be discovered in the literature on fundamental processes.

The following section outlines the main areas in the field which are usually included in a degree syllabus. They should enable the reader to place the subject areas presented in the main text of this book in the context of the scientific discipline as a whole.

1.5.1 Process-based Areas of Research

These approaches include:

- **The biological basis of behaviour** This area of psychology focuses on the **hereditary factors** and the complex **biological systems** (for example, the **nervous system**, the **endocrine system** and the **immune system**) that underlie every aspect of our behaviour and psychological functioning including feeling, thinking, attending, sensing, perceiving and problem-solving.
- **Sensory processes** The study of sensory processes is concerned with how people acquire information about the external world through their **senses** (vision, hearing, taste, smell, and touch) which actively shape information about the outside world helping to create each person's own reality.

- **Perception**   Perception is the process through which sensations are interpreted by drawing on past experiences, including our understanding and knowledge of the world, so that they become meaningful experiences.

- **Memory**   Psychologists have approached the study of memory from biological and psychological perspectives. **Biological** approaches are concerned with the underlying brain and chemical mechanisms whilst **psychological** approaches seek to describe and understand how memory operates, the way in which we reconstruct memories and why we forget.

- **Thinking**   This is an area of cognitive science which is, to a large part, the study of how mental representations are formed, manipulated, and translated into action. Research on thinking in adults has concentrated on **propositional thought**, particularly in relation to **deductive** and **inductive reasoning**, on **problem-solving** and on **decision-making**.

- **Language**   Mainstream psychology has tended to focus on the complex mental processes involved in language in terms of both its production and its comprehension, rather than on its more creative aspects. Psychologists are particularly interested in the structure of language and in the child's development of language.

- **Learning and conditioning**   Learning is involved in practically every aspect of our development: our perceptual, personal, emotional and social development and in the development of our personalities. The study of learning is fundamental to an understanding of human behaviour and has had a central role in the development of the discipline of psychology.

- **Motivation**   This area of psychology is concerned with what people want and with their needs, which may be **biological**, such as thirst or hunger, **social**, such as the need for achievement or power, **biologically based social** as in sexual and maternal behaviour or **curiosity-based**, the need to seek stimulation and actively explore the environment.

- **Emotion**   Psychologists have attempted to study in a systematic way the complex interaction between environment, mind, body and behaviour involved in the experience of emotion. They have seen emotions as a 'call for action' requiring some sort of response to the situation that aroused the emotion.

- **Consciousness**   The term **conscious** is used to describe the contents of the mind that we are immediately aware of. Psychologists have also been interested in **subconscious** and **preconscious** experience and in the study of **altered states of consciousness including** sleep and dreams, meditative and hypnotic experiences and drug-induced states of consciousness.

1.5.2 Person-based Areas of Research

The following areas of research could be included in this category:

- **Personality**   The concept of personality is central to our attempts to understand ourselves and others and is part of the way in which we account for the differences that contribute to our individuality. Psychologists have been particularly concerned with the shaping of the personality in relation to **genetic and environmental influences**, in the **consistency and continuity** of the personality and in **personality assessment.**

- **Intelligence**   Intelligence is a concept that refers to individual differences in the ability to acquire knowledge, to reason effectively and to deal adequately with the environment. Psychologists have been concerned with issues such as the nature of intelligence; the factors (environmental and hereditary) that are responsible for the differences in cognitive skills; the measurement of intelligence, and the question of whether we can predict success or failure in real-life settings.

- **Social psychology**   Social psychology is the scientific study of how individuals think, feel and behave in social situations. It is concerned with the interplay between our own behaviour and that of people around us. This area of psychology covers a vast array of topics including self-perception, self-schema and self-presentation; social perception and attribution; interpersonal attraction and close relationships; stereotype and prejudice; group membership and group structure; roles and role-conflict; attitude and attitude change; social norms, social influence, social power and leadership.

- **Lifespan development**   Developmental psychology was, until comparatively recently, synonymous with the psychology of child development. However, in recent years, there has been a noticeable trend within psychology to adopt a lifespan approach and to incorporate patterns of change and continuity in adulthood into the domain of developmental psychology.

- **Stress and coping**   This area of psychology has examined both the sources of possible stress, and the reactions to stress. Much of the research has centred around ways in which people cope with stress and what factors protect against, or make people more vulnerable to, stress. Another major area of interest is the relationship between stress and health.

- **Abnormal psychology**   The concepts of **normality and abnormality** and issues surrounding the **classification and diagnoses** of psychological disorder are fundamental to the study of abnormal behaviour. This area is also concerned with the major psychological disorders, anxiety disorders, disorders of mood, schizophrenia and personality disorders.

1.5.3 Applied Psychology

Applied psychology is the application of psychological theory and knowledge to a variety of specific, usually 'real-world', contexts. Some examples are listed below.

- **Environmental psychology** which is concerned with the interaction between people and their physical surroundings—our attitudes and behaviour towards the natural and built environment and how the environment, in turn, affects our perceptions and actions.

- **Health psychology** is the application of theories, methods and techniques of psychology to issues of health and illness including attitudes, behaviour and thinking about health. This area includes compliance, doctor–patient communication, the effects of stress on health and the psychological factors associated with physical disorder.

- **Clinical neuropsychology** is concerned with the assessment of memory, perception, attention, language and general intellectual abilities in relation to treatment planning and rehabilitation of people with brain damage or organic conditions that affect their cognitive functioning.
- **Sports psychology** includes the psychological aspects of skill acquisition, team cohesion and performance enhancement. It is concerned with the effect of competitive state anxiety and mood on performance, participation and aggression in sport and also with exercise—motivation, uptake, adherence and dependence.

1.6 PROFESSIONAL APPLIED PSYCHOLOGY (UK)

The term 'psychologist' is not currently legally protected in Great Britain, but the title 'Chartered Psychologist' is. Chartered Psychologists will possess the Graduate Basis for Registration (which normally means they have a first degree in psychology), followed by a training which has been formally approved by the British Psychological Society. All of the specialisms mentioned below have clearly defined routes by which graduates can obtain chartered status and new routes are still being developed (for example, in health psychology).

The British Psychological Society under the terms of its Royal Charter of Incorporation provides a Register of Chartered Psychologists containing names of properly trained psychologists who agree to abide by the Society's Code of Conduct.

Below are some of the specialist areas in which psychologists can become chartered.

- **Forensic psychology** Chartered Forensic Psychologists practise in the field of criminological and legal psychology. They work with offending populations and with the courts, both civil and criminal.
- **Clinical psychology** Chartered Clinical Psychologists are trained in the assessment and treatment of children and adults with mental health problems or learning disabilities. They work with a wide variety of client groups including older adults, clients with neuropsychological problems and people with long-term mental health problems. The majority of Clinical Psychologists work in mental health service settings although increasingly they are moving into other settings such as general hospitals or social services departments.
- **Counselling psychology** Chartered Counselling Psychologists are trained to work psychotherapeutically with clients with a broad range of psychological difficulties and disorders. They work in a variety of settings including primary care (GP surgeries), community mental health teams (CMHTs), social services, clinical psychology departments, private practice, student counselling services and employee assistance programmes (EAPs).
- **Occupational psychology** Chartered Occupational Psychologists are concerned with the performance of people at work and in training, with developing and understanding of how organizations function and how individuals and groups behave at work.

- **Educational psychology** Chartered Educational Psychologists' work includes assessing individual children and recommending a programme of education or treatment; planning special school curricula; advising parents and teachers on children with special needs; advising on aspects of school organization and devising assessment procedures used by teachers.

1.7 OVERVIEW OF THIS BOOK

This book is concerned with the ways in which psychological theory and knowledge can be applied to therapeutic practice. The links and connections between psychology and counselling, which are often less than obvious, are made explicit by the use of explanation, discussion, examples and case material incorporated in the text.

The topics chosen correspond in general to the main research areas in psychology, but with some omissions and with somewhat different emphases and weightings. The reason for adhering to this convention is so that it is possible for the reader, without too much difficulty, to follow up in greater depth any specific area of interest.

After this introductory chapter, the book continues with a chapter on personality. This is to enable the counsellor to understand more about the part background influences play in the shaping of personality; that is, the formation of characteristic patterns of thinking, feeling and behaviour. It could also help the counsellor make explicit his or her own possibly implicit theory of personality. Connections will be made between the approach taken to personality (with each approach having different implications for psychological disturbance) and the approach taken to counselling or therapy.

There then follows four chapters on different psychological processes, the first of which is emotion. The psychology of emotion, which initially seems to be so far removed from what and how people actually feel, provides a wealth of valuable insights into understanding and working with the emotional experience of clients in counselling.

The next chapter, Chapter 4, demonstrates how a knowledge of the processes that underlie memory can help the counsellor or therapist to understand and work with clients' memories; how memories are formed, why we remember, and indeed forget, what we do. Of particular possible interest to counselling is the work on 'reconstructing' memories and also the section on 'false memory' in relation to child sexual abuse.

Chapter 5 on thinking deals with cognition, problem-solving and decision-making. Clients entering counselling often have problems to be solved and decisions to be made. A knowledge of problem solving strategies and decision theory can accordingly enhance or add to the counsellor's repertoire of possible approaches in these situations. However, this topic is not only applicable to working directly with client issues. Even the most client-centred counsellors are constantly making decisions about interventions based on their conceptualizations of clients' presenting concerns. This area of theory and research may provide some insights into this decision-making process; for example, by being aware of some common judgemental errors and pitfalls.

Topics related to consciousness are frequently raised by clients in counselling and therapy. Chapter 6, on States of Consciousness, aims to inform the counsellor on topics such as subconscious processes and preconscious memory, sleep, dreaming, hypnosis, meditation and the effects on consciousness of psychoactive drugs.

The social psychological perspective on the self and relationships is presented in Chapter 7. Here, counsellors are introduced to an alternative approach to understanding clients which, in contrast to the highly individualistic approaches to personality discussed in Chapter 2, takes into account social processes when theorizing about the person. It discusses topics such as self-concept and identity, person perception, interpersonal attraction, relationships and relationship breakdown.

Chapters 8 and 9 take a lifespan perspective to understanding the person. The first of these chapters examines some of the factors in 'normal' childhood development which impact on subsequent development. These include early relationships and attachment, father and sibling influence, social development and family disruption and breakdown. We move on to adolescence and adulthood in Chapter 9 and explore issues related to development, adjustment and change at various stages in adult life. Topics include the development of identity in adolescence, adult relationships, retirement and major loss.

Counsellors have traditionally tended to avoid physiological or clinical perspectives and generally do not conceptualize their clients' experiences in terms of symptomatology. Yet many counsellors will be working with clients who are experiencing the effects of stress or who are extremely distressed. Chapter 10 offers a comprehensive overview of stress and coping in relation to health and ill-health which could contribute to the counsellor's understanding of the processes involved. It may also provide a rationale and direction for counselling. Chapter 11, after discussing concepts of normality and abnormality, outlines the main categories of psychological disorder and discusses the various approaches to treatment. This may be useful to the counsellor when facing decisions about referring on and also when communicating with other health care professionals.

Certain topics which are not so immediately applicable to counselling or therapy have been omitted as chapters in their own right but relevant aspects of the topic will often be subsumed under another heading. For example, there is no chapter on the biological basis of behaviour, but the physiological components of emotion and anxiety are discussed in Chapter 3 on Emotion and in Chapter 10 on Stress, Coping and Illness respectively. Similarly, learning theory is not discussed as a separate topic, but relevant aspects of the subject are presented in the section on Social Learning Approaches to Personality in Chapter 2 and also in Chapter 8 on Lifespan Development and Chapter 11 on Psychological Disorders. In the case of social psychology, the field is too vast to be covered adequately in a volume such as this. We have therefore selected topics within the subject area which are most applicable to the counselling context.

1.8 CONCLUDING COMMENTS

Psychology is often maligned for having little to do with actual people. This is true. As a science, psychology is concerned with general principles, not specific individuals. Ultimately it would be hoped that psychology would find a route back to understanding individual people or events, but what is important in psychology is what any one person or event has in common with others persons or events. Psychology cannot tell us, for example, why John lacks confidence, but it does try to discover some general principles about background influences on current functioning which may contribute to our understanding of John.

This is not to say that counsellors should be psychologists. Counsellors gain and develop their understanding in many ways: through careful listening, to the latent as well as the manifest content; through observation of the moment-by-moment changes that can give some indication of the client's emotional state and by interpreting their own reactions and responses to the client and the client's 'material'. Throughout, the counsellor will be striving to understand and 'make sense of' the client's experience. That is, they will make formulations, psychological formulations. Often these formulations are constructed from our own intuitive understanding and this can be an extremely important and creative process. Indeed, it is often seen as one of the defining features of counselling. What we are suggesting is that psychological understandings can be incorporated into this intuitive process; that formulations can be informed by psychological theory and knowledge and that this, in turn, can contribute to the practice of counselling.

Whether or not the counsellor is trained to, wishes or feels able to apply psychological principles to the practice of counselling, we believe that it is important that those who work in the field of counselling should be aware that a body of psychological literature exists, of what it consists and how it might apply in the context of counselling. This is the subject matter of this book.

2

Personality

CONTENTS

2.1 INTRODUCTION

The task of trying to define what constitutes 'personality' is a very daunting one. How can it be possible to break down into simple statements exactly what it is that makes each of us a unique human being?

Many psychologists have devised theories of personality which attempt to account both for the differences between individuals and also for how any particular individual becomes the type of person that they are; and as we saw in Chapter 1, most people have their own ideas on the subject. Both formal and informal definitions however try to say something about what makes a person recognizable as themselves, and to identify their main and possibly enduring characteristics.

Although much has been written about the development of the personality from a variety of perspectives or theoretical orientations, somewhat less attention has been paid to what may constitute a 'healthy' personality. This is where we start this chapter. We then go on to look at two of the main areas of debate in the psychology of personality. The first concerns the extent to which one's personality is a product of inherited characteristics or innate temperament and how much it is the product of environmental influences and learning. A second area of research and argument is concerned with how much personality can be seen as a relatively fixed and unchanging feature of the individual and how much one's personality is a function of the situations that we find ourselves in, and therefore open to change and development. These two central questions will be examined in turn before looking at the major approaches to personality, the empirical methods they employ to measure and assess personality and the implication of each approach for counselling practice.

2.2 THE HEALTHY PERSONALITY

The question of whether there is a particular personality style, or a number of personality styles, which is more healthy or adaptive than others is a fascinating one. This question however has been little addressed by mainstream psychologists, who have tended instead to give their attention to personality pathology and maladaptiveness. Issues surrounding the idea that there are some individuals with 'personality disorders' are discussed in Chapter 11.

There have been many studies which have examined the role of personality in relation to the development or maintenance of a variety of medical conditions. Risk of coronary heart disease has been found to be associated with a particular personality style called *Type A* (Friedman and Rosenman, 1974). Type A individuals show a pattern of behaviour that includes hostility, feeling time pressured, being competitive and highly achievement oriented. Type B personality is more relaxed and less concerned about deadlines and time pressures. Follow-up studies of individuals who have been classified in this way have found an association between risk of coronary heart disease and Type A pattern. However, attempts to find specific personality patterns that are related to other specific physical disorders have had very mixed and equivocal results (see Section 10.7).

In an attempt to identify a personality type that might be less likely to suffer from physical ill health, some psychologists have introduced the idea of **psychological hardiness** (Kobasa et al., 1979). In Chapter 10 on Stress, we will see how the way in which people construe their world (whether they see events as a 'threat' or a 'challenge') can have a biochemical impact on the body, especially the immune system. The concept of the **hardy personality** is that healthy people can cope with change or stress by view-ing it as a challenge in which they have a sense of personal control and involvement. In studies of various occupational groups, researchers found that those who were able to think about change in this way were less susceptible to ill health.

One of the few psychologists to discuss the healthy personality was the humanistic psychologist Abraham Maslow (1954, 1968). He labelled people whom he thought had a healthy and adaptive personality style 'self-actualizers'. These people were able to successfully meet their needs for security, belonging and esteem. Such a person was characterized by various personality features:

- self-acceptance;
- acceptance of reality;
- concern with external issues;
- desire for solitude;
- independence;
- openness.

Maslow's theory has become very popular with humanistic counsellors and has influenced other humanistic theorists but there has been relatively little in the way of empirical research into these ideas. Nevertheless there are obvious similarities between Maslow's ideas and the idea of the hardy personality.

2.3 NATURE OR NURTURE?

From time to time, stories appear in the media which tell of twin siblings who have been reared apart but then meet each other in adult life. These stories usually highlight the striking similarities between the twins despite their separation. The individuals may have developed the same interests, show similar preferences for hair and dress styles and even choose spouses with similarities.

Psychologists have used this kind of data in a systematic way in order to try to estab-lish how much of one's characteristics may be attributed to genetic inheritance and how much can be thought of as arising from the influence of the environment that a person is brought up in. It is clearly difficult to find examples of identical twins reared apart but some studies of such individuals have been published (Bouchard et al., 1981). The twins in such studies are given a wide range of psychological and other tests.

In general terms, the results suggest that twins show themselves to have equivalent ability levels and to be very alike in their levels of sociability. Goldsmith (1983) has reviewed much of the relevant research and concluded that the evidence was support-ive of genetic influences having a moderate effect on personality. The strongest evi-dence was in those aspects of personality associated with sociability, emotionality and activity levels.

However, it is important to note that even in those aspects of personality where psy-chologists think that there may be some genetic contribution, they never claim that genetics can account for all of the individual differences between people or the level of a particular characteristic within a given individual.

2.4 CONTINUITY OF PERSONALITY

One of the important questions for counsellors is the extent to which a person's personality is an enduring feature of the person and to what extent is it amenable to change. We have seen in the previous section that personality is to some extent genetically influenced, but if it remains a stable and fixed feature of the individual, the idea of trying to help the person to develop and change the way in which they think, feel and behave presents something of a conundrum.

The issue of change and consistency is also linked to how we assess or measure personality. We would not expect a person to answer a personality questionnaire in exactly the same way on every occasion that it was administered. However, we might expect them to show a broadly similar pattern (or else assume that our measure is not actually assessing 'personality'). But does this mean that we should be pessimistic about people's capacity to do other than as they have always done and feel the same emotions whenever they are in similar situations again?

2.4.1 Trait Approaches to Personality

Some psychologists who have written about personality have adopted a dispositional or 'trait' approach. In this model of personality, attributes or dispositions of the individual are viewed as stable and consistent both across time and across situations. In other words, these models have an implicitly conservative view of the kind and degree of change that they think it is possible for people to make in their lives.

However, some psychologists have pointed out that surface inconsistencies may in fact reflect an inner consistency at a deeper level. Allport (1937) gives an example of a University lecturer, Dr D, who is habitually very neat and tidy in his office. However, he does not show these same behaviours in relation to his duties as the departmental librarian. The library is disorganized and untidy. This is not an inconsistency because both behaviours stem from the same underlying personality disposition, i.e. self-centredness. It serves Dr D to be tidy in his own office for his own self-interests but such interests are not served by looking after the library.

Trait theories of personality also share some elements with 'typologies' of personality. These are the theories that suggest that there are a limited number of basic types of persons. One of the most common theories that counsellors may be likely to come across is that of Carl Jung, one of Freud's early associates. This will be discussed later in this chapter.

Trait approaches to personality are similar to typologies in that they assume that individuals show relatively enduring patterns of reaction and behaviour and that such patterns distinguish one individual from another. However, whereas Jung saw introverts and extroverts as two basic personality types, trait approaches would view introversion and extroversion as a continuum, i.e. people will vary in the extent to which they have either trait but do not belong to one category to the exclusion of the other.

Trait explanations of personality are commonly used to account for people's behaviour. For example, if a counsellor has been seeing a client who worries excessively about minor aches and pains or who imagines that they have some, as yet undiagnosed, medical condition then they might find that person has been labelled in various ways by professional agencies that they have come into contact with. An example is given below.

The client is a 33-year-old woman, divorced and living with her two daughters aged four and six years. Ten months ago she was involved in a road traffic accident in which she fractured her arm. She had her arm in plaster for two months, but when the plaster was removed her arm had to be reset. She has now had the plaster off for five or so months, but still her arm does not feel 'right', although she can't explain precisely why. After the accident she also suffered some temporary numbness down the right side of her body which worried her somewhat. She has been told by the hospital that she has no pathological condition.

On her follow-up appointments to the out-patient department of the hospital she has tried to explain to the orthopaedic surgeon her concerns and has also complained (albeit rather apologetically) to her general practitioner on several occasions. However, she feels that they have not taken her seriously, that they were not really interested in her nor really listened to her. On the last visit to her GP, because she became tearful and complained about not sleeping very well, the GP prescribed some anti-depressants. This left her feeling very resentful; the reason she was not sleeping, she had tried to explain, was because of her bad arm, and the reason she had become tearful was because she felt frustrated at not being heard (although she has to admit this is not the first time she has burst into tears recently and she has been finding it rather hard to 'get going' and feeling generally quite 'low'). However, she said nothing about her frustrations about her care and left with the prescription. The GP also made an appointment for her to see a counsellor.

When the counsellor looks at her hospital notes, she finds that the junior doctor in the Accident and Emergency Department has labelled her a 'dependent' personality. On talking to the client's general practitioner, the counsellor learns that the GP sees her problems arising from her 'neurotic disposition' and 'hypochondriacal traits'.

As can be seen from this example, the client's behaviour, that is, complaining of certain physical symptoms and expressing her worries and getting upset about them, is interpreted as a sign of an underlying disposition. However, it is all too easy to make these attributions on the basis of very little evidence and they may reveal more about the person making the attribution than about the client. As Mischel (1986) points out 'A hazard in trait attributions is that we easily forget that nothing is explained if the state *we* have attributed to the person from his behaviour . . . is now invoked as the *cause* of the behaviour from which it was inferred.' Conceptualizing the client's difficulties in this way contributes little in relation to helping the person.

The question still remains however of how stable a particular individual's personal psychological qualities are over time and across situations. Psychologists have distinguished between those traits that are 'source' traits, i.e. more fundamental ones, and those that are 'surface' traits (Cattell, 1965). Other important trait psychologists have included individuals such as Hans Eysenck. It was he (in contrast to Carl Jung) who viewed introversion–extraversion as a dimension rather than two different types of personality. A second dimension that Eysenck has emphasized as a key trait is emotional stability or neuroticism. Eysenck and others have conducted many empirical investigations of these personality dimensions which are viewed as broad traits, which will be seen in many different situations and persist across time. Despite considerable research, there is still no general consensus about which traits are the most fundamental in the personality. There has also been an realization of the complexity of the interaction between the person and their life situations.

Mischel (1986) has suggested that there is not necessarily tension between a 'trait' view of personality and a more 'situational' view. He thinks that it is setting up a false dichotomy to say either personality is stable *or* personality is open to change. Instead he claims, 'The questions rather, are when and how do we find stability, and when and how do we find change, and how can we best understand each phenomenon?'

This view, that behaviour is better explained by elements within different situations rather than by reference to internal traits, provoked controversy in the literature. Some writers pointed out that the situations that we end up in are often partly a matter of our own choice and preference and therefore cannot be seen as entirely independent of our 'personality'.

2.4.2 Assessment of Personality Traits

One of the most common ways in which psychologists have sought to assess personality is via the paper and pencil **personality test**. These are sometimes referred to as psychometric tests. There is a wide range of such tests available and they are often used for specific purposes, such as job selection, by occupational, educational or clinical psychologists. Some tests are restricted so that they can only be used by suitably qualified individuals.

A common approach to assessing personality traits is to use a self report personality test or inventory. In such tests the individual is asked to indicate their agreement or disagreement with various descriptions, e.g. 'I often worry about trivial things' or 'I enjoy meeting people.' Examples of such personality inventories include the **Minnesota Multiphasic Personality Inventory** (MMPI and MMPI-2; Hathaway and McKinley, 1943, 1989), the **Eysenck Personality Inventory** (EPI; Eysenck and Eysenck, 1969), and the **Sixteen Personality Factor Questionnaire** (16PF; Cattell and Stice, 1986).

Such tests obviously assume that personality is stable enough to be measured reliably and validly. However, problems in establishing that such personality measures are indeed measuring what they claim to be means that the results from any personality tests need to be treated with judicious caution.

While the trait approach has led to advances in psychological measurement through the development of various tests and assessment devices, it has been criticized for minimizing the importance of prior learning and current situational factors. It might be that these latter factors could provide stronger and more plausible explanations for a person's ways of thinking, feeling and behaving.

2.5 PSYCHODYNAMIC APPROACHES TO PERSONALITY

The two main psychodynamic approaches with strongly developed theories of personality are those of Freud and Jung. Each will be examined in turn.

2.5.1 Freudian Theory of Personality

Freud thought that the personality was composed of three structural elements: the id, ego and superego. He saw the id as that part which is at the root of the personality and chiefly concerned with the satisfaction of instincts and impulses, and the release of tension. The ego and the superego develop later out of the substrata of the id. The ego is formed as a bridge between the id and the external world; it has to juggle the demands of the id with the constraints of external reality. Freud saw the superego as the internalization of society's and the parents' standards and rules. The superego is sometimes thought to be equivalent to the conscience.

As well as describing the internal organization of the personality, Freud suggested a particular pattern of personality development. He described how there was a series of psychosexual stages that each person passes through. There are four stages or periods in this theory: the oral stage, the anal stage, the phallic stage and the genital stage. In addition he described a 'latency period' between the phallic and genital stages.

During the oral stage, which lasts for about the first 12 to 18 months of life, pleasure and the satisfaction of impulses are achieved mostly through the mouth and the actions of sucking, eating and biting. The anal stage occurs around the second year. This stage is marked by interest in, and gaining pleasure from, the anus and the expulsion of faeces. The phallic stage is between the ages of 3 and 6 years. This is a stage in which the child is interested in obtaining pleasure via their genitals and becomes sexually curious about the opposite gender. This is the period during which the Oedipal complex or Electra complex is thought to occur. In this stage, girls are thought to have a more difficult personality development to achieve. This is because, whereas boys can have a continuity of feelings towards their mothers, girls have to shift their desires from their mothers to their fathers. Following the phallic stage, there is thought to be a latency period until around puberty. In the latency period, sexual desires and impulses are repressed. These impulses re-awaken around the time of puberty when the child enters the genital stage. This is the final stage of psychosexual development. In this stage, a 'mature' personality style is thought to emerge in which the individual is able to relate to others in a way which satisfies both their instinctual needs and also the rules and standards of society. However, in Freud's theory of personality development, the path from one stage to another and to becoming a fully mature personality is not thought to be a smooth one.

The theory suggests that it is possible for the individual to become 'fixated' at any particular stage. This refers to the gratification of sexual impulses through means other than mature genital relationships. Fixation is thought to occur if there has been a degree of conflict at any particular stage. According to Freud, personality change can come about if the individual gains insight, via psychodynamic therapy, into the conflicts that are underpinning their behaviour and their particular pattern of personal adaptation.

Since Freud's time, later psychoanalytic writers have modified his theory of personality in various ways. In particular emphasis has shifted away from the role of sexual impulses towards the role of the ego in the personality. These later theorists have therefore been termed the 'ego psychologists' or neo-Freudians. They also emphasize social and cultural influences rather than focusing only on intrapsychic mechanisms (e.g. Hartmann, 1939; Erikson, 1968).

2.5.2 Jungian Theory of Personality

We have previously touched on some of Jung's views of personality. Jung thought that each individual differed in the way that they habitually experienced the world. He described four basic ways (sensing, intuiting, feeling and thinking) and two attitude types (extraversion and introversion). Jung proposed an elaborate classification of individuals into eight principal personality types. He believed that people could be divided into extraverts and introverts and that in this way people's main characteristic way of acting in life could be described, extroverts being sociable and outer directed and introverts inner directed.

Jung also described four psychological functions: thinking, feeling, sensing and intuiting. The combination of the major orientation (inner or outer directed), plus the four functions, leads to a complex model of personality with eight main types. The eight different psychological types therefore are: the extroverted thinking type, the introverted thinking type, the extroverted feeling type, the introverted feeling type, the extroverted sensing type, the introverted sensing type, the extroverted intuiting type and the introverted intuiting type.

Typologies such as that devised by Jung can have an appealing simplicity and intelligibility about them. It is tempting to adopt a model which provides a convenient category for every possible sort of person. However, the difficulty with such an approach is that it tends to oversimplify what are in fact very complex psychological phenomena and it does not take into account situational, environmental or other influences on personality.

Another important aspect of Jung's theory centres around his rather elaborate view of the 'psyche'. Jung believed that humans possess not only a **personal unconscious** based on life experiences, but also a **collective unconscious** which consists of memories accumulated throughout the entire history of the human race. These memories are represented by **archetypes**, inherited tendencies to interpret experiences in certain ways. Archetypes find expression in symbols, myths and beliefs that have appeared in many cultures throughout history. Some of Jung's notions bear some resemblances to those of modern evolutionary theorists who believe we carry in our genes remnants of our evolutionary history that influence how we perceive, think and act.

For Jung the mature personality was one in which 'both parts of the total psyche, consciousness and the unconscious, are linked together in a living relation' (Jacobi, 1968). Jung called the process by which a person becomes their own unique self and thus self-fulfilled, **individuation**.

2.5.3 Psychodynamic Approaches to Assessment of Personality

Psychodynamic clinicians and researchers generally use the clinical interview and expert judgement as the principal means of assessing the individual's personality and have traditionally not relied on 'paper and pencil tests'. However, some tests, such as the Myers Briggs, which attempts an assessment of the individual's personality in terms of Jungian theory, have developed a certain popular appeal and are used widely by non-specialists.

Psychodynamically oriented researchers and practitioners have sometimes employed **projective techniques** as tools for assessing personality. These are based on the idea that if a person is presented with a stimulus whose meaning is not clear, the person's interpretation of the stimulus will reflect their inner, unconscious needs, feelings, ways of viewing the world etc.

The two most influential projective tests are the **Thematic Apperception Test** (TAT; Morgan and Murray, 1935) and the **Rorschach Psychodiagnostic Inkblot Test** (Rorschach, 1942). In the TAT the individual is shown a series of ambiguous pictures and asked to describe what they think might be going on in the picture, what has gone on before and what might happen next. The individual's responses are then analysed to provide a picture of their underlying unconscious conflicts or motivations.

In the Rorschach the individual is shown a set of cards with 'inkblots' on them and told to say whatever they see or are reminded of by the abstract pattern. Their responses are then interpreted in terms of that person's unconscious processes and personality structure.

Other techniques that may be classified as projective tests include **sentence completion tasks** in which the individual has to complete sentences such as 'I feel . . .' or 'I would most like . . .'.

Although researchers have cast some doubt on the validity of these methods as measures of personality, they are still used by some psychodynamically oriented clinicians for diagnostic or treatment purposes.

2.5.4 Implications of Psychodynamic Theories of Personality for Counselling and Therapy

At first glance it might appear that a Freudian approach to personality development is rather pessimistic and rigid in its approach. According to the theory of psychosexual stages, personality development is virtually complete by the age of six years and the notion of 'fixation' suggests a rather immutable way of relating to the world and obtaining satisfaction from it. However, as noted above more recent psychodynamic theorists have stressed the importance of the ego and the possibility of experiences in adult life having an impact on the personality. These later theorists have incorporated the role of life stresses, culture, immediate environment and cognitive processes into their thinking about personality change (e.g. Arieti and Bemporad, 1978). They therefore do not espouse the view that only intrapsychic factors are important in determining how a person thinks and feels.

Freud thought that personal change occurred in psychoanalysis when the person gained 'insight' into the roots of their problems. These insights were largely to be gained through the relationship, or transference, with the therapist.

The important ideas for counselling arising out of psychodynamic theories of personality are many. In fact, because many of the concepts have entered our everyday language and commonsense and our implicit models of personality, we may find it difficult to recognize when we are employing models that are derived from psychodynamic thinking.

In particular, the idea that personality development in the adult person can only come through insight is one that underpins the majority of counselling approaches. The process of listening, reflecting, summarizing and encouraging free expression of feelings is designed to provide the client with an opportunity to explore their conflictual feelings and arrive at some integration via increasing awareness and insight. The way in which this might be achieved is illustrated by the case of the client we discussed above who presented with the various worries about her physical state after the car accident.

This client has been encouraged by her counsellor to explore her anxieties. In facilitating the exploration of her feelings about not being 'taken seriously' and 'properly looked after' by the medical profession, the counsellor helps the client to make the links between her early experience of 'lack of care' and her current 'neediness'. The counsellor learns that when she was around 18 months old her mother was admitted to hospital for several months. Because she was an only child, she was looked after by her grandmother and her father at this time and saw her mother relatively infrequently.

The client also talks about a number of relationships and situations in which she has never really felt that she is being valued or in any way 'special'. Although she describes her ex-husband as a 'considerate and understanding man' and they had got on well together, she never felt he really loved her or gave her what she needed, although she could not say quite what this was. She also feels that her family and friends take her very much for granted. She sees herself, and is generally seen by others, as a kind and helpful person but she is increasingly feeling 'put upon' by others. She always seems to be the one who ends up helping out (and not just in emergencies). She has fallen out with several friends over this, although she never told them why. She has found it particularly hurtful that nobody has offered to help her out during these last few months after the accident.

From a Freudian model of personality development, it might be postulated that the client suffered deprivation of her instinctual needs during the oral stage of development. This deprivation has left her fixated at the oral stage of development and with a personality that is characterized by pessimism and a belief that her needs will not be met.

If the counsellor was working psychodynamically, she would help the client to focus on other situations, especially her close relationships, where she felt needy or deprived. By clarifying exactly what it is that she, the adult woman, needs and wants and giving her permission to make these desires conscious, it should be easier for her to satisfy her needs herself, to 'reality test' the appropriateness of them and to ask for such help from other people as is required.

2.6 HUMANISTIC AND PHENOMENOLOGICAL APPROACHES TO PERSONALITY

Two contrasting theories will be described here to illustrate the role of models of personality in humanistic and phenomenological theories.

2.6.1 Client-centred Theory of Personality

Carl Rogers' theory of personality that is integral to his person-centred approach to therapy, emphasizes the uniqueness of the individual and the capacity for growth and self-actualization (Rogers, 1951,1961). This theory of personality emphasizes the need for positive regard from others that grows as the child develops self-awareness. In order to achieve the optimum psychological adjustment the child needs **unconditional positive regard**. The self-regard that the child has for itself reflects the regard that it has received from significant others.

Because unconditional regard is so rarely achieved, the child almost invariably grows up with the experience of conditional regard. That is the child only received positive regard conditional upon their 'good' behaviour. Rogers described this as the child having a **condition of worth**. If a child only ever experienced unconditional positive regard then that would lead to the child having a self-regard that was also unconditional. However, because most of us experience conditional regard from our parents and significant others then our self-regard too is a conditional feature. The self develops from our interaction with other people and so do these conditions of worth. The child learns to feel positive about itself only if it is conforming to these conditions. As Prochaska and Norcross (1994) put it:

> When individuals begin to act in accordance with introjected or internalized values of others, they have acquired conditions of worth. They cannot regard themselves positively as having worth unless they live according to these conditions. For some, this means they can feel good about themselves, feel lovable and worthy, only when achieving, no matter what the cost to their organism; others feel good about themselves only when they are nice and agreeable and never say no to anyone. Once such conditions of worth have been acquired, the person has been transformed from an individual guided by values generated from organismic experience to a personality controlled by the values of other people. We learn at a very early age to exchange our basic tendency for actualization for the conditional love of others and ourselves. (p. 131)

The person's experiences in the world are then 'filtered' in terms of how well they match their conditions of worth. Experiences that are congruent with the conditions are perceived accurately but those that are in conflict with the conditions may be denied, distorted or otherwise prevented from coming to conscious awareness. This leads to a gap between the individual's 'self' and their experience, and to the creation of psychological defences.

Rogers posited that personality change can come about via an increase in unconditional self-regard and a reduction in the conditions of worth that the individual imposes on themselves. Because he believed that there is an intrinsic drive toward growth and 'self-actualization' in the individual, Rogers thought that enabling personal growth and change was accomplished by providing the conditions that would allow the organism to pursue this basic tendency. These are the conditions that are hopefully provided in the 'counselling relationship'.

2.6.2 Gestalt Theory of Personality

Gestalt therapy was developed by Fritz Perls (1947, 1973; Perls et al., 1951) who originally trained in psychoanalysis. A number of theoretical influences shaped the theory underlying Gestalt therapy. The most important of these influences were existentialism, Zen Buddhism and humanism. In common with Carl Rogers' theory, Perls emphasized the innate tendency towards actualization in the human person. The person's ability to take responsibility for themselves and their actions is also a core feature of Perls' theory.

Personality development occurs through the natural processes of experiencing need, achieving satisfaction of that need by interaction with the environment, and through assimilation, thus completing a 'Gestalt' or organized whole.

The process of growth or maturation in the child is one of moving from dependency and a reliance on environmental support to independence and reliance on self-support. The child can become stuck if they are over indulged by their parents and never learn self-support. Perls thought that growth often came about through frustration because this leads to the child having to mobilize its own resources to get what it needed from the environment rather than simply having all its needs met by its parents. However, if the parents do not provide enough support before the child is ready for self-support this can also lead to the child becoming stuck in what Perls termed the 'impasse'.

If such growth problems occur, then the individual is unable to organize their behaviour in such a way as to satisfy their organismic needs. Perls thought that the person therefore had to deny or disown parts of themselves thus creating what he called 'holes' in their personality.

Personality change is seen as possible in Gestalt therapy via a process of awareness and integration. The person has to become aware of their needs, their patterns of avoidance and to make authentic contact with their environment in order to satisfy their needs via self -supporting strategies.

2.6.3 Humanistic and Phenomenological Approaches to Personality Assessment

Assessment of personality, in the phenomenological and humanistic schools, has tended to eschew the self-report inventory approach. Since such psychologists do not believe in a measurable 'objective reality', they have tended to adopt procedures which allow for the intensive and individualized assessment of the individual.

For example, they have often used clinical interview material which has then been subjected to qualitative and quantitative content analysis. In this way they have used self-descriptions as a main source material rather than monitoring specific behaviours or enquiring about traits. Other techniques employed by this group of clinicians and researchers have included the **Semantic Differential** (Osgood et al., 1957), the **Role Construct Repertory Test** (Kelly, 1955), and **Q SORTS** (Stephenson, 1953).

2.6.4 Implications of Humanistic and Phenomenological Theories of Personality for Counselling and Therapy

The emphasis of the two approaches described above on the subjective reality of the individual, their optimism about the possibility of personality growth and the focus on the organism as an entity has had a profound and extensive influence on counselling practice. In particular, Rogers' focus on change and growth has been a very motivating model for practitioners. Rogers' model suggests that changes in behaviour are brought about by changes in the way that the person experiences themselves and, in particular, changes in their self-concept.

Although there are many shared elements between these two theories, the practical application of them can be strikingly different. However, for present purposes we will examine how the previously mentioned client's difficulties might be viewed from a humanistic and phenomenological perspective in terms of her personality development.

In working with the client, the counsellor finds that during the period when her mother was in hospital, and afterwards, she was rewarded by praise and attention for being a good girl. Being good meant not being demanding, complaining or giving her parents any cause for anxiety. She felt that because of her father's worries about her mother's health, she had to be docile and conforming and not 'cause any trouble'. She therefore kept many of her childhood anxieties and desires to herself so that she didn't cause any upset.

From a Rogerian view of personality development, the client failed to get the necessary degree of unconditional positive regard from her parents. This may have been in part because of her mother's ill health and self-preoccupation and in part because of her parents' belief that their positive regard should be contingent upon her 'good' behaviour. She would then have internalized their view and come to believe herself that it was a condition of her own self-regard that she should be 'good', that is, docile and undemanding. However, this has led her to deny her ongoing needs for positive regard and attention. Because she is not aware of her own needs in intimate relationships, she allows herself to give her partner's needs priority. However, over time, her own needs come to the foreground and emerge in the form of her intense demands to be 'special' and to be 'looked after'. Here, the Rogerian counsellor or therapist would provide, through the therapeutic relationship, the 'conditions of worth' necessary for the client's personal growth and development.

From the viewpoint of Gestalt theory, the client may have had her parental support withdrawn too early before she was ready for self-support. She then had to discover her own neediness as a child and these unfulfilled needs are carried as 'unfinished business' into her adult life. Personal change in the Gestalt theory would come about by the client becoming aware of her needs and taking responsibility for satisfying them rather than trying to manipulate the environment to provide her with support.

Both of these models, although more especially the Rogerian approach, have been widely adopted by counsellors and therapists. The client-centred approach sees the provision of positive regard, warmth and empathy being crucial ingredients in allowing the person to explore their personal problems and to then move on to a more healthy level of functioning.

One criticism that is levelled at both models is that they tend to underemphasize and underestimate the role of the social, cultural and immediate environment of the individual. Also, since they play down the individual's biography, they can appear to be tackling the more 'superficial' aspects of personality rather than deeper personality structures.

2.7 SOCIAL LEARNING AND COGNITIVE APPROACHES TO PERSONALITY

The role of internal cognitive processes is the key element in social learning and cognitive approaches to personality. This approach grew out of a dissatisfaction with earlier behavioural theories which viewed personality as a set of learned behaviours and attempted to specify the conditions under which particular patterns of behaviour are developed, maintained and changed. Learning was said to occur through the process of **classical conditioning**, involving the pairing of an unconditioned stimulus with a previously neutral stimulus, and **operant conditioning**, in which behaviours are influenced by consequences, such as **positive reinforcement** that occurs after the behaviour.

2.7.1 Social Learning Theory of Personality

Although Albert Bandura's **social learning theory** (Bandura, 1986) recognized the importance of positive reinforcement, punishment and other consequences in influencing behaviour, he believed that humans are more than passive responders to external stimuli. They can learn in other ways, for example by solving problems 'symbolically' in their heads without having to resort to trial and error. Also, very importantly, people learn vicariously: they learn through observing other people, or **models**.

The importance of having models for behaviour and the relative impact of different models is stressed. Models who are seen as powerful and prominent are more likely to influence behaviour. Whether the child then performs a particular behaviour and under what circumstances is seen as a function of both reinforcement (the consequences) and **internal expectancies**. Expectancies are the internal beliefs about what outcomes will follow from one's behaviour and the value that an individual places on those outcomes. Expectancies will vary according to the situation that people find themselves in. This means that social learning theorists, unlike trait theorists, do not necessarily expect behaviour to be consistent across situations. Other social learning theorists such as

Rotter (1972) have also given a central role to cognitive expectancies and learned behaviour rather than attributing causality to intrinsic dispositional factors.

For personal change to occur, Bandura (1982) thinks that the critical factor is the person's expectancies of **self-efficacy**. Such self-efficacy expectancies can be enhanced by experiences of mastery and success: 'Change is mediated through cognitive processes, but the cognitive events are induced and altered most readily by experiences of mastery arising from successful performance.' (Bandura, 1977) Difficulties in personal adjustment are seen by this theory as being specific problems in behaviour and expectancies which result from the individual's learning and reinforcement history.

Cognitive theorists have taken the assumptions behind some of Bandura's ideas further and elaborated therapeutic approaches based on cognitive models. One of the best known is Aaron Beck. Although Beck (1976) originally trained and practised as a psychoanalyst, he developed a model of therapy which puts how and what people think at its centre. It has a somewhat sketchy description of how particular patterns of thought and behaviour develop in the individual. Experiences, either early in life or of a sufficiently critical nature, give rise to assumptions or **schemas** which determine the way the individual perceives and interprets their world. Thereafter it is not so much what happens to an individual that is important but how the individual *perceives* what happens to them.

2.7.2 Personal Construct Theory of Personality

Another important cognitive personality theorist was George Kelly (1955). Kelly's model has been very influential, especially his method for assessing personality—the Role Construct Repertory Test. Kelly was similar to the phenomenological theorists in that he did not hold that there was some external, objective reality that could serve as a reference point but rather he stressed the importance of the way in which the individual made sense of their world.

The things that interested Kelly therefore were the ways in which a person saw their world, interpreted their world and meshed these interpretations with their existing beliefs. Kelly called these interpretations that a person made about themselves and the world constructs. He held that there were **core constructs** which were central to the individual's habitual way of dealing with the world and also **peripheral constructs** which were more easily changed. The person's personality can then be thought of as their overall **construct system.**

In order to change, Kelly thought that it was necessary for the person to have a spirit of experimentation. This is exemplified in the key metaphor that Kelly employed of 'man as scientist'. That is someone who treats their own view of the world as a theoretical position which is capable of modification or refutation through observation and experimentation. One therapeutic strategy arising from this model is that of **fixed role therapy.** The person is encouraged by the therapist to act as if they were a different kind of person, the kind of person that they might prefer to be.

This emphasis on behavioural experiments and cognitive processes suggest a rather different style and focus in therapy than that adopted by the phenomenologists such as Rogers.

2.7.3 Social Learning and Cognitive Approaches to Personality Assessment

Many of the assessment techniques discussed in relation to the phenomenological and humanistic approaches are also applicable to the social learning and cognitive approaches. In particular **Kelly's Role Construct Repertory Test** (or the Rep Grid Test as it is sometimes referred to) is a way of getting at those constructs that the individual uses to understand themselves and their environment. This assessment method has been very widely used, both quantitatively and qualitatively, for a wide range of clinical and research purposes.

2.7.4 Implications of Social Learning and Cognitive Theories of Personality for Counselling and Therapy

An emphasis on cognitive processing styles and particular patterns of cognitive beliefs or 'schemas' is the hallmark of these approaches. The individual is thought to have a set of core assumptions about the world (e.g. 'I must be perfect or no-one will love me', 'The world is a dangerous and unpredictable place', 'My future is in my own hands') which shape the way in which that person perceives, interprets and appraises their experiences. (See also Section 11.5.3. on Models of Depression and Implications for Treatment.)

The task of the counsellor, in this model, is to elicit these core beliefs, help the person to examine the advantages and disadvantages of holding such beliefs, to challenge any maladaptive beliefs and to help the person find more adaptive ways to think about the world.

Because these models stress the role of the person's environment, and especially their social environment, in shaping their cognitive beliefs, the counsellor might also help the person look at what aspects of their current situation might be reinforcing or maintaining a 'faulty' thinking style. These models are therefore relatively optimistic about the possibility of change in the person, which can occur by targeting either environmental factors or cognitive factors. We will now see how a counsellor might work with and conceptualize the client's difficulties from a cognitive perspective.

The same client and the counsellor work together to identify any maladaptive beliefs that she might have which could help them to understand her particular patterns of behaviour. In examining her tendency to finish relationships because she feels undervalued as a result of her special needs not being recognized, they find that there are certain assumptions that she holds about relationships. She realizes that these assumptions have led her to be generally compliant and uncomplaining in relationships and to put her own needs second. She also rarely makes it explicit what she does need. She has then tended to become increasingly resentful about the way in which others respond to her and has broken off relationships rather than try to negotiate a more reciprocal arrangement.

*Both the client and counsellor agree that these assumptions bring more disad-
vantages than advantages and start to explore more adaptive beliefs about relationships that would help her to have some of her needs met within the relationship.*

Because of her early history of 'lack of care' and needing to be a docile child, The
client has developed beliefs such as 'If I put other people's needs first, then they will
love me,' 'If someone really cares about me, they will understand what I want without
my having to ask for it.'

Working in a cognitive way, the counsellor might encourage the client to devise various 'homework' experiments to test her core beliefs. For example, she might try being
more explicit about her needs with her close friends, and then examine the outcome of
this 'experiment' with the counsellor. Thus change in the client's personal style is seen
as coming about through a combination of behaviour change and change in her belief
system.

2.8 IMPLICATIONS OVERALL FOR COUNSELLING PRACTICE

In the previous sections we have touched upon some of the main theoretical ideas on
personality and illustrated some of the implications for counselling practice. Because of
the restrictions on space, the various theories have been simplified and summarized.
The counsellor needs to keep in mind that the distinctions drawn between the various
theories of personality may be somewhat artificial in practice where counsellors and
therapists often draw upon more than one model.

However, it might be useful at this point to draw together the various elements in order
to compare across the different theoretical positions. Each theory has implications for: (i)
assessment of the client; (ii) definitions of psychological maturity; and (iii) scope for personality change and development. Table 2.1 illustrates these points in summary form.

Table 2.1   Main approaches to personality: implications for counselling and therapy

	Trait	Psychodynamic	Humanistic/ phenomenological	Cognitive
Assessment of the client	Focus on typical behaviours and feelings	Focus on childhood experience and intrapsychic factors	Focus on client's immediate experience	Focus on client's construing
Psychological maturity	Good fit between disposition and environment	Having satisfactory relationships and occupational life	Taking responsibility for oneself and valuing oneself	'Realistic' view of self and world
Personality change	Limited by disposition	Via insight into conflicts	Via awareness and self-acceptance	Via changes in beliefs and expectations
Role of the counsellor	Not applicable	Guide and facilitator	Facilitator and collaborator	Collaborator

Theories of personality are ways in which writers have tried to make sense of the great diversity among individuals and the complexity within any one individual. Because these different theories are attempts to summarize processes across all individuals they are necessarily often oversimplified and over-generalized in their descriptions. No single personality theory could ever encompass every single human type. However, each of them can be useful in helping us to understand a particular person who comes for counselling. It may be the case that in some circumstances one theory will be more useful and fruitful than another for the purpose of understanding and assessing a particular client. However, this is not to say that any particular theory is more 'true' than another.

It may also be the case that conceptualizing a person's difficulties as arising solely from their personality is less than helpful, both for the client and for the counsellor. This is especially true if there are important situational factors that are having an impact on a person's behaviour. It may be that aspects of the person's situation are better predictors of their behaviour than aspects of their personality. Social and cultural factors may also need to be taken into account when trying to understand a person and their behaviour. For example, aggressive and impulsive behaviour in a young man may be viewed as normative for someone of that age and gender but for a young woman might be taken as evidence of some personality problem.

The role of the assessment of personality in counselling and psychotherapy is not necessarily straightforward. In practice, therapists or counsellors may use several different methods of personality assessment with clients: direct observation, psychometric tests and the clinical interview. Some methods require specialist training in administration and interpretation of results. Each of these methods has limitations and drawbacks which the counsellor must be aware of and sensitive to.

Because of the limitations of both psychometric and projective techniques for assessing personality, many professionals are sceptical about the usefulness of such measures. Also humanistically oriented practitioners may feel it antithetical to their philosophy to try to sum up someone with the relatively crude tools that are available. The more behaviourally oriented practitioner may prefer to use procedures such as self-monitoring or observation which do not require any inference about internal dispositions.

Sometimes counsellors adopt assumptions about personality and personality change without really being aware of the underlying theories from which such assumptions are derived. However, as we saw in the first chapter, it may be that we unconsciously communicate our implicit views about the nature of personality and the possibility of personality change to clients. It is therefore important for the counsellor to appreciate what assumptions or implicit models of personality are guiding their work.

Mischel (1986) has described the approach that uses different theories for different purposes as a 'constructivist' approach. As he describes it:

> The constructivist view holds that there is no single correct reality, no one truth that exists 'out there', waiting to be discovered. Rather, we invent or construct theories and concepts, very much like lenses, through which we view a complex and ever-changing world. What we see and find, then, depends on the particular lenses we have created and on where and how we look through them.

2.9 CONCLUDING COMMENTS

Interest in 'personality' among psychologists has waxed and waned over the years as different personality theories have become more, or less, popular. One important off-shoot of this interest has been the development of a range of methods (questionnaires, projective techniques and phenomenological methods) of assessment. These assess-ment devices can be used in a pragmatic way in therapeutic practice as a means of help-ing the client conceptualize and verbalize their feelings, attitudes or beliefs. However, the uncritical acceptance of the 'results' of such measures needs to be guarded against otherwise we run the risk of reifying what are dynamic, interactive processes.

Whilst trait theorists have put personality at the centre of their concerns, other psy-chologists have equally embedded their ideas about personality within wider theories of human development and psychopathology. This is why some writings on personality tend to merge into texts about clinical phenomenon, or abnormal maladaptive person-ality styles. In the past, a certain therapeutic pessimism tended to be associated with the attribution of the cause of a person's behaviour with their personality. However, the above schematic review of theories of personality will hopefully suggest that personal-ity theorists themselves have not adopted such a view. Rather they have tended to see personality theory as a means of understanding the person in order to facilitate personal change and development.

3

Emotion

CONTENTS

3.1 INTRODUCTION

Emotions colour our world, give meaning to our lives. Our capacity to experience emotions—love, joy, anger, enthusiasm, jealousy, yearning—lies at the heart of being 'human'. Indeed, it is our emotions which we think of as differentiating ourselves from non-human life forms (who could forget Mr Spock—although for one memorable episode of *Star Trek* they did let him fall in love!) and, of course, from androids (e.g. Dick, 1972).

Many clients will have entered into counselling because of disturbances in their emotional state; they feel unhappy, dissatisfied, frustrated, angry or confused. Their emotional state has alerted them to the fact that something in their lives is wrong or very unsatisfactory and they have consequently sought or accepted help in order to alleviate the distress.

Most counsellors would see exploration of the client's emotional world as crucial to gaining an understanding of the person and that person's experience. Counsellors will recognize there are marked individual differences in the degree to which clients are aware of, can conceptualize, and can express their emotional states. Some clients present a considerable richness, depth and intensity of emotional experience whilst others appear to have great difficulty identifying or articulating their feelings.

We all intuitively *know* what emotions are like, but emotions are so much a part of our everyday world, so much taken for granted that we rarely stop to think about why they may be important, what they mean or what they do. These are some of the questions that psychologists have been interested in; not so much, as counsellors are, at an individual level. But at a more general level they have tried to understand how, and why we feel as we do.

Psychodynamic theories of personality have a great deal to say about how emotions develop, are expressed and are defended against. Freud saw emotions as mere shadows of fiery sexual and aggressive instincts which become distorted by necessary defensive processes. However, much of the psychological research on emotion comes from more mainstream experimental psychology. At first glance, this literature appears somewhat limited and unidimensional when comparing it with first hand or fictional accounts of emotional experiences. This is, in part, because psychologists have, until recently, in the interest of scientific rigour, tended to study emotion in the laboratory. Laboratory experiments have, however, contributed significantly to our understanding of some of the basic processes involved in emotion and can provide us with valuable knowledge and insights which can be applied to the real world of individuals, including those in distress.

3.2 THE ROLE OF EMOTION IN OUR LIVES

Although there are probably times in most people's lives when they wish they weren't feeling as they were, and, indeed, when they wonder why they have to feel at all, for the most part we take feelings for granted and accept that it is just part of being human.

Psychologists, however, have seen emotions as having a number of important functions in helping us to adapt to the world. The two possibly most important will be discussed here. Firstly, emotions signal that something important is happening, they rouse us into action; and secondly, our emotions communicate something important about ourselves to others. We shall be discussing below how these functions relate to counselling and therapy.

3.2.1 Emotion as Motivation

Some emotions, such as anger and fear, are relatively easily defined and identified by most people. Others such as guilt, pride, hope or shame are often more complex and sometimes more difficult to describe. Our emotions can also be mixed and contradictory, and accordingly difficult to label. For example, the woman who, after hearing about a rail accident, discovers her husband is safe but her son is injured may not know what, or how, she is feeling.

Emotions, however, generally have **valence**; they are usually experienced as either *positive*, such as contentment, enthusiasm, hope, happiness or satisfaction, or *negative*, such as anxiety, shame, sadness or jealousy. Generally, we would want to act in ways which would promote or enhance our experience of positive feelings and ways likely to avoid or eliminate the negative ones. Emotions can therefore **motivate** us to take some action. Obvious examples of this are the feelings of fear on a narrow precipitous mountain path which would lead us to take steps to avoid the danger; the feelings of frustration at work which may stimulate us into doing something to make things more satisfactory or even to look for a new job; and the feelings of achievement we get from passing an exam which may motivate us to continue to work hard. In this way, the experience of emotion has been important to our survival, in the evolutionary sense, and also has particular significance for our well-being (Izard, 1990).

Emotions are always, according to Lazarus (1991a), related to personal 'meaning' or our own individual 'goals'. So, for example, we would only feel achievement at passing the exam if the event was personally relevant to us; if it helped us in some way to move forward; or if we had failed miserably at school, or underachieved. If passing the examination had no personal meaning then we would be unlikely to attach much importance to it and consequently feel little about the result.

How strongly we experience the emotion, that is, the **intensity** of the emotion, is also related to motivation. The stronger the feelings are, the more likely we are to take some action. So if we feel only mild irritation about a situation at work, we may decide to let it pass, but if we feel extremely annoyed about something we will probably try to do something to resolve the situation.

There are also, as noted in the previous section, individual differences in the intensity with which emotions will be experienced. Some people's emotional intensity seems naturally to be very low and nothing seems to get them very upset or excited. An extreme lack of emotion, however, would make it difficult or impossible to function normally. At the other end of the scale, too much emotional arousal can also cause problems and an overly emotional person may find it difficult to concentrate or to coordinate thoughts and actions effectively. Although emotional intensity can be affected in the shorter term by psychological disturbance, such as depression (see Section 11.4) it is usually viewed by psychologists as an aspect of temperament which, as we discussed in Chapter 2, seems to be genetically based, although social learning plays an important part (Eisenberg and Fabes, 1992).

If, as suggested above, emotions are important to our physical survival and our psychological well-being, it follows that we need to pay heed to them. With some emotions in certain contexts, our responses would be difficult or impossible to ignore, such as the feelings of fear on the mountain path mentioned above. Other emotions give us less urgent messages. The messages they communicate nevertheless are important. As we have pointed out, we would be unlikely to experience any intensity of feelings unless those feelings had some inherent meaning for us. Our emotions act as a signal to us that something important is happening; something related to our deeper values and needs. Our emotional responses therefore provide us with an important source of **feedback** to ourselves. This does not mean, of course, that we should always act on our feelings. But if we consistently ignore them, then we deny important aspects of ourselves and we may become discontent, alienated and unhappy. Suppression of emotion can also have an adverse effect on mental and physical health (see Sections 3.7 and 10.7 on Stress and Health).

This 34-year-old man is an example of someone who had consistently ignored the feedback from his emotions. He had been referred to the counsellor because of symptoms of moderately severe depression. He is married, lives with his wife and dog, and works for an insurance company. He has been on sick leave for the past four weeks.

As a young child he spent several periods of three to four weeks in hospital. He subsequently became very attached to his mother and they remained extremely close until her death two years ago. He admired his father enormously, although he did find it difficult sometimes to live up to his very high standards, even though he felt his father never had particularly high expectations for him. He reported that he had always been a 'good' child, but he also talked about occasionally having quite violent rages.

Life as a teenager was a little difficult when his older sister and his younger brother both 'rebelled'. He felt he had to make up for them and decided he would never give his parents any cause for concern. And indeed, although he sometimes resented it, he never did. He was conscientious, responsible and hard-working at home, at school and then at work. Apart from a brief engagement to a girl deemed by his parents to be 'unsuitable', he always did what was expected (although he has, on more than one occasion, had fleeting feelings of resentment and anger over his parents' interference in the matter; but he had to admit that they were right). He subsequently married a 'girl' of whom his parents approved, he cleaned the car on Saturdays and mowed the lawn on Sundays. On Friday evening he would take his wife to the supermarket, on Tuesday evening put out the rubbish. He was always on time at the office and left each evening half an hour after the office closed.

This was the life that he thought he wanted for himself. He got on well with his wife and he wanted a conventional well-ordered life. So why, he wondered, could he not be happy? Going to the supermarket 'knotted him up inside'; he would inwardly 'rage' as he mowed the lawn; he would fantasize about killing his fellow commuters.

A year or so ago a colleague he never particularly liked was promoted above him. This person has made a number of changes and the client finds it infuriating the way in which the colleague seems to be challenging any initiatives which he has taken, even in his own area of expertise. However, as always, the client got on with things without making a fuss; as always, he adopted an affable and pleasant manner and was never bad-tempered, uncooperative or surly. Nor did he confront the person in question or make any attempt to resolve the situation.

But underneath, the client knew things were very wrong. He was subject to 'internal rages', often found it extremely difficult to get up in the mornings and quite fre-

quently thought about suicide. He had also begun to think more and more about his mother, and was aware that he had not been able to grieve for her. However, on the surface, he carried on with his life as before. He ignored the feedback from his emotions and made no attempt to make sense of what this might mean to him.

In counselling, he began to 'listen' more to this feedback and to explore what this was 'telling' him, rather than trying to persuade himself what he 'ought' to be feeling. This has led to what are, to him, quite significant changes in his life. The lawn has been partly paved over and what remains is not as neat as it was, sometimes he and his wife go to the pub instead of the supermarket, and he has taken to using the car wash even though it is not as good as washing it himself. He has also taken himself off fishing a few times by himself. Although these adjustments, on the face of it might not seem to be particularly far-reaching or profound, the process of change has been difficult and painful for the client. Indeed,it has challenged the whole foundations on which he had based his conscious life.

It has also had some obvious implications for others. His colleagues and boss do not find him quite so easy-going; he can be quite 'prickly' on occasions. His wife has had to make a number of adjustments herself and his father has realized he did not know his son quite as well as he thought he did. Happily, his relationship with the dog has remained unchanged. The re-negotiation of his other relationships has, however, on the whole been positive for the people concerned and the client is now functioning in a way more consistent with maintaining his psychological (and physical) well-being.

The client in the above example desperately wanted to feel happy with the life he had created for himself. He wanted to enjoy mowing the lawn, washing the car etc. But emotions are not something we can make happen. Unlike actions, which are initiated by the person, emotions 'happen' to us; in this way they are **passions** not actions. We cannot decide to experience happiness or joy. Nor can we determine when to feel grief or sorrow. We may feel we 'ought' to feel happy, appreciative, even angry. Indeed it is something counsellors frequently hear from their clients. For example, 'She's so good to me, I really do try to be appreciative, but all I feel is irritation.' 'I thought that now the pressure was off and I'd found a new job that I'd be really happy, but it's not like that.'

Although emotions seem to just happen to us, this does not mean that we have no control over them. This is because emotions, as we shall see, can in part result from our cognitive appraisal of the situation; that is, the way in which we think about and interpret what is happening. (See Chapter 2 and Section 3.4 below.) But if we do not make any changes in the way in which we think or act, and the emotion remains unresolved, the physiological changes that accompany particularly anger and fear (which mobilize us to fight or flee), when maintained too long can exhaust our resources and can even cause physiological damage. A chronic state of high arousal can therefore take its toll on physical health (see Chapter 10).

But in a counselling context it is not only clients' awareness and response to emotional feedback that is at issue. Our own emotional responses as counsellors or therapists to the client and the client's 'material' can provide an important source of information for ourselves. In psychodynamic terms, this would be seen as an aspect of what is termed

counter-transference, the interpretation of which requires a high level of self-aware-ness and understanding on the part of the counsellor. Therapists from other theoretical orientations would probably not disagree. This, of course, is why some training courses in counselling (and most in psychotherapy and all in counselling psychology) require their trainees to undergo a period in counselling or personal therapy themselves.

3.2.2 Emotion as Communication

Emotions, as we have seen, tell us, or remind us that something important is happening to ourselves. Our emotions are also important ways of communicating to others infor-mation about our internal states and intentions. Indeed, people can make broad inter-personal judgements with a high degree of accuracy from videotaped samples of expressive behaviours (Ambady and Rosenthal, 1992). The signals we give, therefore, are interpreted, and in turn influence the response of others, including their emotional response. For example, expressions of sadness and distress evoke empathy and helping behaviour from others (Izard, 1989) and parents report feeling disturbed, distressed, irritated, sympathetic and unhappy on hearing their babies cry (Frodi et al., 1978).

If people do not communicate their feelings to their friends, partners, relatives, col-leagues etc. and others are left to 'guess' what they are feeling, then they may guess wrongly, or possibly even worse, fail to notice. This is likely to lead to misunderstand-ings and a breakdown in communication. Failure to communicate feelings can therefore lead to the individual feeling unacknowledged, misunderstood and unimportant as well as leaving the other person baffled and confused.

Of course, there may be many reasons why someone does not express openly what they feel and this is an area which the counsellor may need to explore with clients who are emotionally unexpressive.

A 37-year-old woman, who has suffered several episodes of severe depression in her adult life is talking about her relationship with her husband.
Client *The trouble is, whenever I try to talk about something, particularly what I feel about something, unless I know before I start what I'm going to say, he just launches in—he always seems to get there first—says he knows what I mean, knows what I must be feeling.*
Counsellor *Sort of one jump ahead.*
Client *Yes, but he's not. He* doesn't *know what I'm feeling, and the problem is once he starts, I'm not sure I do either . . . I just shut down. It's not worth it. Now I don't bother. I haven't really bothered for years.*

(Earlier in the session the client had recounted an episode between her father and her 11-year-old daughter. Her daughter had expressed an ongoing concern to her grandfather that they had so much to eat when there were so many hungry and starv-ing people in the world. He responded to this by telling her that this was ridiculous and she shouldn't be so stupid. This ended with the little girl in tears and the grand-father apparently unconcerned.)

> *The client went on to recount many episodes when she felt her own opinions and feelings were ignored or overruled by her father. It seems that she was still experiencing, or 'in touch' with her emotions, but possibly as a result of her childhood experiences of feeling 'put down', had given up trying to communicate. Being more emotionally assertive subsequently became a major focus of the counselling for this client.*

As noted above, it can also be difficult and frustrating living or interacting with someone whose expressive signals are weak. A session with the client's husband confirmed this.

> *'I've no idea what she feels. Sometimes it comes out later, usually in a roundabout way. It makes it so difficult to plan things, even to enjoy myself when I don't know what's going on in her. I do try to understand.'*

At the opposite extreme, people can be overly emphatic in the way in which they communicate their feelings. This too can cause problems, the recipient often feeling overwhelmed and powerless.

> *'As soon as she comes into the room I know what sort of mood she's in. It completely throws me—takes me over. I then don't know what I'm thinking or feeling myself. It's only when she goes away that I can really be myself and get on with things'.*
> *This particular client went on to explore with the counsellor ways of 'protecting' himself, for example, by engaging in distracting behaviours in order to avoid the stimuli (his wife's overly expressive behaviours) to which he was responding.*

A particular method of psychological therapy which directly addresses the subject of emotional expressiveness is **social skills training**. This is a form of cognitive behaviour therapy developed to 'train' interpersonal and emotional skills. This involves helping the individual both to develop social and emotional behaviours and also to interpret the emotional responses of others (Wilkinson and Canter, 1982). Although the training has traditionally been carried out in groups following structured 'programmes' the methods can be adapted for working with individual clients and can, with care, be integrated into counselling sessions. For an example of how this might be done, see Section 7.4 on Social Skill and Relationships.

3.3 COMPONENTS OF EMOTION

People express their experience of emotion in many different ways. For example, one person may say, 'I was absolutely furious, just shaking with rage', another might say, 'I was absolutely furious, particularly because I knew he was lying', and yet another, 'I was absolutely furious, I just yelled at him at the top of my voice'. Each person has conceptualized anger differently: the first in terms of **physiological sensations**, the second in relation to a 'weighing-up' of the situation, often referred to as **cognitive appraisal**, and the third in terms of **expressive behaviour**. There is a considerable body of psychological theory and research on these three 'components' of emotion.

Emotions, though, do not occur in a vacuum but in response to eliciting stimuli. We usually are angry *with* someone or something, happy *about* something, fearful *of* someone or something. The eliciting stimuli need not be external but can be in the form of memories or images. Most of us can recall situations which elicit feelings of anger or happiness when we think about them. Much of the time we are aware of the 'triggers', but not always. People sometimes feel irritable or anxious without really knowing why and it appears that some emotional responses are triggered more or less automatically with little conscious awareness on our part. We will be looking at this in more detail in Section 3.5.2 on Unconscious Appraisals.

Although in the above example the three responses were attributed to three different hypothetical people, the physiological, cognitive and expressive components of emotion are by no means mutually exclusive and can all be experienced by one individual in response to a particular stimulus.

> *A father is describing his feelings about his new-born son. 'Whenever I think about him I get a funny sort of warm glow inside (physiological). I feel he's all the more precious because we waited so long for him (cognitive). I haven't been able to take the grin off my face for three days now!' (behavioural expressive).*

In this example the feelings being expressed were relatively straightforward. However, as noted above, emotional experience can be extremely complex and often mixed or contradictory. It is therefore hardly surprising that clients frequently find it difficult to assign particular labels to them. This is why the question 'what are (or were) you feeling' is often inappropriate. Below, the therapist used her knowledge of the components of emotion to explore the client's experience rather more broadly.

> *The client is a 36-year-old woman who, as a child and young adolescent, was sexually abused by her father. She has brought along to the session some photographs of him.*
> **Counsellor** *What happens to you when you look at them?*
> **Client** *My mouth goes dry, I'm cold, I'm sweating . . . I took them out. I couldn't handle them. (Voice breaking, breathing heavily) I can't handle them—in any shape or form. I can't handle them. I can't cope with them. (Crying, head in hands, sobbing)*
> **Counsellor** *What do you think when you look at them?*
> **Client** *I don't think anything at all. I can't think. I want at this moment not to be able to see his hands and his eyes when I close mine—his skin . . . I know I've got to face the photos.*
> **Counsellor** *What do you feel you want to do?*
> **Client** *I want to destroy him. (Said angrily. She takes up one of the photographs and tears it in small pieces) The sodding bastard. I want to get rid of his face, his body, smashing his face. There isn't a single part of his body which when I picture it doesn't fill me with horror, with fear. . . (voice dropping and trailing off) whatever.*

(She stands up, paces the room) My mind and my body—thinking about it—It's close to chaos and hell.

In this extract, the therapist has focused in on the concept of emotion being something which 'happens' to the person ('What happens to you when you look at the pictures?'), on the cognitive components ('What do you think when you look at them?') and on the behavioural expressive ('What do you feel you want to do?').

The client has conceptualized her emotional experience in terms of physiological responses ('My mouth goes dry' etc.), cognitive elements ('I want not to be able to see his hands' etc.) and the behavioural expressive aspects ('I want to destroy him'). It is interesting to note that the only time the client attempts to express the emotion in the more straightforward 'feeling' sort of words of 'horror' and 'fear' that she loses some of the momentum of the expression, as if the words were inadequate to express the intensity of her experience.

Body, mind and behaviour therefore play a major part in our feeling lives. The physiological, cognitive and behavioural components of emotion, however, are not the emotions themselves. Emotions are not physiological sensations, nor are they specific thoughts or overt behaviours. Emotions are subjective experiences. What psychologists have been particularly concerned with is the way in which the components of emotion relate to this subjective experience of the feeling, and how the components relate to each other.

3.4 THE PHYSIOLOGICAL COMPONENT OF EMOTION

3.4.1 The Autonomic Nervous System

When we experience an intense emotion many parts of the body are involved and a number of bodily changes occur, some of which were described by the client in the example above. The degree to which we are aware of these changes varies. Sometimes we are only too aware; at other times the changes may be less apparent. Most of the physiological changes that take place during emotional arousal result from the activation of the sympathetic division of the autonomic nervous system (see Figure 3.1).

The **autonomic nervous system** is a subdivision of the nervous system and controls the glands and the 'smooth' muscles of the body, which include the heart, the blood vessels and the lining of the stomach and intestines. Many of the activities the autonomic nervous system controls are autonomous and self-regulating, such as digestion and circulation. There are only indirect connections between the autonomic nervous system and those parts of the brain involved in consciousness. We are not, for example, immediately aware that our stomachs have secreted gastric juices, but we may hear our stomach grumbling. Similarly, we can only indirectly influence autonomic activity by physical methods, such as holding our breath and straining our muscles to increase blood pressure, or by cognitive means by, for example, imagining ourselves in an exciting situation.

There are two divisions of the autonomic nervous system, the **sympathetic division**, which gears the body for action, or **fight or flight**, as it is sometimes referred to, and

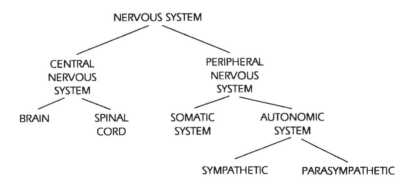

Figure 3.1   The organization of the nervous system

the **parasympathetic division**, the energy-conserving system which, as the emotion subsides, takes over and returns the organism to its normal state. These activities of the autonomic nervous system are themselves triggered by the regions of the brain: the hypothalamus and the limbic system.

The state of arousal produced by the activity of the sympathetic branch of the autonomic nervous system and by hormones from the endocrine system causes a number of changes (all of which need not happen at any one time) which include:

- more rapid respiration;
- increase in heart rate and blood pressure;
- increase in perspiration;
- decrease in secretion of saliva and mucus;
- dilation of pupils;
- quicker clotting of blood in the case of wounds;
- decrease of motility in gastrointestinal tract;
- diversion of blood from the stomach and intestines to the brain and skeletal muscles;
- increase of blood-sugar levels to provide more energy;
- goose pimples due to hairs on skin becoming erect.

These kind of changes in physiological functioning occur in relation to emotions which require the body to be prepared for action, such as anger or fear, although some of the same changes might also occur during sexual arousal or experiences of joy. Some bodily processes may be depressed or slowed down, however, during emotions such as grief or sorrow.

3.4.2 Autonomic Arousal and Emotional Experience

One of the earlier theories of emotion, the **James–Lange theory**, argued that the emotions we experience result from our perception of these bodily changes (increased heart-rate, sweating etc). That is, when we encounter an 'emotion-arousing' stimulus, our bodies react and our brains interpret our responses and tell us we are afraid, in love, annoyed etc (see Figure 3.2). This, on the face of it, seems to be entirely the wrong way round; we usually think that our heart is beating quickly *because* we are afraid, and not we are afraid because our heart is beating quickly.

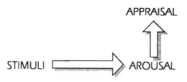

Figure 3.2   James–Lange theory

If feedback from bodily sensations associated with autonomic arousal tells us what we feel then we would expect to find that interference with that feedback would affect our subjective experience of emotion. Some evidence for this comes from studies where drugs have been used to increase or decrease arousal such as adrenalin and Beta-adrenergic blockers (Fonte and Stevenson, 1985). In these studies, subjects have reported feelings consistent with the artificially induced arousal.

It might also be expected that patients who have suffered from spinal injuries who do not receive autonomic feedback will report some decrease in emotional experience or intensity. Although early studies reported that this might indeed be the case (Hohmann, 1962), more recent research, with a population who had been encouraged to adopt a philosophy of active coping, has found no evidence of decrease in emotional experience (Chwalisz et al., 1988). These findings have cast doubts on the claim that arousal feedback from the body is absolutely necessary in order to experience emotion.

Although the evidence in support of the James–Lange theory of emotion is somewhat inconclusive, our physiological responses nevertheless play a crucial role in our experience of emotion. It is therefore reasonable to suppose that, in the counselling context, methods that sensitize client to their own autonomic arousal may help them gain access to the emotional state, as the following extract demonstrates.

The client is a 34-year-old man who is a supervisor in a small factory. He has always appeared to his friends and colleagues as a really kind and good person, 'someone who would do anything for anybody'. His wife also describes him as someone who does tend to take things very much to heart'. He reports a good relationship with his boss for whom he has a great deal of respect. Over the past few months the company has had several large orders and everyone has been under a lot of pressure at work. However, the client knows that the company is struggling to survive, and at least he is in work.

Several days before this session he had walked out in the middle of an appraisal interview with his boss and left the building. He has been off sick since.
Counsellor   *What was happening to you just before you walked out?*
Client   *I don't know. It's all a muddle. I just had to get out.*
Counsellor   *Do you remember what was happening in your body?*
Client   *No, not really—just wanting not to be there.*
(The counsellor notices that the client's breathing has become quite rapid and that he is clenching his fists)

Counsellor *What's happening in your body right now?*
Client *I can feel my heart thumping. I could feel it then. Do you know—no, I couldn't have done—I think I wanted to hit him, although I didn't think it at the time, not like that, but somehow that's what I wanted to do. But that's ridiculous—I like the man and he's as pushed as I am. And I'm not the sort of man to do a thing like that.*

Here the client, by becoming aware of his autonomic state, begins to articulate feelings which he finds somewhat baffling and of which he was scarcely aware himself.

3.5 THE COGNITIVE COMPONENT OF EMOTION

Cognitions also play a vital part in our experience of emotion and a particular event may evoke different emotions depending on how we view or **cognitively appraise** it. This will depend on a number of factors including our own system of values and personal goals, past experiences, prior knowledge and personal beliefs. These beliefs, as we noted in Section 2.7, on Social Learning and Cognitive Approaches to Personality, can be irrational and self-defeating. (See also Section 11.4 on Cognitive Theories of Depression.)

If we are walking along the street and see a neighbour, who we know has been ill, cross to the other side of the road, we may interpret this as the person wishing to avoid us. We must have done something to offend them. Maybe we should have visited them, sent some flowers, etc. This may result in feelings of anxiety and discomfort. Alternatively we could interpret the situation as the neighbour, who is only just up and about, being distracted, not noticing us and needing all her attention to carry out her necessary tasks. In which case we may feel pleased for her, that she is out and about, but a little concerned about her health.

The **personal beliefs** about the situation in the first appraisal are, 'It must be my fault', and in the second, 'People who have been unwell will not "be themselves" '. Personal beliefs are in turn affected by our past experiences. It would come as no surprise to discover that the person making the first appraisal had, in the past, been exposed to hypercriticism or made to feel inappropriately personally responsible for events outside of her control. We can therefore see how **past experiences** can affect how we feel. Past experiences affect our beliefs which then influence our appraisal of a situation and subsequently the emotion we experience. We shall be looking at the role of personal beliefs and cognitive appraisal in relation to depression in Chapter 11.

3.5.1 Cultural Learning and Appraisal

We have seen how personal beliefs affect the way in which we appraise a situation, and we might expect that these, in turn, would be influenced by **cultural beliefs**. If this were the case then we would find differences in the way in which people from different cultures appraised situations. This has not, in fact, been the case. Considerable similarities were found between cultures, particularly in appraisals of events that evoked joy, fear, anger, sadness, disgust, shame and guilt (Wallbott and Scherer, 1988). A more recent study led to similar conclusions (Mauro et al., 1992); the few cultural differences that

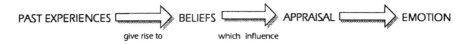

Figure 3.3   The relationship between past experience and emotion

did emerge were related to personal responsibility for events. American subjects, as compared with the Japanese, reported that in order to experience pride, they would need to feel a higher degree of personal control over the outcome of events.

3.5.2 Unconscious Appraisals

We are not always aware of the appraisals that underlie emotional responses (Lazarus, 1991a). An adult who, as a child, experienced some painful sessions with a doctor which were preceded by sitting in the hospital waiting room, may experience anxiety in similar settings. In this case the adult experience is not the result of the current interpretation of the situation but (in behavioural terms) of inappropriate learning (Zajonc, 1984). (See also Sections 4.5 on State-dependent Memory and 4.6 on Childhood Amnesia.)

Psychoanalytic theory has been particularly concerned with unconscious processes in relation to emotion. Freud suggested that there is both **conscious processing** (appraisal) and **unconscious processing** of emotional information. More recent psychobiological research has given some support to this view by suggesting that unconscious emotional reactions may occur because of structural characteristics in the brain. This has led Lazarus (1991b) to propose that people are capable of having two simultaneous emotions in response to the same event; a conscious one (occurring as a result of **cortical activity**) and an unconscious one (created by direct input from the senses to the **amygdala**, part of the limbic system) before the information reaches the cortex, where conscious processing takes place).

We may indeed, as Freud suggested, sometimes not really *know* what we feel at a deeper, inaccessible level, although we may be behaving in a way that is consistent with that feeling. This may help to explain why certain aspects of our emotional lives are puzzling and why behavioural reactions sometimes seem at odds with the emotion that is being experienced at a conscious level. For example, 'I'm being really aggressive to her and I don't know why. I don't really feel angry.' This area of theory and research has considerable implications for counselling, although there is a continuing debate on the degree to which it is possible to gain access to these sorts of unconscious processes.

3.5.3 The Relationship between Cognition and Arousal

Whereas the James–Lange theory discussed above viewed the experience of emotion as resulting from appraisal of our physiological responses, Schaachter and Singer (1962)

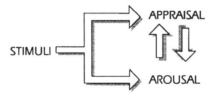

Figure 3.4   The Schaachter–Singer theory of emotion

argued that both physiological arousal and cognitive appraisal are important in the experience of emotion. That is, our experience of emotion is based on our appraisal of the *situation*, our physiological responses to the situation, and our appraisal of these bodily responses.

According to this theory, the **intensity** of the physiological arousal tells us how strongly we are feeling something, but we **label** emotion as fear, anxiety, anger or whatever on the basis of the situation we are in. The labelling depends on **attribution**, or identifying the cause of some event. People may attribute the same sensations of physiological arousal to different causes, depending on the situation. If we are watching the cup final we would probably attribute a racing heart and rapid breathing to excitement, and label the emotion as such, but if we were about to sit an examination, we would probably attribute the same sensations to nervousness, and again, describe the emotion in those terms. Whether we label what we feel as being 'upset' or being 'angry' will also sometimes depend on our appraisal of the situation.

Schaachter and Singer also hypothesized that if we are in a state of physiological arousal which is unrelated to an emotion-provoking event, for example as a result of physical exercise, we will try to attribute our aroused state to something in the immediate environment, with the result that the feeling becomes intensified. This might help to explain the client's actions in the example below.

A child care worker in a residential children's home had just returned from a run and had leapt up two of the three flights of stairs when a resident (a fourteen-year-old boy) put out his arm to stop him to give him a 'phone message. The client grabbed his arm and threw him to the floor. This constituted an assault. It would seem that the care worker had appraised the situation as confrontational, an interpretation that was consistent with his high level of arousal. That is, his response may have resulted from emotion generated by exercise-induced arousal rather than from his appraisal of the situation itself.

People can also remain physiologically aroused much longer than they are aware of, and arousal from one experience can be carried over into another, quite different situation. This is called **transferred excitation** (Reizenzein, 1983) and occurs when the overt signs of arousal subside, but the sympathetic nervous system is still active. Most of us will have experienced having been in a distressed or angry state and 'taking it out' on someone or something else.

3.6 THE BEHAVIOURAL EXPRESSIVE COMPONENT OF EMOTION

So far, emotion has been described from the 'inside', as people experience their own emotions both physiologically and cognitively. The third component of emotion is concerned with the outward expression of feelings. When we are happy, we probably laugh or smile, withdraw when frightened and possibly get aggressive when angry. Why do we do these things and what effect does it have on ourselves and others? We have already discussed emotional expressiveness as communication. In this section we shall be examining this in a little more detail, and also looking at the way in which the expression of feelings may contribute to the subjective experience of emotion.

3.6.1 Facial Expressiveness

Although many parts of the body can communicate feelings, facial movements and expression play a primary and fundamental role in communicating emotions; it is the face on which we generally focus our attention in social interactions. The human face is capable of generating between 6000 and 7000 different expressions (Izard, 1971); indeed, an eyebrow need only to be raised almost imperceptibly to communicate quite significant information. It is hardly surprising that psychologists have made facial expressions the focus of much of their research into emotional expressiveness.

We have discussed above how the experience of emotion can be important to our survival, warning us of danger, or preparing us for the fight. Many theorists maintain that the *expression* of emotion, similarly, is of evolutionary significance. Looking frightened may warn people of danger, and looking angry may signify that the person may become aggressive. Darwin (1872) maintained that certain facial expressions seem to be universal and innate, regardless of the culture in which the individual is raised.

This idea has been tested out by asking people from a range of very different cultures, including members of remote preliterate tribes who had no contact with western culture, to look at photographs showing facial expressions of surprise, sadness, anger, happiness, disgust and fear. These people had no difficulty in identifying the facial expressions correctly. This was also the case when American college students judged the emotional expressions of Fore natives from videotape, although there was a tendency to confuse fear with surprise (Ekman, 1982).

Further evidence for the argument that some facial expressions are innate comes from the fact that babies, even blind babies who cannot imitate adults, do not need to be taught to smile in pleasure or grimace in pain (Eibl-Eibesfeldt, 1973). However, even though babies begin with an innate set of emotional responses, they soon learn to imitate facial expressions and to use facial expressions to express a developing range of emotions.

3.6.2 The Effect of Culture on Emotional Expressiveness

If certain facial expressions are innate, as suggested by Darwin and the research discussed above, does culture have any part to play? It would seem that it does. As children grow, they learn the **display rules** of their particular culture; that is, the rules (and
norms) that govern what emotions are appropriate in what circumstances and what
emotional expressions are acceptable. These 'rules' may vary within and between cultures and also over time. In one experiment designed to explore cultural commonalities
and differences in facial expressiveness no differences were found between American
and Japanese students whilst viewing a highly stressful film in private. However, when
interviewed about the film the Japanese students presented a 'happy' face throughout,
and the American students clearly registered disgust and anxiety on their faces.

Cultural rules therefore specify the particular ways in which emotions are expressed.
This is a kind of 'language' of emotion, over and above the basic expression of emotion; a language that is recognized by others within a culture. For example, sticking
your tongue out in China expresses surprise and the Masai tribe of Africa consider
being spat on a great compliment.

Thus biological factors play an important role in how people respond emotionally,
but cultural display rules can influence how, when and where they express their feelings. This seems to apply also to the expression and communication of emotion through
variations in voice pattern, particularly variations in pitch, timing and emphasis. Some
of these variations appear to be universal, for example a sharp increase in pitch indicates fear, and others to be more culturally specific.

Clearly when working with clients from different cultures it is essential to be sensitive to the cultural context, both from the point of view of understanding what the client
may be experiencing and expressing and also in relation to possible behavioural change
which may result from the counselling.

3.6.3 Gender Differences and Emotional Expressiveness

There is considerable evidence that females are more non-verbally expressive than
males particularly with respect to facial display. (They are also, across cultures, better
judges of facial expression; Ekman, 1982.) It has been suggested that the underlying
feelings of men and women may in fact be similar, and that the differences in emotional
expressiveness result from differences in gender-based display rules. That is, it is more
acceptable for women to express emotion than for men (LaFrance and Banaji, 1992). In
one study, however, although females were found to be more facially expressive in
response to emotional material, they showed significantly less autonomic arousal than
males, who expressed little facially, but conveyed more physiologically (Buck et al.,
1974). Does this mean that the suppression of external display enhances physiological
arousal whilst expression of the emotion reduces it? The finding is somewhat controversial in the light of other data discussed below which show positive associations
between physiological and expressive measures.

3.6.4 Facial Expressiveness and Emotional Experience

Facial expressions, in addition to communicating feelings, also contribute to our experience of emotion. This is called the **Facial Feedback Hypothesis** (Adelmann and Zajonc, 1989; Izard, 1977, 1990). Facial muscles feed messages to the brain, and this feedback combines with the other components of emotion to produce a more intense experience (Laird, 1974).

In addition to contributing to the intensity of our emotions, it would seem that facial expression can determine the quality of emotion. Strack et al. (1988), found that subjects rated themselves as feeling more pleasant when they held pens in their teeth, which activates muscles in smiling, than when they held pens in their upper lips, which activates muscles involved in frowning. Subjects also rated cartoons as funnier while holding pens in their teeth than when holding pens in their lips, providing more evidence for the idea that facial expression can contribute to the intensity of emotion.

In another study, comparisons of the subjective experiences of subjects who pronounced different sounds such as 'ee' and the German 'u'. Saying the 'ee' sound, which activates smiling, was associated with more pleasant feelings than pronouncing the 'u' sound, which activates muscles involved in negative facial emotions (Zajonc et al., 1989).

It has been suggested that facial expressions may have an indirect effect on emotion by increasing autonomic arousal. This was demonstrated by Ekman et al. (1983) who found that subjects producing particular emotional expressions showed changes in heartbeat and skin temperature. This provides further evidence in support of the James–Lange theory discussed above, which holds that emotion is the perception of certain bodily changes.

Of what relevance is the facial feedback hypothesis to counselling? This area of theory and research seems to be so far removed from the real world of emotional experience, yet it provides some physiological support for some of the more creative and innovative psychological therapies. **Gestalt therapy, psychodrama** and **social skills training** have all recognized the importance of facial expression and have suggested, either explicitly or implicitly, that 'acting' or exaggerating emotional expressiveness, including facial expression, can enhance the experience of emotion and even generate different feelings.

3.7 EMOTIONAL EXPRESSION AND COUNSELLING

Many counsellors will see facilitating the client's expression of emotion as an important part of their counselling work. But what is the evidence that this is, in fact, beneficial? Two areas of theory and research are particularly relevant to addressing this issue. The first of these is the work of James Pennebaker and his colleagues on the role of emotional expression in overcoming the effects of trauma and the second is concerned with the effects of the expression of aggression on subsequent arousal.

Those who have been the victims of trauma frequently experience intrusive thoughts and vivid, disturbing memories of the event. These are some of the symptoms of post-traumatic stress disorder (see Section 11.6). Research evidence (e.g. Wegner et al., 1990) suggests that it is unassimilated emotions that drive these memories to the surface of consciousness (Harber and Pennebaker, 1992). Furthermore, attempts to suppress unwanted thoughts lead to a 'boomerang effect' with the suppressed thoughts entering consciousness with even greater force.

Pennebaker and his colleagues conducted a number of studies examining the effects on arousal, health and well-being, of writing or talking about traumatic events (e.g. Pennebaker et al., 1988, 1989). From these studies, it would appear that disclosure is a remarkably powerful process. Although subjects often reported that writing about upsetting experiences was painful and would leave them feeling initially distraught, these same people reported that six weeks to six months later they felt happier (than the controls in the studies). There were also improvements in health (with significantly fewer health centre visits) among the experimental subjects. In a subsequent study in which subjects were asked to write the facts about a traumatic episode without reference to their emotions, writing only about the 'cold facts' did not appear to be psychologically or physically beneficial (Pennebaker and Beall, 1986).

More recent studies have focused more specifically on the role of emotional expressiveness during the disclosure of personal traumas. It has been found that those who convey the most emotion in their voices had the greatest reduction in physiological arousal during their disclosure (Pennebaker et al., 1987). In studies of Holocaust survivors, those people who exhibited the greatest reduction of arousal when talking about their traumatic experiences were also significantly healthier a year later (Pennebaker et al., 1989).

But although trauma victims undoubtedly seem to benefit from talking and expressing their feelings about the event, and indeed often have a natural urge to do so, listeners (friends, colleagues and relatives) will often seek to avoid hearing about such experiences. This reluctance may be an attempt by the listener to avoid the vicarious effects of the trauma, but it makes it even more difficult for the victim.

We have discussed how the expression of feelings in relation to traumatic events can lead to a reduction in arousal and improved health. But is it always the case that it is beneficial to express our feelings? Does the expression of intense anger and rage similarly lead to a lowering of arousal or does it, as the work on facial expressiveness discussed above might suggest, serve to intensify the feelings? The theory and research on aggression, and more specifically the debate between aggression as an innate drive and aggression as a learned response, might provide us with some clues.

Psychoanalytic theory maintains that we have an **aggressive drive** or instinct. When our efforts to attain a goal are blocked or frustrated, this drive acts as a motivation to injure the obstacle or person causing the frustration, and will persist until this is achieved.

Social-learning theory rejects this idea of aggression as an instinctual drive. It proposes instead that aggression is a **learned response** acquired through observation or imitation and that the more often it is reinforced, the more often it is likely to occur. There are, according to this theory, a number of responses to frustration other than aggression, and people will choose the response that has relieved the frustration successfully in the past.

If aggression is an innate instinctual drive then the expression of aggression should be cathartic, and the intensity of the aggressive feelings or actions should be reduced. If, on the other hand, aggression is a learned response, the expression of aggression, if reinforced, would be expected to lead to an increase in aggression.

Currently the evidence would seem to favour the view that aggression is a learned response and that the expression of aggression would not act as a catharsis, or 'purging'. But what happens when people express angry feelings which would normally not be conceptualized as 'aggressive'? Research evidence suggests that the expression of angry feelings can, in fact, also stimulate more anger. In one study, workers who had been made redundant were interviewed about their feelings, and subsequently asked to describe their feelings in writing. If aggression were cathartic, it might have been expected that those who had expressed a high level of negative feeling in their interviews would have 'got it out of their system' and would have expressed less when asked subsequently to write down their feelings. The results, however, showed the opposite; that those who expressed aggression verbally, expressed even more in their written reports. 'Fuming' or 'ranting and raving' in their verbal reports may have stimulated the angry feelings rather than dispelling them (Ebbesen et al., 1975). There would also, of course have been individual differences in emotional expressiveness which might have accounted for these results.

So how can the psychological literature inform or guide the counsellor or therapist? What the research indicates is that the expression of emotion in relation to difficult, painful or traumatic events or situations is beneficial to both psychological well-being and health. It also suggests that as counsellors and therapists, we should be aware of the possible consequences of facilitating the expression of anger. It could act to fuel the anger, and the arousal may then be carried over as transferred excitation and be expressed outside of the counselling session.

This does not mean that all clients should therefore be discouraged from expressing their negative feelings in counselling sessions. The expression of anger may make the person *feel* better. It may make them feel stronger, more powerful and more in control. It may motivate them to take some positive action in their life. The expression of anger by a client who is frightened of his or her own anger may also serve to desensitize them to the fear of losing control. Finally, the facial feedback hypothesis discussed above would suggests that 'acting' angrily, particularly through the facial muscles, would increase the subjective feelings of anger. This may be useful in working with clients who experience low emotional intensity and may also improve the behavioural skills important in communicating feeling. Very importantly, the counsellor needs to make a careful assessment of the client and their situation when working directly with angry or aggressive feelings and to be clear about the purpose, rationale and possible consequences of the intervention.

Finally, of course, we need to remember that the experienced emotion may be the result of inappropriate appraisals. We may feel upset because we have quite erroneously appraised a remark as a slight. In these instances, it might be more useful to explore the issues surrounding the appraisals rather than encouraging the expression of the resulting emotion.

3.8 CONCLUDING COMMENTS

In this chapter we have seen how psychologists have attempted to increase our under-standing of emotion. It would seem that emotion has three main components: a physio-logical, a cognitive and an expressive component. How these interrelate, relate to our experience of emotion and may be relevant to the counselling situation that has been discussed. On the one hand it appears that we know quite a lot about emotion and about why might we experience it, but on the other we may still be left wondering what exactly it is. Early work, as we have discussed, viewed emotion as no more than autonomic arousal. Theories are constantly being developed or modified in the light of fresh research evidence. For example, one of the more recent theories conceptualizes the experience of emotion as an unconscious form of **self-perception** resulting from cues of arousal, expressive behaviour, action and the situation (Laird and Bresler, 1992) and this seems like a promising way forward.

Another difficulty with the psychological approach to emotion is that most of the studies have been conducted in the laboratory and have been concerned with manipu-lation of variables involved in the more obvious or basic emotions such as anger, dis-gust, pleasantness etc. This has enabled psychologists to find out a great deal about the various aspects of emotion and something about emotional processes but little about emotions themselves. This is probably because psychology is still a relatively young discipline and has been rather anxious to consolidate its scientific position. As a result, psychology has missed out on the often lengthy and systematic observation of phenom-ena in its natural state that, in the natural sciences, has preceded any form of manipu-lative control.

The situation is changing. Researchers are moving out of the laboratory and apply-ing the theory and knowledge gained therein to the study of more complex emotions in natural settings, for example, hope in the dying (Dufault and Martocchio, 1985).

For the counsellor, no amount of theory and research will provide information about what the client is feeling and experiencing. A knowledge of the psychological processes involved in emotion can, however, help the counsellor to be aware of the various dimensions involved in emotional experience and may inform and guide the process of counselling.

4

Memory

4.1 INTRODUCTION

Life without memory would be meaningless. Imagine what it would be like if all our memories were wiped out. We would have no knowledge, no life history, no recognition of friends, family or enemies, no identity. It could be argued that we are our memories; for the very notion of 'self' depends on a sense of continuity that only memory can bring.

The memories clients bring to, and uncover, during the process of counselling can therefore contribute to their sense of self. Memories also, of course, help to place the clients' current difficulties in the context of their life history. This is important in developing an understanding of how and why the person responds and reacts to current situations as they do.

Although most clients can provide a reasonably comprehensive overview of their backgrounds, they will generally be telling the counsellor *about* their childhood or adolescent experiences. It will be an account and possibly an explanation based on memories, but given from the client's current perspective, with the benefit of hindsight. It will, importantly, probably be an account of what the client him or herself feels is relevant; it may also be coloured by what the client thinks the counsellor may want to know.

But it is often the experiences which have been forgotten, or considered insignificant, that can provide important clues and valuable insights in building up a 'picture' of the client and their experiences.

Going back in memory to specific episodes can also engender similar feelings to those originally experienced. In the case of traumatic experiences, painful emotions may have been repressed or denied as a way of coping. Confronting traumatic memories (as we discussed in the previous chapter) is an important aspect of recovery from trauma (Harber and Pennebaker, 1992).

Because specific memories always seem more 'real' than mere descriptions of events, it is tempting to give them the status of accurate accounts. However, in remembering past events, what we may be accessing is a memory of a memory, practised and rehearsed a number of times in the intervening period of time. We may therefore not have been remembering the events themselves, but our later interpretation of them.

Even working with clients on previously unremembered and relatively unprocessed memories is no guarantee of accuracy. Memory, the psychological research would suggest, does not just act as a 'storehouse' of information, but as an **active information processing system that as well as storing information, also receives it, organizes it, alters it and recovers it**. Psychologists have accordingly been particularly interested in what takes place between the exposure to new information and later recall.

Psychologists have also been concerned with identifying and exploring different *types* of memory. Different memories are used to store information for short and long periods and also to store different kinds of information (for example, we seem to have a particular type of memory for skills and another type for autobiographical facts). Although much of the research on memory has, like so much of psychological research, taken place in the laboratory, memory is increasingly being studied in real-world settings (e.g. Tulving, 1983).

This chapter will examine the work on the structure (sensory, short-term and long-term memory), the process (encoding, storage and retrieval) and the content of memory (concentrating on biographical memory) before focusing on areas of the topic which will be of particular relevance to counselling. These include the effect of personal and situational factors on memory, the way in which we 'reconstruct' the past, false memory in relation to child sexual abuse and very importantly, how and why we forget.

4.2 THE STRUCTURE OF THE MEMORY

It is useful to think of memory as involving at least three steps. Incoming information from the senses is first held for a second or so by sensory memory. Selective attention then controls what is transferred to temporary storage in short-term or working memory which can hold material only for a few seconds. If it is transferred into long-term memory, it becomes relatively permanent, although, as we all know, retrieving it may be a problem (see Figure 4.1.).

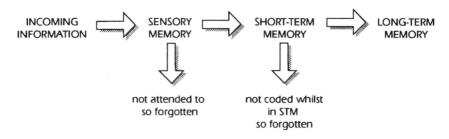

Figure 4.1 The memory system

4.2.1 Sensory Memory

Sensory memory holds for a second or so, an exact copy of the stimulus just long enough for recognition to occur (Baddeley and Logie, 1992). If your attention wanders as a friend or partner reaches the end of a list of tasks that need to be done or items to be bought you may automatically ask, 'What was that last thing?' and then realize almost simultaneously that you know what the answer is. This is because it has been held in the auditory sensory memory.

Without further processing these sensory memories simply fade away. The process of **selective attention** controls what is transferred into the second memory system.

4.2.2 Short-term (Working) Memory

Generally speaking, short-term memory is memory for things that are the focus of attention at the moment (Goldman-Rakic, 1992). It acts as a temporary storehouse for small amounts of information. Unless the information is important, it is quickly discarded from short-term memory and is lost forever. Short-term memory prevents our minds from being cluttered up with useless information: names, dates, telephone numbers that we no longer need (Miller, 1956).

Short-term memory can hold information for a few seconds, some say up to 30 seconds, but the amount it can hold is limited. Many studies using different kinds of memory tasks indicate that people can hold no more than five to nine meaningful items in short-term memory (which is why, with long telephone numbers, unless we 'rehearse' them in our mind or 'chunk' some of the numbers together or attach some meaning or significance to a part of the number we will probably not be able to recall it).

Although it is of limited capacity, our short-term memory is crucial, and is where much of our thinking takes place. In order for this to happen we need to refer to information from long-term memory which allows us to interpret the material in short-term memory. If the information is important or *meaningful*, it is transferred into the third memory system, long-term memory.

4.2.3 Long-term Memory

Long-term memory acts as a relatively *permanent* storehouse of information and contains everything we know about our world. Whenever we speak, read, play tennis or recognize people we know we refer to our long-term memory system. Yet there seems to be no danger that we will run out of space in long-term memory; that it will get 'filled up'. On the contrary, long-term memory seems to have an almost limitless storage capacity and in some sense, the more we know the easier it becomes to add new information to memory. This is because when new information enters short-term memory, it is related to knowledge stored in long-term memory. This gives the new information meaning and makes it easier to store in long-term memory. However, it can also be the case that it is difficult to assimilate new information which does not 'fit in' with our existing ideas or views.

In order to understand why we remember some information far better and for far longer than other information we need to look at how the information is 'processed'; how we form memories (**encoding**), how we maintain them (**storage**) and how we access them (**retrieval**).

4.3 INFORMATION PROCESSING CONCEPTS

4.3.1 Encoding

Although long-term memory capacity is vast and seems to have infinitely more storage space than the largest of libraries, its contents, like those of a library, must be organized in terms of specific 'codes' if the information is to be available when we wish to retrieve it. In some instances, as when trying to memorize information for an examination, the organization of the material often takes place at a conscious level, and there are various techniques for doing this. But for the most part we do not deliberately try to organize incoming information for the purposes of subsequent retrieval, and our memories are formed without any sort of conscious processing. We now know, however, that a considerable amount of processing, or coding does, in fact, take place when information enters long-term memory store. There are different types of coding for different types of information but the most common forms of coding are semantic coding and sensory coding.

Semantic coding

Whereas with short-term memory it is usually the individual sounds, whether numbers or words, that are encoded, it is usually the *meaning* or general *ideas* rather than specific details that are encoded in long-term memory. So after hearing a sentence, most of what you can recall or recognize is the sentence's meaning. If you heard the sentence, 'The author sent the committee a long letter', two minutes later you would not be able to tell whether you had heard that sentence or one with the same meaning: 'A long letter was sent to the committee by the author' (Sachs, 1967).

We are continuously encoding meanings in real life. When people report on complex social, domestic, emotional or political situations, they may misremember many of the specific details, who said or did what to whom, at what point someone entered or left the room etc. but can reasonably accurately describe the basic situation and the 'gist' of what took place.

What we construct in memory therefore seems to be a broad-based 'theme' that describes the meaning of the episode, rather than a precise record of what happened during the episode. The theme in turn is guided by a **schema**. This is a mental representation of a class of people, events, situations or objects (Fiske and Taylor, 1991; Greene, 1992). Because information stored in memory is often encoded and organized around schemas, what is eventually remembered will depend, in part, on the nature of the individual person's schemas.

Every counsellor who has worked with couples or has interviewed a member of a client's family will have come across the situation of different versions of the same episode. This is probably accounted for by the fact that the situations which clients report on in counselling may have been encoded according to a particularly high degree of personal meaning and so may be remembered differently by the different parties involved. This is something counsellors need to be aware of, not only when working with couples or families, but with individual clients too. We also need to be aware of the fact that it is not only the client that is doing the encoding! Counsellors are also encoding the clients' accounts according to their own personal meanings. This is particularly important to be aware of when writing case notes or reports about particular clients.

Sensory coding

Although long-term memory normally involves semantic coding, people can also encode visual images, sounds, tastes and smells into long-term memory. So the distinctive, personal, poignant smell of someone who is no longer here, who has maybe died, remains in memory; not to be recaptured in words, not to be recalled by olfactory 'triggers'; it remains nevertheless.

When both semantic and sensory content have been encoded, usually referred to as **dual coding,** subsequent recall is often improved. (This is why when writing out a shopping list you should try to visualize it before you forget to take it with you.)

4.3.2 Storage

Although as noted above, long-term memory capacity is vast, it is unlikely that everything we ever learned or experienced is still there in memory waiting to be retrieved. Some information is almost certainly lost from storage (Loftus and Loftus, 1980).

As new memories are formed in long-term memory a process of **consolidation** takes place over a period of months or longer. (It is this process that seems to be interrupted by electroconvulsive therapy (ECT) given to alleviate severe depression, although retrieval can also be affected.) When new information is received, the information is **recoded** and related to other contents in memory. **Networks** are built up by association and a changed pattern of total information within the storage system is created. *Older memories are accordingly often updated, changed, lost or revised* (Baddeley, 1990).

Updating memories is called **constructive processing**. Research has shown that gaps in memory, which are common, may be filled in by logic, guesses or new information (Loftus, 1980). It is even possible to have 'memories' for things that have never happened. These are often called **pseudo-memories** or **false memories** (see Section 4.7 on Memory as a Reconstructive Process).

4.3.3 Retrieval

Our ability to remember depends, in part, on how well the information was encoded in the first instance and partly how effectively we are able to search and access the memory store.

The more actively or 'deeply' we process or organize incoming information and form associations with other memories, the better our long-term recall will be (Craik and Lockhart, 1972). Counsellors, of course, are constantly processing incoming information, locating it in a theoretical framework (explicitly or implicitly) and probably relating it to other similar information or instances drawn from their experience. This may be one of the reasons that experienced counsellors often report very good memories in relation to their clients, even after many years of non-contact.

Stimuli that help people access appropriately encoded information logged into long-term memory are called **retrieval cues.** A retrieval cue is usually part of the code that is laid down when the memory was classified. Counsellors can explore aspects of the client's experience by the careful use of retrieval cues. A **semantic retrieval cue** is one that is presented verbally. With a client who reported that there had been absolutely no physical contact between him and his father, the retrieval cue 'bed-time' brought back a flood of memories of sitting on his father's knee begging for yet another story.

Retrieval cues can be sensory as well as verbal. **Visual images, smells** and **tastes** can all be powerful sources of recollection for many people.

The more similar the retrieval cues are to those that were present when the memory was encoded, the more likely they are to evoke the memory. This is known as the **encoding specificity principle** (Tulving and Thompson, 1973). Returning to the school you attended as a child may awaken many memories because the sights and sounds you encounter on your return visit were likely to have been present in the environment when you originally encoded the memory. It has also been demonstrated repeatedly that it is easier to remember information in the environment in which it was acquired. For example, one study found that students remember better when tested in the classroom in which they learned the material than in a different classroom (Smith et al., 1978). This is known as **context-dependent memory.**

Describing an environment, rather than actually revisiting it, can also evoke previously unrecalled memories. In the example below the counsellor 'tests out' her hypothesis that the client had been subject to some racial comments/abuse as a child (and that this would have had some bearing on her current interpersonal style). She uses the semantic retrieval cue 'first school' and goes on to ask the client to describe details of the playground, classrooms, fellow pupils which provide, albeit in an indirect way, visual retrieval cues for recall.

The client is a 39-year-old professional woman of mixed race with an Asian mother and father of Afro-Caribbean descent. She was brought up in a small village in the west country by her mother and step-father. She has no recollection of her biological father.

Although highly successful at work, she has a history of getting into confrontations with colleagues and friends. She has had several boyfriends but the relationships have all been fairly volatile and ended in conflict. She has become concerned by what her boss has called her 'aggressive style', particularly because to her, it seems inconsistent with the sort of person she is. It is also making her life extremely difficult for her.

Exploration of possible background factors revealed that apart from her mother, she was the only non-white person in her village and also at her first and middle schools. However, although she had always been aware of being a little different, she had always felt loved and accepted and could not remember ever being on the receiving end of any racial comments or abuse. Or maybe, she added, there was the occasional comment, but nothing, she thought, that amounted to much.

Working on specific memories of school revealed quite another picture. The comments were frequent, and they hurt. When she reported these to her mother, she (her mother) laughed it off; told her she'd just have to learn to cope, as she had done.

She did learn to cope, and very effectively. She is rarely the butt of such remarks now. As she said, 'No-one would dare!'

Research has shown that because we generally encode material in a number of different ways (verbal, visual etc.) dual or multiple cues, which can provide more points of access to a new memory, are more effective in enhancing recall than single cues (Baddeley, 1993).

4.4 TYPES OF MEMORY

When we talk or think about memory in a counselling context, what we are generally referring to is our memory for events in our lives or those of our clients. This type of memory is usually known as **episodic** or **autobiographical** memory. This is one of three types of memory that have been identified by various theorists. The other two types are **semantic** memory, which is concerned with our knowledge of the world and language, and **procedural** memory or memory involved in how to perform some skill.

4.4.1 Episodic (Autobiographical) Memory

Episodic memory is an **autobiographical** record of our personal experiences. It is the store of information about past experiences; what happened, when and where. It records life events day after day, year in and year out. Episodic memory is constantly changing; information is rapidly lost (although it may be retrieved with the right cues) as new information comes in.

As one might expect, older memories tend to be more generalized than more recent ones, when quite specific details of events etc. can be recalled (Pillemer et al., 1988). However, it has been found that emotionally disturbed people have difficulty retrieving specific memories, regardless of the age of the memory, and tend to retrieve only general classes of information about themselves or their families (Williams, 1992).

Taking a cognitive–behavioural view, Williams suggests that counsellors and therapists could help their clients to identify and challenge negative generalized memories, such as 'I was always unhappy at school' and 'I never had any friends'. By remembering specific events, the client can then re-evaluate their experience in a more realistic, and hopefully less negative way.

Avoiding specific memories may also serve as protection from the full impact of traumatic events. In the previous chapter (Section 3.6 on the Expression of Emotion and Counselling) we discussed the therapeutic advantages of talking or writing about distressing events. Although this can undoubtedly be extremely painful, it has been suggested that the process of describing such events and the accompanying expression of emotions facilitates the assimilation of emotional distress and is of considerable benefit to psychological and physical health.

Clients sometimes, then, will talk in a generalized quasi-'objective' way *about* the experience, thereby to some extent distance themselves from the painful emotions.

In the following account, the counsellor gently but directly confronts the client about his experiences of sexual abuse from a close family friend. He has previously told the counsellor, in an unemotional way, that the abuse took place regularly over a period of four years between the ages of eight and twelve. Although he says he has recently had vivid recollections of what took place, he has never previously revealed to anyone what happened to him. He has tried to put all this to the back of his mind, but it refuses to stay there.

The client starts with a generalized memory. By the use of direct closed questions the counsellor encourages the client to focus on specific events.

Counsellor   Tell me what you actually remember from that time.

Client   I remember him getting me under his wing.

Counsellor   Is there anything you can actually remember?

Client   Frequently taking me from my home.

Counsellor   Do you remember a particular occasion?

Client   He'd changed his car—took me for a ride—took me to his house. I don't recall how he got me into his bed. But I remember the act—took me into his bed—kissing me repeatedly.

Counsellor How did he do this?

Client With his tongue – ugh – I can feel it now. Pushing my hands down to stroke him.

Counsellor Where?

Client On the genitals. We'd carry on until he went to the bathroom. I never knew why. There was so much I didn't understand. The same thing happened again and again.

Counsellor Can you go back to a particular time it happened?

Client On one occasion he took me down with a couple of friends to . . . (a long way away)—camping. He arranged for them to be in a different tent so I ended up with him. Intense kissing. I remember—I kissed his genitals. I thought he'd like it. I wanted to. That's what's so awful now. He told me never ever to do that again. I remember now how I felt. Disgusting, humiliated. Do you know I've never been able to kiss my wife. Not even on the cheek. I'd never realized why.

It was only when the client described 'from memory' his experiences that he expressed any emotion he felt about what had occurred. The counsellor then proceeded to work in a more non-directive way, responding to the emotional aspects rather than the actual content of the client's memory.

A particularly distinctive type of episodic memory is the phenomenon known as **flashbulb memory**. These memories are usually related to very significant, and often traumatic events in our lives. They are characterized by their vivid detail and the fact that they are likely to be maintained over long periods of time. This is because the events remembered in 'flashbulb' tend to have evoked strong emotional reactions at the time of encoding and have probably been repeatedly recalled in memory and in subsequent conversations with friends or family (Bohannon, 1988).

One such flashbulb memory reported by a fifty-three-year-old client was of her father lifting her up onto a horse when she was six years old. She remembered quite vividly what she was wearing, the name and the colour of the horse and what it felt like to be aloft such a huge animal. That night she remembers her father coming into her bedroom, as usual, to kiss her goodnight. She also remembers what he said. It was 'Goodnight darling. I want you to look after Mummy'. She remembers thinking at the time that this was a little odd, but that he must be making one of his trips which she did not know about. That was the last time she saw him. That night, he hanged himself.

4.4.2 Semantic Memory

Semantic memory contains all we know about the world. In contrast with episodic memory, it is relatively organized and stable. It contains all the knowledge we need to converse, read or solve problems. Most importantly, it contains the 'tools' for thought: the words we use, the concepts, schemas and the grammatical rules for constructing sentences and presenting coherent arguments. We will be discussing some of these processes in the next chapter on Thinking.

4.4.3 Procedural Memory

We use our procedural memory when we type a letter, ride a bicycle or throw a ball. Procedural memories are learned skills. Unlike the contents of episodic or semantic memory which can be verbalized, and are sometimes referred to for this reason as **declarative**, procedural memories are used for *doing*, rather than describing. We do not consciously have to think how to ride a bicycle, for instance. Indeed it would be quite difficult to describe how we do it; we just do.

4.5 THE EFFECTS OF STATE AND MOOD ON MEMORY

The effect of context on memory has been discussed above. But context is not always external, as in physical locations. What is happening inside, our internal state, is also a part of our context. Like the external environment, our internal psychological environment can be encoded as part of the experience and can subsequently act as a retrieval cue.

When a person's internal state can aid or impede retrieval, memory is called **state-dependent**. The most extreme examples of this come from studies of people's memory under the influence of alcohol or drugs. Most people have heard about the person who had to get drunk again in order to find the wallet they lost whilst under the influence! Although this is often told as a joke, it has been found that if people learn new material whilst under the influence of alcohol, marijuana or other drugs, they tend to recall it better if they are tested under the influence of the substance in question again (Overton, 1984; Eich et al., 1975; Eich, 1989).

Mood is also an aspect of our internal environment that can act as a retrieval cue for previously encoded material. This phenomenon is known as **mood-congruent recall**.

It was on their honeymoon that this client first experienced her husband's violence. He had had rather more to drink than he would normally have done, and when they were alone in their room, he 'turned on her', accusing her of flirting with one of the waiters. When she vehemently denied it he started punching her. She became extremely frightened and suddenly memories of her drunken father lurching into her bedroom at night came flooding back. She remembered how she would, as a small child, be frightened to go to sleep; she remembered cowering behind the bedroom door when she heard him coming in from the pub; she could almost 'hear' the tirade of abuse and accusations of having committed some trivial misdemeanour, and 'feel' herself covering her head to protect herself from the inevitable blows which would fall before her father would 'comfort' her. These memories were, for her, almost as distressing as her husband's actions.

Evidence for mood-congruent recall comes from studies which have demonstrated that college students remember more positive incidents from their diaries or from their earlier life when they are in a positive mood at the time of recall (Bower, 1981). It also seems to be the case that more negative events tend to be recalled when people are in a negative mood (Lewinsohn and Rosenbaum, 1987)

When depressed people are asked to recall autobiographical memories, they tend to recall unhappy incidents; the more depressed the individual, the more rapidly the unpleasant experience is recalled (Baddeley, 1993). The difficulty with interpreting this finding is that people who are depressed may genuinely have had more negative experiences to remember as compared with people who do not suffer from depression. Indeed, the negative experiences that they recall may have been significant in causing the depression.

In one study designed to disentangle this, patients were selected whose depression fluctuated during the course of the day. During 'sad' periods, they were consistently less likely to produce happy memories than at other times. Indeed, as anyone who has been depressed, or who has had contact with someone who is depressed, will know, people who are in a depressed mood will have difficulty retrieving any pleasant memories and will be likely to recall mainly unpleasant incidents from the past, further lowering self-esteem and intensifying the depression. This is something that cognitive behavioural psychologists would see as part of the aetiology of the condition. That is, the negative thinking which is present during depressive episodes is part of a cognitive 'style' and may have preceded and been causally related to the onset of depressive symptoms.

Cognitive approaches to the treatment of depression often involve helping the person gain access to the less depressing memories and negative aspects of their lives, and to revalue the more positive areas of their experience which tend to be hidden in the downward spiral of negative thoughts.

4.6 FORGETTING

Sometimes it seems that we remember things we would rather forget and forget the things we would like, or need, to remember. But although forgetting can be very frustrating, it is also very necessary. Imagine what it would be like if we remembered absolutely everything we had ever seen, heard, read or experienced since we were born. Forgetting protects us against the nightmare of such information overload: it can also be useful in protecting us temporarily from painful traumatic experiences.

But how do we forget? Is it like pulling the plug out of a bath, causing information to be lost at a constant rate to make way for new incoming information? Does memory fade as the memory traces decay over time as a result of disuse? This is the traditional theory of forgetting but whilst it may be intuitively appealing, there is little evidence that this is, in fact, what happens; at least not to information in long-term memory.

The notion of disuse fails to explain why some unused memories fade, while others are carried on for life, nor why elderly people may forget what they told you five minutes ago but remember 'as clearly as if it were yesterday' some apparently trivial incident from their pasts. There is also experimental evidence from a number of studies (e.g. Ebbinghaus, 1885) that information loss is very rapid at first, and then levels off. There are, however, a number of plausible explanations for forgetting.

4.6.1 Encoding Failure

The most obvious cause for forgetting is often the most commonly overlooked. In many cases we 'forget' because a memory was never formed in the first place. A great deal of information from the environment we do not need; so, having been processed by our sensory registers and entered into short-term memory, it may be discarded rather than encoded into long-term store. (However, when you have forgotten to carry out some request made by your nearest and dearest and you explain, 'Honestly, I didn't forget, it was merely an encoding failure', you cannot expect your plea to be greeted with the understanding you had hoped for.)

4.6.2 Interference

Memories sometimes cannot be retrieved because other information in memory interferes with the retrieval process. **Proactive interference** occurs when material learned in the past interferes with recall of material learned later. **Retroactive interference** is the opposite, when newly acquired information interferes with the ability to recall information learned earlier.

There is a great deal of support for the interference theory and many cognitive psychologists view interference as the primary reason for forgetting. Most of the work in this area has been carried out in relation to semantic memory. Its relevance to episodic memory, which is probably of more interest to counsellors, is less clear.

4.6.3 Emotional Factors in Forgetting

We have already discussed in Section 4.5 how mood can affect retrieval of memories, with pleasant memories being 'forgotten' by people who are depressed or whose mood is low. Emotion can affect our ability to remember in other ways.

Anxiety and forgetting

Many of us have experienced the kind of panic which sets in when taking an exam about which we are not very confident. You read the first question; it's about something on which you have done some revision, but not a lot; your mind goes blank. You look at the next question. It may not be particularly difficult but the anxiety which set in on reading the first question transfers to this one. By the time you get to the end of the paper you can hardly remember who you are, let alone the subject of the examination!

It has been suggested that what happens in such instances is that it is not so much the anxiety itself that causes the memory failure. It is the intrusion of extraneous thoughts that usually accompany anxiety; thoughts such as, 'There's no way I'm going to pass', that interfere with the retrieval process (Holmes, 1974).

Repression

Repression is close to the extreme end of retrieval failure associated with emotion. Freud suggested that a good deal of everyday forgetting has its origins in the repression of everyday events associated with anxiety. He also proposed that some emotional experiences in childhood are so traumatic that becoming aware of them in adult life would cause the individual to be totally overwhelmed by anxiety. Such traumatic experiences are believed to be stored in the unconscious, or repressed, and can only usually be restored by therapeutic means, when some of the emotion associated with them has been diffused. This notion of active 'blocking' is qualitatively different from previously discussed ideas of forgetting.

Repression has proved difficult to study in the laboratory. There are clearly ethical problems involved in exposing subjects to traumatic events and 'measuring' repression. The studies that have come nearest to this by exposing subjects to mildly upsetting experiences would seem to lend some support to the repression hypothesis (Erdelyi, 1985). Further evidence in support of repression comes not from normal forgetting, but from the pathological forgetting associated with neurosis: hysterical amnesia.

Hysterical amnesia

It has long been recognized that major trauma can result in hysterical loss of memory. During World War II *150* of the first thousand soldiers admitted to hospital were diagnosed as such (Sargent, 1967). Very occasionally one also hears of someone who is undergoing an emotional crisis 'losing their memory'. They may be found wandering many miles from home, unaware of who they are, where they came from or how they got there. Usually with care and attention memory comes back within a few days (Baddeley, 1993) and, providing they confront the source of their anxiety, they are unlikely to relapse.

> One very unfortunate 27-year-old client suffering from amnesia was not found wandering about anywhere (as is frequently the case with people suffering from amnesia). She woke up in a hospital bed and found to her astonishment that the previous day she had given birth prematurely at 26 weeks to a baby girl, and that she had had major abdominal surgery for the removal of her colon resulting in an ileostomy and the necessity to wear an ileostomy bag. Although she knew who she was and remembered being pregnant, she had no recollection of becoming ill with acute abdominal pain, of going into hospital, giving birth, nor of having surgery for a perforated bowel. These two days and the two days on either side were completely missing.
>
> She reported that she had always been a nervous sort of person. 'Terribly phobic', she said, 'particularly about hospitals and being ill'. She had been prescribed diazepam (Valium) by her general practitioner some four years ago and she had taken them for six months. She had been delighted when she became pregnant, although somewhat anxious about whether she would cope. The first few weeks of her pregnancy were fine. Then she started to have some rectal bleeding. She visited her doctor who reassured her that she was suffering from haemorrhoids. What no one knew was that she was, in fact, suffering from acute ulcerative colitis.
>
> It is hardly surprising, particularly in view of her long-standing fear of illness and hospitals, that she had no memory for the traumatic events of the previous four days. It was all too much for her to process.
>
> As the client began to work with the counsellor on her distress, particularly on the anger she felt at having 'missed out' on the birth of her daughter, and as her

health improved, so her memory for those four days began to return. For her, the memories, painful as they were, caused her less distress than the idea of having 'lost' four days of her life.

4.6.4 Childhood Amnesia

Hysterical amnesia is fairly extreme and not very common. One type of amnesia we all experience is childhood amnesia; virtually no-one can remember events that took place before they were three years old. Some people *think* they can but it is very difficult to be sure that these are really memories and not reconstructions. Most of us are told 'stories' of ourselves or have seen pictures of our early years so what we may be remembering is the story or the image encoded in long-term memory.

Freud (1905), of course, viewed childhood amnesia as the repression of sexual and aggressive feelings that the young child experiences towards the parents. The problem with this explanation is that it is not just sexual and aggressive thoughts and feelings from that period that are repressed; it is everything.

A more accepted explanation is that children do not remember because of the way information is encoded into long-term memory. In Section 4.4 above we discussed how new information is processed and classified according to meaning and encoded in relation to the existing contents of long-term memory. Young children will not have developed these associative networks. They will encode their experiences without connecting them to related events. Once a child begins to form associations between events and to categorize those events, early experience becomes lost (Schactel, 1947). Language development of course plays an important part in this process. We also know that the very young child is unable to consolidate memories because the brain structure involved in this process, the **hippocampus**, is not mature until the child is about one to two years old.

There is no doubt, however, that children can learn and in some sense remember from the earliest months of life, but such 'memories' are implicit, rather than explicit. They are reflected in behaviour but remain outside awareness, so cannot be expressed verbally.

4.7 MEMORY AS A RECONSTRUCTIVE PROCESS

It will now be obvious that retrieving information from long-term memory bears no resemblance to viewing a taped replay on a video-recorder. Often our memories are sketchy and incomplete, even though we may sometimes think otherwise. You will realize this if you have ever tried telling a family 'story' with other members of the family present; 'No, it didn't happen like that,' 'It was the year we went to Bournemouth, not Bognor,' 'I wasn't even there at the time,' 'Yes you were, I remember you wore that blue swimming costume you hated so much.' In these sort of situations we may **reconstruct** a reasonable memory by embellishing directly retrieved memory with plausible elaborations.

We also have generalized ideas, or **schemas**, about how certain events happen. We use these schemas to organize, and in some cases to reconstruct memories. The schema in the above example would have been something like 'seaside holidays'.

In a classic experiment of reconstructive memory, Bartlett(1932) got his subjects to read stories, including a North American Indian tale which included a strong supernatural element. When Bartlett's English subjects retold the story, they reconstructed it in a way that made sense to them, in relation to their own specific cultural schemas; for example the hero was 'fishing', not hunting seals, and 'the war party' became 'the enemy'. Also the longer the time interval between reading and retelling the story, the more the story changed to fit in with English culture.

We use schemas to help us make sense of the world and our experience. Another device we use for this purpose is **inference**. But inferences can also affect memory and play a part in the construction of **false memories**.

To illustrate this point, Loftus and Palmer (1974) showed subjects a filmed road traffic accident. Afterwards some of the subjects were asked how fast the cars were going when they 'smashed' into each other, and for other subjects the word 'smashed' was replaced by 'bumped', 'contacted' or 'hit'. A week later, all the subjects were asked whether they had seen any broken glass. Those asked earlier about the cars that 'smashed' into each other were more likely to say 'yes', even though no broken glass was shown in the film. The new information 'smashed' had been encoded into subjects' long-term memories after viewing the film and had subsequently altered them.

Some cognitive psychologists believe that post-event information can permanently alter an individual's original memory so that the original memory can never again be retrieved (Loftus et al., 1978). Others are not so sure that memory is permanently altered (McCloskey and Zaragoza, 1985). However, what is generally agreed is that memory can be significantly influenced by post-event information.

4.8 RECOVERED MEMORIES AND CHILD SEXUAL ABUSE

The term **recovered memory** is used to refer to memory, usually of childhood events, of which the adult has previously had no conscious recollection. The cases which have aroused the most public interest are those in which memories of childhood sexual abuse have been 'recovered' by clients in therapy, sometimes by therapists employing 'memory recovery' techniques, such as hypnosis.

Freud in the early years noted a number of his patients reported memories of childhood sexual abuse. Although he initially accepted these claims as true, he later viewed them as fantasies representing the sexual attraction a child feels for the parent of the opposite sex; fantasies which are unacceptable and become 'repressed' until they appear as 'memories' in therapy.

In recent years it has become all too apparent that sexual abuse is no fantasy. Estimates of the frequency in the adult population in Great Britain vary with the samples and the definition of abuse. One survey found that 6 per cent of women in a representative sample reported child sexual abuse involving physical contact, but some estimates are several times larger (British Psychological Society, 1995).

Compared to the numbers of people who have suffered child sexual abuse, those reporting recovered memories from complete amnesia are relatively rare (British Psychological Society, 1995). They are, however, very significant in terms of the consequences for the individuals involved, for their relatives and, where the person has been in therapy, the therapists in question.

Because of the increasing number of allegations made against parents by adult children, the False Memory Syndrome Society was set up in the USA in 1992 and the British False Memory Society in Britain in 1993 as parents' support groups. They maintain that the recovered memories have been implanted by therapists who believe that a wide variety of psychological problems and symptoms (such as depression, eating disorders, self-destructive behaviour, low self-esteem, difficulty in making relationships) indicate sexual abuse in childhood.

On the other hand, some therapists and members of the survivors' movement have pointed out the fact that some recovered memories have been substantiated. Members of this 'camp' allege that the false memory groups could possibly act as a refuge for perpetrators who join the society for protection.

Some therapists and counsellors maintain that it is not the therapist's job to question the authenticity of recovered memories; what the client experiences is what is crucially important, not what actually did happen.

This approach raises two obvious problems. Firstly, if the therapist automatically and uncritically accepts the client's recovered memories of abuse, he or she may be colluding with a false belief which may have considerable implications for the family of the client and in turn, for the client herself (or himself).

Secondly, in the USA, as many counsellors are aware, recovered memory is increasingly moving out of the consulting room and into the law courts. It may only be a matter of time before this happens in Britain. If and when it does, the validity of the claim of sexual abuse becomes significant.

Counsellors and therapists therefore may need to be aware of the scientific evidence surrounding the phenomenon of recovered memories. The areas of psychological research particular relevance to this issue are childhood amnesia, reconstructive memory, repression, hypnosis and suggestion.

4.8.1 Childhood Amnesia and Reconstructive Memory

We have already discussed childhood amnesia; that children do not remember events before the age of about three years. However very young children clearly learn and possess memory in some form for early events, but as noted above this memory is implicit and cannot be accessed verbally.

We have also seen from the research how memories can be reconstructed, as a way of trying to make sense of our experiences. If some traumatic episode (such as hospitalization) had been experienced before the age of conscious memory it could be hypothesized that 'memories' of sexual abuse might be reconstructed in an attempt to make sense of the earlier trauma. If this were the case, however, we must ask why when so many children experience traumatic events at an early age, so few adults experience recovered memories.

4.8.2 Repression and Child Sexual Abuse

As we have noted above in Section 4.6.3, it has long been recognized that major trauma can result in hysterical loss of memory. Baddeley (1993) reports that 30–40 per cent of criminals convicted of violent crime are unable to recall the crime, particularly when there are close emotional or familial ties with the victim. However, another study based on the memories of victims rather than perpetrators found no evidence for repression in children who had seen a parent killed (Malmquist, 1986). It has recently been suggested that repeated or extended severe trauma is more likely to lead to extreme amnesia than a single episode.

In relation to child sexual abuse, surveys report that between one third and two thirds of survivors had experienced some period of amnesia for the abuse. Unfortunately the results of most of the surveys are difficult to interpret. This is partly due to the fact that the mechanisms that underlie repression are still poorly understood.

Hypothesized mechanisms in repression have included the active inhibition of previously clear conscious memory for events; 'blacking out' at the time of the trauma so that the memory has never been consciously available; that the memory is not part of the person's self-schema; the memory has come to mind in whole or part (flashbacks etc.) but was interpreted as something different; the memory has not come to mind because the relevant retrieval cues have not been encountered and that event memory has been compartmentalized or 'dissociated' so that certain events can only be recalled when the person is in a particular state of mind.

Only one study of survivors of sexual abuse made explicit the distinction between total and partial forgetting, reporting a rate of 19 per cent total amnesia and the two studies which have addressed corroboration of the abuse did not look separately at cases where complete amnesia had been reported (British Psychological Society, 1995). Clearly there is a need for further work on repression and recovery of memories of abuse.

4.8.3 Suggestion and Child Sexual Abuse

A number of complaints have been made about therapists suggesting strongly to their clients that sexual abuse might have occurred if memories are missing or hazy. Indeed in one guide for survivors of child sexual abuse (Bass and Davis, 1988), which is often also used by counsellors, it states quite explicitly, 'If you are unable to remember any specific instance . . . but still have a feeling that something abusive happened to you, it probably did' (page 21) and, 'So far no one we've talked to thought she might have been abused, and then after discovered she hadn't been . . . If you think you were abused and your life shows the symptoms, then you were' (page 22). The symptoms the authors refer to are low self-esteem, suicidal or self-destructive thoughts, depression and sexual dysfunction.

Although we know that because episodic memory is often fragmentary we tend to reconstruct to fill in the gaps, is it possible that an entirely false memory can be created by suggestion? Both Baddeley and Loftus, two of the most eminent workers in the area of memory, think it can.

Baddeley cites the recording of an interrogation by police and a psychologist of a man accused of ritual sex abuse. After the man had confessed to the abuse, the psychologist presented the man with an invented incident which he stated the man's children had reported. After initially reporting no memory of the incident, the man subsequently recalled vague pictures of the scene and the following day wrote a detailed account of his 'memories'. The memories, however, could have had a similar status to a false confession. That is, the individual may be well aware of their provenance, but provides the evidence which will enable him to temporarily escape from the situation (the interrogation).

In a study reported by Loftus, certain adults and adolescents were made to believe that they had been lost when young in a particular shopping mall. They then went on to 'remember' details of the mythical incident.

There are also, of course, a number of reports of individual cases of apparent false beliefs being created after extended directed therapy. In spite of what we know, and indeed, do not know, about the complexities of memory it is rather surprising to find in the British Psychological Society's report on Recovered Memories (BPS, 1995) the statement, 'overall we agree with Lindsay and Read (1994) in a recent comprehensive review: *There is little reason to fear that a few suggestive questions will lead psychotherapy clients to conjure up vivid and compelling illusory memories of childhood sexual abuse* (page 294; emphasis added)'.

The authors of the report fail to take into account the sometimes powerful nature of the transference relationship. The 'few suggestive questions' which in any other context would be harmless, taken together with the dynamics of the therapist–client relationship and a client who may be vulnerable for reasons other than having been sexually abused as a child may provide the conditions which could be interpreted as highly persuasive.

4.8.4 The Effects of Hypnosis on Memory

Popular belief has it that hypnosis holds the key to our forgotten memories (see also Section 6.6). This belief has been fuelled by seemingly impressive accounts in the press of witnesses under hypnosis vividly recalling previously unremembered details of accidents and crimes. It is also believed by many that gaining access to childhood memories will help us to understand and cope with our current lives. It is hardly surprising then that hypnotic regression has been seen to be an obvious choice of some therapists working with suspected survivors of child sexual abuse.

The use of hypnosis to enhance memory is based on the video-taped model of human memory; that everything we have experienced is somehow recorded 'in there' and can be accessed in its original form given the 'right' conditions for recall; that is, hypnosis.

As we have seen, this is a totally erroneous view of memory. It will come as no surprise then to learn that research has shown that a hypnotized person is more likely than under normal conditions to use imagination to fill in the gaps in memory; that is, to reconstruct memories. It has also been shown that 'leading' questions asked under hypnosis can alter memories (Sanders and Simmons, 1983), and also when subjects are given false information, they tend to incorporate it into their own memories (Sheehan and Statham, 1989).

Hypnosis undoubtedly uncovers more information (Watkins, 1989) but it also increases false memories more than it does true ones. In one study, 80 per cent of new memories produced by subjects under hypnosis were *incorrect* (Dywan and Bowers, 1983). What is perhaps the most worrying feature of all is the confidence that the hypnotized person feels in the accuracy of these false memories; confidence that can be unshakable (Laurence and Perry, 1983).

Where does this leave the counsellor? There is no doubt that child sexual abuse occurs and it seems highly probable that memories of the abuse in some cases are repressed. It also may be the case that some memories have been reconstructed or are false.

We clearly need to be alert to the dangers of suggestion but sometimes clients will arrive in therapy having recovered memories either with another therapist or in the course of their daily lives. Much of the counselling 'work' is conducted in the context of a trusting alliance between counsellor and client. We as therapists want to trust our clients as much as we want them to trust us; but we need to be aware that counter-transference can operate as powerfully as transference. We may *want* to believe our clients and lose our sense of perspective and our judgement on the matter.

As well as recognizing the difficulties and personal demands of working with recovered memories it is important to recognize that our capacity for distinguishing genuine repressed memories from reconstructions and inventions is extremely limited. We should never, however, forget that whether the recovered memory is literally true, partially true or completely false, it may be equally traumatic for the client and could have considerable repercussions for the client's family. What we need to do is to find ways of taking the client seriously, whilst avoiding drawing premature conclusions about the 'truth' or otherwise of the recovered memory.

4.9 CONCLUDING COMMENTS

This chapter has attempted to demonstrate how a knowledge of the processes that underlie memory can help the counsellor to understand and work with the client's memories.

As we have seen, we have come a long way from the early formulations of memory as a sort of video-taped recording of events located in our heads. We have seen that memory is a dynamic process with new information being added to, and changing, what was in the existing store with new memories constantly updating and replacing the old.

By understanding how memories are transferred from short- to long-term memory and how they are encoded and stored, we can begin to understand why people remember what they do, and how they forget. It also helps to explain the fascinating areas of reconstructive memory and recovered memory. The process of repression however, so important in counselling and therapeutic work, is still relatively poorly understood. It is to be hoped that future work in this area may uncover some of the mysteries and help us understand this phenomenon better.

5

Thinking: Information Processing, Decision-making and Problem-solving

CONTENTS

5.1 INTRODUCTION

We spend a great deal of our lives thinking. Sometimes we let our minds 'wander', as when we daydream; and sometimes our thinking is more focused, as it is when 'thinking through' a particular issue or problem, or trying to come to some decision or course of action. This process is often so much part of our everyday life that it requires little conscious effort, such as deciding whether or not to take an umbrella when we leave the house. But at other times a greater degree of conscious planning may be required, and we will be aware of 'turning our minds' to the problem; in deciding, for example, what to do about impossibly noisy neighbours, how to handle a particularly tricky situation at work, or in working out ways to cope with the various and sometimes conflicting demands of home and professional life.

Clients often enter counselling or therapy at times when they are confronted by particular problems which they have found difficult or impossible to work through themselves; they may also be faced with making decisions which could have a considerable effect on their lives and possibly the lives of others.

Counsellors also are constantly faced with 'problems' to be solved and decisions to be made: 'What approach is going to be most beneficial for this particular client with this particular difficulty?' 'Is counselling going to be helpful or would joining a peer support group be more appropriate?' 'Might this client benefit from anti-depressant medication so be advised to discuss it with the GP, or shall I speak to the GP myself?'; 'How many sessions will be needed and at what intervals?' Even the most non-directive of counsellors make decisions about what 'material' to respond to and at what emotional level.

Although when we engage in this type of thinking we are not aware of the underlying mental processes, these have been extensively studied by psychologists working in the field of cognitive psychology. Indeed, cognitive psychology has been concerned primarily with how people think, and with what takes place between the stimulus (such as the state of the sky) and the person's subsequent response (taking an umbrella or not, as the case may be). This is usually referred to as **information processing**. As we shall see, the stimulus need not be external; we can also respond to internal stimuli (such as our beliefs that others would think badly of us if we appeared looking like a drowned rat).

Cognitive psychologists have used the concept of information processing in attempting to understand and study the way in which people solve problems and make decisions. Although there are a number of counselling models that adopt problem solving and decision-making approaches (e.g. Egon, 1986; Janis and Mann, 1977), a knowledge of the 'groundwork' and the foundations on which these are based will enhance the counsellor's understanding of these models and enable them to take a more informed approach and to locate their work within a wider theoretical framework.

We accordingly start this chapter with looking at the **information processing model** and also at some of the factors that can affect the way in which we perceive and make sense of stimuli. We will also discuss some of the 'errors' which can occur in processing information. The next section is concerned with the work on problem-solving, and we demonstrate how this might apply to an actual 'case'. We also include a section on creative problem-solving which counsellors might find useful in working with clients or in relation to themselves. The final section focuses on decision-making and how to improve it, and once again, we have concentrated on the work which is of particular relevance to real-life settings and problems.

5.2 INFORMATION PROCESSING

In order to understand, make sense of and respond to what is going on in the world around us, we are constantly 'processing' information. If we are driving along the road and the traffic signals turn from green to amber as we approach them we perceive a complex pattern of incoming stimuli which we evaluate before making a decision and acting. Although this all occurs so rapidly it can seem to be automatic, a number of stages occur between the presentation of a stimuli and the execution of a response.

In the first stage of this process, information about the stimulus (the traffic lights, the state of the road, the layout of the junction, the other traffic etc.) reaches the brain by way of sensory receptors.

In the second stage the information must be attended to, perceived and recognized and this requires matching the perceived pattern to a pattern in long-term memory. So we make sense of the stimuli by relating it to what we already know (what the changing pattern of lights means, what we know about speed and braking distances, how this might be affected by weather conditions, possible penalties for infringement of the law etc.). This process demands progressively more attention.

The information may simply be stored in memory, but if, as with this example, a decision has to be made to take some action, a response must be selected (to brake, or to 'jump' the lights) before moving on to the fourth stage, the execution of the response (actually doing it). The effect of the response on the environment is then fed back as new information to be processed. (You crash, hear the police sirens or, with a sigh of relief, realize you have got away with it.)

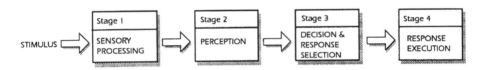

Figure 5.1   Information processing model

We can see from the above example that attention, pattern recognition and memory each play an important part in information processing. These three areas of theory and research, and how they relate particularly to the perceptual and recognition stages of processing information, will be discussed below with reference to a particular 'case'.

The client is a 54-year-old man who has been experiencing severe marital difficulties. (His wife has refused to attend either joint sessions or to come to sessions on her own.) He has been married for three years, his first marriage having ended apparently reasonably amicably some seven years previously. He reports that his wife is 'insanely' jealous of his relationship with his grown-up children and has now 'forbidden' him to have contact with them. He describes her losing her temper with him and 'screaming and ranting and raving' at him. He deals with this by trying to pacify her and reassure her that he loves her. He had thought that the situation would improve when, six months ago, her eight-year-old son, of whom he is very fond, came to live with them. It didn't, and recently the outbursts have become more frequent and now occur almost daily.

In the third session the client has been exploring alternative ways of managing the situation at home and seemed to be reasonably optimistic about trying them out. Having confirmed his next appointment, the counsellor opens the door for him and

notices her next client pacing up and down in the waiting room. As he is leaving, the
client she has been seeing says in a conversational tone, 'Well thank you very much,
I'll look forward to seeing you next week, if I'm still around. I am worried though.
It wouldn't be the first time, you know, she's had a go at me and I've had to hide the
kitchen knives. But thank you anyway.'

Here we shall regard the stimulus as the closing remarks of the client and discuss
attention, pattern recognition and memory in relation to this example.

5.2.1 Attention and the Selection of Information

The information processing model suggests that attention is necessary particularly
during the perceptual and decision stages of processing. Counselling requires a very
high level of attention and counsellors are trained to attend much more carefully and
intently than is normally required in conversation. They are also trained to attend to
paralinguistic cues as well as to the verbal aspects; to the latent as well as the manifest content. But even the most highly trained and experienced counsellor cannot
attend to everything, otherwise they would be overwhelmed by sensory messages
from the environment. Only a few of these messages register on awareness; the rest
are 'filtered out' and perceived either dimly or not at all. This is called **selective
attention**.

In the example above, the counsellor had perceived and recognized the conversational tone of the client's remarks and had shifted her attention away from him onto the
waiting area where she noticed her next client. Her attention was brought back sharply
to focus on the client only when she heard the words 'knives'.

Results from laboratory experiments have demonstrated that we cannot attend completely to more than one thing at a time but we can shift our attention back and forth
rapidly enough to get the sense of two different messages (Sperling, 1984).

5.2.2 Pattern Recognition and Concept Formation

The information processing mode suggests that we recognize a 'complex pattern of
incoming stimuli' and that this pattern is matched or compared to similar instances in
long-term memory. This enables us then to categorize the stimuli. The process of developing these patterns in long-term memory is called **concept formation**. Some concepts
are relatively straightforward and the boundaries of the concept fairly clear. Most people in western cultures would agree, for example, on the concept of 'fruit' (that is, until
you asked them about tomatoes!). So when we encounter a new strange object, we recognize what aspects it has in common with, and how it is different from other instances
included in our concept. We may also refer to our **prototype** of the concept, that is, the
part of the concept that contains the properties that describe the best examples of it.
Whether or not we categorize this object as a 'fruit' or not depends on the outcome of
this process.

The relevance of this to counselling becomes clear when we turn again to the example of the ending of the session outlined above. In the same way as we form concepts of fruit, so we form concepts and prototypes of 'dangerousness' and 'dangerous situations'. But how do we recognize, for example, situations as dangerous and what is included in our concept of dangerousness? Does it include a man feeling it necessary to remove the kitchen knives during an argument with his wife? Clearly there will be considerable differences between individuals in this respect and how the concept is formed will be determined by a number of factors such as background experiences and cultural context. Ultimately, how the counsellor in this case decides to act will depend, in part, on their concept of dangerousness.

5.2.3 Memory and Information Processing

We have discussed above the role of memory in processing information. In addition to concepts and categories, permanent memory includes memory for events, images, and words. When the counsellor hears the words 'worried' and 'knives' she will probably be searching in her memory for other references to potentially violent behaviour which the client might have made.

Long-term memory also includes more complex structures such as **schemas** (which we discussed in Chapter 4 on Memory) and **scripts**. By a schema we mean a set of beliefs and expectations that can help to organize past experience and provide us with a framework for understanding future experience. The term script refers to a schema related to an event or social interaction.

Many counsellors and therapists will be familiar with the client who self-discloses right at the end of the session and will accordingly have developed a schema of such a phenomenon, referred to by one colleague as the 'coat-rack' phenomenon (on account of the fact that it occurs just as the client takes his coat ready to leave). We may even have developed a script about responding to such behaviour; to ignore it, to confront the person at the start of the next session etc.

Schemas and scripts therefore exert a powerful influence on our subsequent choice of action. This can be very useful, particularly in situations when we know it is relatively 'safe' to operate on 'automatic pilot'. If, however, such mechanisms are guiding us as counsellors and therapists, we need to be aware of this possible influence and, it could be argued, be actively engaged in trying to identify our own particular schemas and scripts which may be influencing how we conceptualize our clients' experiences and which may, in turn, be influencing our own therapeutic decisions.

5.2.4 Errors in Information Processing

As soon as we start discussing attention, concept formation and memory in relation to information processing, we can immediately see how easy it could be to 'get it wrong'. These errors can fundamentally influence the way in which we interpret situations and affect our subsequent actions.

Attention

As noted above, it would be impossible for us to pay attention to the multitude of stimuli to which we are constantly exposed. We therefore attend selectively in order to avoid 'sensory overload'. We do this, firstly, by focusing on particular stimuli, and secondly, by filtering out incoming information.

Attention is also strongly affected by both the nature of the stimulus and personal characteristics. If we perceive or conceptualize a situation as 'dangerous', it is more likely to catch and hold our attention. But if, in the above example, the counsellor had not classified the situation as such, her attention might have switched to focus on her next client, particularly if he had appeared in some way disturbed; and although it is possible to switch attention quite rapidly between competing stimuli, we cannot attend to two things at once. Some information would accordingly be lost.

Focusing on particular stimuli helps to filter out irrelevant information from the environment. This filtering process can, it has been suggested, act as a defence to protect us from anxiety that might be aroused if we allowed ourselves to perceive stimuli which we saw as threatening. As with most defences, this can at times be very useful, but it can also be damaging, particularly if it forms part of our 'perceptual style'. Finally, stress can lead to a narrowing of attention and we may miss features of the stimulus.

Concepts

Difficulties may arise because the person may not recognize the situation as belonging to a particular 'class' of situations because they may not have developed sufficiently robust relevant concepts. Alternatively their concepts may be over-inclusive (too much is included so almost everything becomes 'dangerous') or under-inclusive (the concept of dangerous is limited to violent criminals). Problems can also arise if the assigning of events, etc., to categories is overly rigid. An example of this would be if the counsellor immediately ascribed the client's closing comments as 'coat-rack comments'; that is, something that clients tend to 'throw out' at the end of the session. If the remarks were classified as such, then the subsequent actions of the counsellor would probably be consistent with their script for this type of situation.

Memory

The information process relies on information stored in long-term memory. But information relevant to the present situation may not have been committed to long-term memory; and even when information has been 'stored' there may be problems of retrieval. Memory, as we discussed in Section 4.7, may also involve the construction of material, as much as it involves the retrieval (see Chapter 4).

5.3 DECISION-MAKING

In the preceding section we saw how the way in which we perceive and conceptualize, or process information, will affect our subsequent decisions and actions. We have, until now, been concerned more with the moment-by-moment processing involved in day-to-day functioning than with the sort of life decisions which confront us all and which often concern clients. A young adult must make a choice of career, or an older one whether to retire; a patient has to make a decision about elective surgery or a client about how to deal with an abusive partner. And, of course, the counsellor in the first example in this chapter must decide how to respond to his client's revelation. We will now look at how people make these sort of real-life decisions, a subject that has been studied extensively by social psychologists.

Decision-making always occurs in the context of uncertainty, otherwise there would not really be a decision to be made. Ultimately, we are concerned with probabilities which in real life are often not clear cut. Evaluating these probabilities can be crucial. The young adult must assess the probability of a particular college course helping him to get a better job at the end of it; the older one the probability that taking early retirement and living on a reduced income will be better than staying the course until he is 65, thereby increasing his pension. The patient contemplating elective surgery must do their best to weigh up the relevant risks involved against the possible benefits; a client may need to evaluate the likelihood of being more content if she left her husband and family home. Going back to the first example, the counsellor must estimate the probabilities of the client's wife responding violently.

Janis and Mann (1982) have suggested that in making decisions we should 'spend the necessary time and effort seeking clarification of the issues involved, striving to be open-minded when deliberating, searching for relevant information about consequences of the alternatives, making contingency plans, and taking other specific steps in order to arrive at a decision that will not be regretted' (p. 49). But even the 'best' decisions can sometimes lead to unsatisfactory outcomes because the world is full of uncertainties. Decisions of this sort made when the outcome is uncertain are usually referred to as **risky decisions**, or **decisions under uncertainty**. But psychologists have discovered many other reasons why human decisions may lead to unsatisfactory outcomes. Some of these are described below.

5.3.1 Difficulties in Decision-making

Estimating probabilities

When making decisions in real life we are very unlikely to know what the exact probabilities are of a particular event happening so we make use of various **heuristics**, or 'rules of thumb' to help us estimate likelihoods. Heuristics underlie much of our everyday decision-making, but their misuse, as we shall see, can lead to serious errors (Tversky and Kahneman, 1973).

One of the most common heuristics employed in decision-making is the **availability heuristic**, which leads us to base our decisions on the availability of information in memory. Availability may be a function of a number of things. People tend to notice the unusual or atypical which can lead them to overestimate the probability of an event occurring. For example, when people were asked to estimate the likelihood of being victims of a violent crime, they estimated it at a one in four chance. It is, in effect, more likely to be one in two hundred.

Another factor affecting availability of information is **salience**. The GP in the example in the first chapter made the decision to advise his patient to put more into her relationship probably because this approach that had worked for him was both recent (and therefore readily available to him) and important (and therefore striking).

Another way in which we often estimate probability is by employing what is known as the **representativeness heuristic.** This involves judging the extent to which something is similar to our ideal or model (prototype) of that particular concept and whether it fits into that class or category.

For example, if you encounter a man who is tidy, small in stature, wears glasses, speaks quietly and appears somewhat shy, and you were asked if this man was more likely to be a librarian or a farmer, you might well, like the subjects in an experiment by Tversky and Kahneman (1974), choose 'librarian'. But the chances are that this answer would be wrong. Although this description is probably more similar to most people's prototype of a librarian than their prototype of a farmer, there are very many more farmers in the world than librarians and probably more farmers who match this description than librarians. Therefore a man matching this description is more likely to be a farmer than a librarian. If the counsellor had employed a representativeness heuristic to the episode described in the previous section, she may well have classified the situation as representative of a coat-rack situation and acted accordingly.

When using this heuristic it can be seen how easy it is to confuse representativeness with probability; to ignore the overall probabilities and focus instead on what is representative or typical of the evidence available.

Yet another way in which we can make errors of judgement in evaluating probabilities comes from **confirmation bias**. Much research has shown that people generally seek evidence or information to support their beliefs. A consequence of this is that erroneous beliefs may be maintained indefinitely by selecting and generating evidence supporting those beliefs and avoiding or re-interpreting evidence which may disconfirm them.

For instance, someone who believes that women are poor drivers may be more critical of women drivers and remember those instances when a woman drove badly. Additionally, these instances may be organized as a (semi-)coherent concept, thus being easier to remember when called for. He or she will probably not consider the relative occurrence of poor driving by males.

5.3.2 Cognitive processes involved in evaluating options and outcomes

Decision-making involves searching for relevant information about consequences of alternative courses of action, or options. Each option will probably have positive and negative features, or **attributes.** Deciding on which college to attend, whether or not to leave home or move house are all examples of **multi-attribute decision-making** (Edwards, 1987).

One of the reasons multi-attribute decisions can be difficult is because the limited storage capacity in short-term memory does not allow people easily to keep in mind, combine and compare all the attributes of all the options (Fischoff et al., 1977) and people seem unable to keep in mind more than a few 'chunks' of information at any one time (see Section 4.2.2 on Short-term Memory).

People also tend to short-cut the essential stages of search and appraisal when they become aware of undesirable consequences to be expected from whichever choice they make (Janis and Mann, 1977). They are often inclined to deceive themselves into thinking they have conducted a complete information search after brief contact with a so-called 'expert', maybe the counsellor, and perhaps a few informal discussions with friends or acquaintances.

Other studies emphasize different flaws and limitations in information processing, such as the tendency of decision-makers to be distracted by irrelevant aspects of the alternatives, which lead to erroneous estimates of predictable outcomes (Abelson, 1976). Another source of error is the illusion of control, which makes for over-optimistic estimates of outcomes that are a matter of chance and luck (Langer, 1975). People's confidence in their predictions has been shown to be consistently greater than their accuracy (Fischoff and MacGregor, 1982). The moral of this is to be wary when people express confidence that a forecast of a decision is right. They may be wrong more often than they think.

5.3.3 Uncertainty and stress in decision-making

As noted above, decisions, by their very nature, are required where there is uncertainty present. Uncertainty has been found to be an important element in whether or not events (or anticipated events) are perceived as stressful (for example, Fleming et al., 1991). High uncertainty is also likely to result in loss of self-esteem, as counsellors who work with clients with illnesses where the prognosis is uncertain will be well aware.

There are a number of factors in addition to uncertainty that can lead to high levels of stress in the decision-maker. The task may be too complicated to manage; there may be little time available in which to make the decision and the decision-maker may become harassed and the consequences of the decision may involve potential material losses or damage to the person's self-esteem. Stress tends to lead to a narrowing of attention which may have a significant effect on information processing, particularly in relation to information search and in considering possible alternatives.

It has been suggested that another source that can hinder decision-making arises from what has been termed **decisional conflict** (Janis and Mann, 1982). The person finds it difficult or impossible to make a decision because of 'simultaneous opposing tendencies within the individual to accept and at the same time to reject a given course of action. The most prominent symptoms of such conflicts are hesitation, vacillation, feelings of uncertainty and signs of acute psychological stress' (p. 50). Janis and Mann suggest some basic maladaptive patterns people adopt when trying to cope with the stresses of such situations. One obvious example of decisional conflict is the man or woman who faces a decision about whether or not to leave their partner, and where there may be another relationship involved. Many counsellors will have seen clients with this sort of motivational conflict.

- **Unconflicted adherence**   The decision-maker complacently decides to continue whatever he or she has been doing, ignoring information about risks and losses.
- **Unconflicted change to a new course of action**   The decision-maker uncritically adopts whichever new course of action is the most prominent or most strongly recommended.
- **Defensive avoidance**   Here the decision-maker escapes the conflict, at least temporarily by procrastinating, shifting responsibility to someone else, or constructing wishful rationalizations to bolster the least objectionable alternative, remaining selectively inattentive to corrective information.
- **Hypervigilance**   Here the decision-maker searches frantically for a way out of the dilemma and impulsively seizes upon a hastily contrived solution that seems to promise immediate relief. They may overlook the full range of consequences of the choice as a result of emotional excitement, perseveration and cognitive construction (manifested by reduction in immediate memory span and simplistic thinking). In its most extreme form, hypervigilance is referred to as 'panic'.

5.4 IMPROVING DECISION-MAKING

The most obvious way of improving decision-making is to develop strategies to avoid the problems and difficulties highlighted in the section above. The counsellor should be sensitive to the operation of the various heuristics and biases identified in his or her own thinking and judgement, understand how cognitive processes operate in the search for and appraisal of information concerning the possible options and outcomes, recognize and acknowledge the relationship between uncertainty and stress and identify and work towards avoiding or eliminating maladaptive coping strategies.

In addition to avoiding the pitfalls of decision-making, there are a large number of models, theories and strategies which have been developed to facilitate effective decision-making. Two of the most relevant to the counselling context are the **conflict-theory model** of Janis and Mann (1982) and the **expectancy × value theory** (Brehm and Self, 1989; Weiner, 1992).

The conflict-theory model maintains that there are five basic patterns of coping with the stress generated when we are confronted by having to make a vital choice. Four of these are the defective patterns listed above. The fifth, this theory maintains, will generally lead to decisions that meet the basic criteria for 'high quality decision-making'. This fifth pattern is:

- **Vigilance**   Here the decision-maker searches painstakingly for relevant information, assimilates information in an unbiased manner and appraises alternatives before making a choice.

Janis and Mann suggest a number of ways in which counsellors can help their clients to foster vigilance and avoid defective coping patterns, and thus improving decision-making. These include an 'awareness-of-rationalizations' procedure, role playing in structured psychodramas, a balance-sheet procedure devised to evoke awareness of a full range of consequences and stress inoculation for post-decisional setbacks.

An approach derived from **expectancy × value theory** can also help people make effective decisions under motivational conflict. In this procedure, clients are helped to identify the alternative courses of action available to them and the positive and negative consequences that might result from each. They then assign numerical values to each consequence in terms of how likely it is to occur (expectancy) and how positive or negative it is (value). These scores can then be multiplied to produce an expectancy × value score for each pair of decision alternatives. The person can then use this score as a basis for making a rational decision.

The counsellor and client should not, however, be tempted to treat this 'score' or the numbers from which it has been derived as being any more than an indication of the direction of the person's thinking. Even so, clients will sometimes change their minds.

The results of conducting such an exercise with one particular client trying to decide whether or not to return to her war-torn country and possibly face political charges indicated that she should not go back. The following session, however, she told the counsellor how helpful this had been, thanked her and said 'Goodbye'. The process of doing the exercise had sharpened her thinking and enabled her to come to a decision which she felt was the 'right' one. She knew, she stated, that she had to go back and somehow had found the courage to make the decision. Subsequent communication with the client confirmed that although the consequences of going back had been very distressing for her, she still felt it had been the right decision.

5.5 PROBLEM-SOLVING

If we avoid all the errors and pitfalls mentioned above, it would seem from the information processing model that human behaviour would be all smooth efficiency and we could, without too much difficulty, make the appropriate decisions sailing effortlessly through life. But often, as we all know, the decision is not clear cut. Sometimes we are in situations that are very unsatisfactory. We are not where we would like to be at all, but the path between the problem and the solution is not at all clear.

There has been a considerable amount of research on problem solving but much of this has been centred around laboratory experiments designed to study the underlying processes involved in, for example, deciphering anagrams and finding solutions to various geometric problems, often where there is a 'right' answer. These underlying processes, according to cognitive psychologists, include understanding (or diagnosing) the problem, devising a plan to solve the problem, executing the plan and evaluating the results (Polya, 1957). The problem-solver goes through a sequence of internal steps which are directed towards a goal, the solution of the problem.

One of the main research techniques in studying problem-solving has been to get subjects to 'think aloud' whilst attempting to solve a problem. This has enabled psychologists to study how subjects have used **reasoning** (the process by which people evaluate and generate arguments and reach conclusions), **logic** (the mental procedures that lead to valid conclusions) and **heuristics** (a mental short-cut or 'rule of thumb') in problem-solving.

Heuristics is the area of problem-solving theory and research particularly relevant to understanding and facilitating the kind of problem-solving generally encountered in counselling situations.

5.5.1 Problem-solving Heuristics

Most people attempting to solve real-life problems adopt a heuristic, or 'rule of thumb' approach. Heuristics typically reduce the number of alternatives a thinker must consider. They guide the person's judgements about what events are probable, but they can, as we shall see, be biased.

Heuristic strategies include:

- Identifying, defining and reframing the problem (diagnosis). This can be helped by formulating hypotheses which can then be eliminated or selected and tested.
- Having some idea about where you would like to be (the goal or solution).
- Reducing differences between the current state and the goal state.
- Exploring possible solutions and relevant knowledge.
- Working backwards from the desired goal to the starting point or current situation.
- If the goal cannot be reached directly, identifying an immediate goal or sub-problem that at least gets you closer to the desired outcome.

The following case illustrates heuristics in action.

The problem

Mrs C is a 32-year-old woman in the fortunate position of living in a fairly large, comfortable house in the country with her two children and their ponies, a labrador and the usual number of assorted pet rodents in cages. She is also, however, in the very unfortunate position of having a husband who sticks objects, including beer bottles, up her vagina two or three times a week. This usually occurs when he has returned late from the pub which he frequents, but it also happens when he has not been drinking. Mr C refuses to discuss either his sexual or his drinking habits with Mrs C or anyone else for that matter.

The background to the problem

Mrs C is the daughter of fairly well-off parents and attended boarding school from the age of eleven to eighteen. During her last two years at school she suffered from anorexia and spent a period of three months in hospital. (Her eating and weight are now normal.) Her academic work subsequently suffered and she took only two out of the usual three 'A' levels, for which she received reasonable grades, but not sufficient for entry into higher education. She did a secretarial course and married when she was aged twenty.

When she was aged twenty-three she was raped at a party by her husband's best friend. Although she was extremely distressed, her husband seemed unperturbed and told her she should not have gone into the garden with him in the first place and anyway, he was an old school friend and a good mate of his. It was the aftermath of this incident for which Mrs C had originally sought counselling, some eight years after its occurrence.

Mr C works in the city and has recently suffered considerable financial losses and has talked about the necessity of selling the house. He drinks socially, has a couple of lagers at lunchtime and three or four times a week goes to the pub in the evening where he drinks four or five pints of beer.

Diagnosing the problem

One of the important tasks of counselling is often identifying and defining (diagnosing) the problem(s). This may involve a certain amount of **reframing** or **restructuring**. Often clients will present with problems of mood or functioning: they feel depressed, angry, demotivated, they feel worthless or cannot carry on the tasks of daily life, cannot sleep etc. In the above example, quite a lot of reframing has already taken place in the process of the counsellor working with the client on dealing with the distress of the rape and exploring her relationship with her parents, husband and children.

One strategy for facilitating 'diagnosis' in this sense, is through the **formulation and testing of hypotheses**, or potential solutions. These can be both explanatory and predictive. That is, hypotheses can both explain how something has come about, and predict possible outcomes. Ideally this would involve the following three stages:

Stage 1—Determining what explanations will be considered. This is usually referred to as establishing the initial hypotheses. (The client may well have started to do this before they came to counselling but it is important that the client and counsellor do not uncritically adopt this frame).

Let us look at some of the hypotheses generated by Mrs C:

- **Hypothesis 1**   He does it because I'm a useless wife. If I were a better wife and more exciting in bed he would not do it (abuse her sexually with objects).
- **Hypothesis 2**   He does it because he's been drinking. If I could get him help for this he would not do it.
- **Hypothesis 3**   He does it because there's something wrong with our relationship. If we went to marriage guidance he would realize his behaviour was unacceptable and change.
- **Hypothesis 4**   He does it because he thinks I'm a slut for allowing myself to be raped by his friend and is trying to punish me. If he would talk about this or seek help then he would not do it any more.
- **Hypothesis 5**   He does it because he's quite disturbed in that area. I don't know why because he won't talk about it. If I were not around he couldn't do it to me.

Stage 2—Determining which of these explanations are consistent with the evidence that has so far been observed and ruling out any explanations that do not fit the evidence. This is called evaluating the hypotheses against the evidence.

> *Having completed the first stage, Mrs C went on to rule out hypotheses 1 and 2 because the evidence did not fit. Hypotheses 3 and 4 also had to be discarded but for different reasons. Mrs C felt that she had already tried to test these and had done all she could to encourage her husband to talk or to seek expert help. This left hypothesis 5.*

Stage 3—Testing the hypotheses that remain. Is there any test that would give one result if one hypothesis were true and another result if another hypothesis were true? If so the test can be made and the hypothesis evaluated again in the light of the evidence from the test. This stage involves further information gathering and requires certain types of information to be actively sought, especially information that would challenge the hypothesis. This is essentially what scientists do when they design experiments. The purpose of this is to rule out hypotheses, not to prove they are true.

> *In this case there was only one hypothesis to be tested out—Hypothesis 5, 'He does it because he's quite disturbed in that area. I don't know why because he won't talk about it. If I were not around he couldn't do it to me'. This hypothesis also gave her an idea about where she wanted to be; that is, it provided her with her goal or solution.*

The goal or solution

The solution tells you where you *want* to be, not how to get there. How goals are framed is of considerable importance to our perception of choices, as research on the framing of potential outcomes demonstrates. When half the subjects in a particular experiment were told that there was a 50 per cent success rate and the other half told there was a 50 per cent failure rate in a new experimental treatment that removes cancerous cells, the '50 per cent success' group rated the treatment as significantly more effective and expressed a greater willingness to have it administered on a family member than did the subjects in the '50 per cent failure' group (Kahneman and Tversky, 1979). Framing a choice in terms of positives and negatives has this effect because people tend to assign greater costs to negative outcomes than they assign value to positive outcomes, as the example of Mrs. C demonstrates.

> *Mrs C's solution was to get herself into the situation in which her husband could no longer sexually abuse her. If she had framed it in terms of leaving her husband her thinking would in all probability have followed something like this: 'I'd have nowhere to live, my husband would become really difficult over the children, they*

would have to leave their private schools, what about the animals, my children would be deprived of their father, friends, their ponies, my husband might get custody of them. I can't do this to them, I'll just have to put up with it until they're grown up'. By framing the desired outcome in a more positive way, Mrs C was able to proceed further with her problem-solving.

Working backwards

The next stage is to work backwards from the desired outcome and to identify intermediate *sub-goals*, thereby lessening the gap between the current situation and the goal in question. This is how the process went in the case of Mrs C.

- To put herself in a position in which her husband could no longer abuse her she would need to be financially independent (even though she would be entitled to some maintenance).
- To be financially independent would necessitate some training.
- In order to undertake any training at the level at which she would clearly be capable she would need to take another 'A' level (to obtain entry into higher education).
- In order to get used to studying she would need to start with a less demanding course.

The outcome

With this approach the goal is not something which necessarily has to be achieved, but is there to give a sense of direction, something to work towards. The first sub-goal, to start a less demanding course, was fairly low-level, requiring little 'cost' to the client so did not require any major decisions to be made. Although Mrs C understandably was concerned about how she would cope with her family and further training, and although she was still extremely distressed by her husband's behaviour she continued to work through her sub-goals.

What we often tend to forget, when making these sort of long-term plans, is that life will take its course anyway. Things happen over which we have little or no control so trying to think of every eventuality at the planning stage is not particularly productive. If Mrs C had done this she would once again have got bogged down in issues like 'How will I manage if I have to go on a placement as part of my training?', and she would never have started that first course.

Today, Mrs C is has successfully completed her first degree and is in her final year of her professional training. As her self-esteem increased, her husband's sexual abuse decreased. The marriage did break up, the ponies were sold, the children did move to state schools, there was an extremely difficult period of uncertainty when Mrs C feared the family would be split up as they had nowhere to live. The cost has been high in material terms, but Mrs C feels that she is now where she wanted, and wants, to be; she has a good relationship with her children and feels overall that they have benefited from the adjustments they have had to make.

5.5.2 Problems with Problem-solving

There are an number of problems, errors and pitfalls which are often encountered during problem-solving, although most of them occur at the beginning or diagnostic phase.

Fixations

One of the most common barriers to problem-solving is **fixation** or **mental set**. This is the tendency for the person to be blinded by one particular hypothesis or strategy which they continue to apply even when better alternatives should be obvious. (This is an example of what is known as an **anchoring heuristic**.) They get fixated on wrong solutions or are oblivious to alternatives. Somewhat unfairly, though, the greater the motivation towards a solution, the stronger the mental sets are towards the problem. This is fine if the set is appropriate, but hard to break out of if not (Glucksberg, 1962). The creative problem-solving techniques discussed in Section 5.6 can be used to encourage people to break out of rigid mental sets.

Generation of insufficient hypotheses

People often begin to solve a problem with only a vague notion of which hypothesis to test and fail to generate a sufficient number to facilitate effective problem-solving. They may get fixated on one particular one or they may consider only the one that comes most easily to mind. (This is known as the **availability heuristic**.) Several characteristics might make one hypothesis easier to remember than others; for example, simplicity, emotional content and how recently it was experienced (Tversky and Kahneman, 1974). In counselling or therapy, clients can be encouraged to generate and explore new hypotheses to be tested.

Confirmation bias

People often have a tendency to confirm, rather than to refute, their chosen hypothesis, even in the face of strong evidence to the contrary. They are quite willing to perceive and interpret data that support their hypothesis, but they tend to ignore information that is inconsistent with it (Adams, 1989). This is more likely to be the case if the person is 'fixated' on one particular hypothesis and has not explored alternatives.

Ignoring negative evidence

Sometimes what does not happen is as important as what does happen. The fact that symptoms are not present can be important in disconfirming the original hypothesis. For example, some people will hypothesize that it is all their fault in spite of any evidence to support this assertion. Compared with symptoms that are present, however, symptoms or events that do not occur are less likely to be noticed (Hunt and Rouse, 1981)

Problems with logic

If a hypothesis is derived from a process of faulty reasoning then it will not be valid. The most common errors involve faulty premises (assumptions) or faulty logic. The following examples, called **syllogisms**, demonstrate this:

- *Syllogism 1*
     Major premise: *All teenagers today are likely to encounter drugs.*
     Minor premise: *My son is a teenager.*
     Conclusion: *Therefore he is likely to encounter drugs.*

     The premise of this syllogism is true; the logic is valid; this means the conclusion is true.

- *Syllogism 2*
     Major premise: *Only youngsters from unhappy or broken homes take drugs.*
     Minor premise: *My daughter is not from an unhappy or broken home.*
     Conclusion: *My daughter can't be taking drugs.*

     The major premise on which this syllogism is based is faulty, so that even though the logic is valid the conclusions are not.

- *Syllogism 3*
     Major premise: *My parents are dying and need me to stay close by.*
     Minor premise: *I want to move forward in my life by leaving this provincial town and going to live in London.*
     Conclusion: *Therefore by saying I want to move to London, I'm saying I want them to die.*

     Here the premises are valid, but the logic is faulty therefore the conclusions are wrong.

It can therefore be seen that challenging faulty premises or faulty logic in the context of problem-solving may be a particularly important task for the counsellor.

5.6 CREATIVE PROBLEM-SOLVING

The creative thinker comes up with a solution that is both novel and relevant to the problem in consideration. According to first hand accounts, critical insights usually occur at unexpected times and places: in the bath, going to pick the children up from school, walking the dog, pottering about in the kitchen or garden. They do not seem to happen to order, when we would like them to; when we find time to sit down and really think about the problem; when we allocate time to trying to find a solution.

These sorts of 'inspired' solutions seem to occur out of the blue and involve some kind of conceptual reorganization. There is usually a period of concentrated cognitive activity, when the person is immersed in the problem. There then typically follows a period of **incubation**, when the person 'puts it on one side' but does not turn away from the problem altogether; they continue to work on it unconsciously. It has been hypothesized that this allows inappropriate mental sets to be broken, giving new solutions a chance to emerge.

It requires some mental discipline to stop 'worrying' at a problem, but if, after a period of trying to work through to a solution, it can be put on one side, then the problem-solver may be rewarded by fresh insights.

Another way in which creative problem-solving may be facilitated is by **delayed evaluation**. Various studies suggest that people are most likely to be creative when they are free to play with ideas and solutions without attempting to evaluate them or to assess the consequences. Worrying about the appropriateness of solutions seems to inhibit creativity (Amabile, 1983). This approach has led to the technique of **brain-storming**.

Although brainstorming was developed as a group technique, it can be applied to individual problem-solving and to counselling. The essential feature of this method is that production and criticism of ideas are kept separate. The main idea is to encourage **divergent thinking** (thinking that produces many ideas or alternatives, a major element in original or creative thought). The problem-solver, or each person in the group, produces as many ideas as possible without fear of criticism or evaluation (Haefele, 1962; Buyer, 1988). Ideas should be produced without regard for logic, organization, accuracy or practicality. One idea triggers another, and only when an exhaustive list has been made are the suggestions on the list reconsidered, evaluated, modified, combined, rejected or accepted.

Like all creative approaches to problem-solving, brainstorming operates on the principle of breaking out of rigid mental sets.

5.7 CONCLUDING COMMENTS

The aim of this chapter has been to give an overview of the psychological work on decision-making and problem-solving in order to help the counsellor understand some of the basic psychological processes involved. The relevance of this work to problems and decisions facing both counsellor and client has been demonstrated by the use of examples.

One of the limitations of presenting illustrative case material in this context is that it all looks so neat, tidy and clear cut. We all know that life is not like that, nor is counselling and therapy. Take the example of Mrs C. There were, of course, many emotional issues, conflicts and difficulties which were addressed during the course of the counselling. There were also many different leads and strands that were followed. None of this has been presented here. Instead, you are seeing what amounts to a skeleton which, for much of the time, is held in the counsellor's awareness and brought to the client's attention at relevant times during counselling.

Any intervention in counselling or therapy must take place in the context of the therapeutic relationship and the therapeutic process. Problem-solving and decision-making procedures are no exception. It is essential that the counsellor remains sensitive to the client's internal world and to their emotional needs and states. Counsellors should therefore avoid the rigid adherence to any of these approaches or strategies but use them in a creative and flexible way to create a framework for interventions that will help their clients to achieve their chosen objectives.

6

States of Consciousness

CONTENTS

6.1 INTRODUCTION

We all intuitively know what it is to be conscious, and most of us are aware of when consciousness fluctuates (as when we pass from wakefulness into sleep, for instance), when it is disturbed (when we might say, for example, 'I really don't feel myself') or when it is altered (such as by alcohol). What consciousness is, and quite how to define it, is another matter, and is something that has baffled philosophers, psychologists and neurologists for many years.

People throughout history have pursued ways of altering consciousness. Some altered states are sought primarily for pleasure, such as through drug intoxication, but many cultures regard changes in consciousness as pathways to enlightenment. Ways of achieving this include fasting, meditation, prayer, isolation, sleep loss, whirling, chanting and psychedelic drugs.

Modern psychology started in the 1870s with the study of consciousness, mostly by methods of introspection. However, as the new scientific discipline progressed, psychologists increasingly turned their attention to studying only observable stimuli and responses. Introspection and, with it, the study of consciousness accordingly fell out of favour. The study of behaviour has dominated psychological research for much of this century, but by the 1950s, some psychologists felt that something was missing; that behaviourism was too confining. Eventually mainstream psychology widened to once again include the study of consciousness with an emphasis on what is termed altered states of consciousness. These have included sleep and dreams, relaxation and meditation, hypnosis and the effects of psychotropic drugs.

Although psychologists do not agree about the definition of consciousness, for most purposes it is considered to be our moment-to-moment awareness of ourselves and our environment; of our thoughts, feelings and our perceptions. Consciousness is a property of these mental processes, rather than a process in its own right. Thus perceptions, for example, can be conscious, but consciousness is not perception.

Many aspects of consciousness are relevant to the counselling context. Counsellors and therapists will often be dealing with preconscious memories, subconscious, and maybe unconscious processes and possibly divided consciousness in the form of dissociation. The area of sleep is also of interest to the counsellor and this chapter will look at patterns of normal sleep, as well as sleep disorders, some of which are quite common in people whose lives are disturbed or disrupted and who are distressed.

Dreams, of course played a central role in Freud's conceptualization and treatment of psychological disturbance. His ideas on dreams will be discussed and some of the more recent cognitive and neurological theories and research on dreaming will be introduced.

Clients often ask about hypnosis and some counsellors may practise it. Questions such as 'What is it?', 'How can it be explained?' and, 'Can it help?' have all been addressed by psychologists and some of this work is outlined in this chapter. Similar questions have also been asked about meditation. Again, the psychological work in this area is briefly reviewed.

Finally the effects of various psychoactive drugs on consciousness will be discussed. These drugs include anti-depressants, stimulants, hallucinogens and cannabis.

6.2 FUNCTIONS OF CONSCIOUSNESS

The awareness of ourselves and our environment is important for our survival in that it gives us information to which we may need to respond. But we could not possibly monitor and process all the available stimuli and so our consciousness focuses on some stimuli and ignores others. Events that are important to survival have top priority; if we are in the middle of an important interview and we become conscious of the smell of smoke our attention is immediately drawn to doing something about it and it would become impossible to concentrate on the meeting in hand.

Another function of consciousness is to help us to plan, initiate and guide our actions, whether the plan is simple such as arranging a picnic with friends, or complex, such as planning a complete career change. Such activities which involve attention and conscious effort are said to involve **controlled processing**. But a wide range of mental activities do not seem to require our conscious attention and involve **automatic processing**. These activities include the knowledge of structures that are used to understand and produce language, to commit information to memory and to carry out certain motor tasks, such as driving a car whilst daydreaming about something else (see Section 4.4 on Memory).

Because a great deal of complex cognitive activity can, through automatic processing, take place outside our conscious awareness, we often make appraisals of which we are completely unaware. We may not even know why we have made them (see also Section 3.5.3 on Unconscious Appraisals). Automatic processing, which has also been termed **mindlessness** (Langer, 1989), can therefore have its disadvantages. It can keep us unaware of problems we may have, prevent us from challenging old ways of viewing the world and from finding new ways of approaching problems and difficulties, as we discussed in Section 5.5.2 on Problems with Problem-solving.

6.3 LEVELS OF CONSCIOUSNESS

Automatic and controlled processing relates to the degree to which we are aware of our mental processes; how conscious we are of a stimulus, whether it be a thought, perception or feeling. This may vary from being acutely aware to being completely unaware. Psychologists often use a classification scheme that specifies four levels of conscious awareness.

6.3.1 Consciousness

The term **conscious** is used to describe the contents of the mind that are in our immediate awareness. These include what is going on in the environment as well as within our own bodies. For example, you are conscious of what you are reading at this moment. If you are unfortunate enough to suffer from back problems, you may also be conscious of physical discomfort or pain.

6.3.2 Subconscious Processing

A considerable body of research indicates that we register and (as we have discussed elsewhere) evaluate stimuli that we do not consciously perceive (Kihlstrom, 1987). So objects or events that are not the focus of attention can still have some influence on consciousness. These are said to operate at a **subconscious** level. For example, you may not have been aware of a clock beginning to strike the hour, but after a few strokes, when you become conscious of the sound, you 'know' how many times it has already struck. This kind of everyday example gives us some insight into the sort of processing that operates at a subconscious level of awareness.

6.3.3 Preconscious Memories

The term **preconscious** refers to thoughts and memories which are outside of conscious awareness, but can be recalled under certain conditions. Preconscious memories include specific memories of personal events which are often the focus of counselling or therapy as well as information accumulated over a lifetime.

6.3.4 The Unconscious

Thoughts, feelings and memories that cannot be brought into conscious awareness under ordinary circumstances are referred to as **unconscious** material. According to psychoanalytic theory emotionally painful memories or desires are relegated to the unconscious, or **repressed**, but may continue to influence our actions in indirect or disguised ways, through dreams, for example, or irrational behaviour or slips of the tongue. The goal of psychoanalytic therapy (as we discussed in Section 2.5.4 on The Implications of Psychodynamic Theories of Personality to Counselling and Therapy) is to draw the so-called repressed material into consciousness and in so doing, to improve psychological health and functioning.

Most psychologists would accept the notion that we have memories of which we may have no conscious awareness. However, many would not agree with Freud as to the reason for this and have tended to focus not so much on reasons for, and hypothesized content of such memories, but on mental processes upon which we constantly depend in our everyday lives but to which we have no conscious access. Such processes would include our knowledge of the structures used to understand and produce language, as discussed above.

These four concepts of consciousness, subconscious processes, preconscious memories and the unconscious (of repressed material and of mental inaccessible processes) are widely used in psychology. However, it should be noted that there is some debate about these definitions and different theorists interpret them somewhat differently.

We will now turn to the phenomena of consciousness that are both in the forefront of psychological research and of particular relevance to counselling and therapy: sleep and dreaming, hypnosis, meditation and drug induced altered states of consciousness.

6.4 SLEEPING

We devote a considerable amount of time, effort and resources to the management of the strange state of semiconsciousness called sleep. In western cultures about one third to a half of usable space in any private house is taken up by special rooms devoted to this purpose, for the most part people do not do it in the kitchen, bathroom or dining room. We put on special sleeping garments and we engage in specific rituals, such as emptying the bladder, cleaning the teeth and getting into purpose-built sleeping furniture (Empson, 1993). Yet in spite of a vast amount of research into the subject, quite why we spend 30 to 40 per cent of our lives asleep is still something of a mystery (Ellman and Antrobus, 1991).

The most prevalent theories of sleep suggested fall into two broad categories: those which emphasize its evolutionary function, and others the restorative. Evolutionary theories maintain that the sleep cycle keeps organisms inactive, and possibly hidden, during the period of day or night when they would be particularly vulnerable to predators (Webb, 1974). Restorative theories suggest that when we are fatigued, sleep gives our bodies a chance to recuperate. Some evidence for this view comes from the fact that most of the body's supply of somatotropin, a growth hormone that aids in protein synthesis and tissue regeneration, is produced during deep sleep. However, other findings do not support this restorative view. For example, our bodies use the same amount of oxygen and glucose during sleep as during relaxed wakefulness (Horne, 1988). Therefore, although the restorative view of sleep is intuitively appealing, the question of why we sleep remains unanswered.

6.4.1 Stages of Sleep

Analysis of patterns of brain waves by **electroencephalogram** (EEG) suggests that sleep involves five stages: four depths of sleep and a fifth stage, known as **rapid eye movement** (REM) sleep, when we dream.

As the eyes close, breathing becomes slow and regular, the pulse rate slows and the body temperature drops.

- **Stage 1**   As you lose consciousness and enter light sleep your heart rate slows even more, breathing becomes even more irregular and the muscles relax. This sometimes triggers off a reflex muscle contraction called a **hypnic jerk**. Muscle spasms in the legs that occur later during sleep are called **myoclonus**, also known as **restless leg syndrome**. Someone awakened during stage 1 sleep may not say they were asleep.
- **Stage 2**   As sleep deepens, the body temperature drops even further. After about four minutes of stage 2 sleep, most people who are awakened would say they were asleep.
- **Stage 3**   This involves deeper sleep and further loss of consciousness.
- **Stage 4**   Deep (slow wave) sleep is reached about an hour after sleep begins and the sleeper is in a state of oblivion. If a loud noise sounds during this stage, the sleeper will awaken in confusion and not remember the noise.
- **REM sleep**   After the adult has been asleep for an hour or so another change occurs when it is possible to observe the sleeper's eyes move under their eyelids.

It is a period of high emotion. Heart rate increases to its daytime level and the brain appears (from EEG) to be more active than at its daytime level. Furthermore, during REM sleep we are virtually paralysed. Whereas non-REM (**NREM**) sleep is dream-free 90 per cent of the time, sleepers awakened during REM sleep almost always report having had a dream. During periods of stress and emotional crisis the proportion of REM sleep increases, giving some support to the view that psychological restoration occurs during this type of sleep.

Sleep cycles

The various stages of sleep alternate throughout the night (see Figure 6.1). Sleep begins with non-REM stages and consists of several sleep cycles, each containing some REM and some NREM sleep. As you can see, the person goes from wakefulness into a deep sleep (stage 4) very rapidly. After about 70 minutes, stage 2 recurs, immediately followed by the first REM period of the night. The deeper sleep (stages 3 and 4) tend to occur during the first part of the night, whereas most REM sleep occurs in the last part. There are usually four or five distinct periods of REM sleep. This is a typical pattern for a young adult. The pattern, however, varies with age.

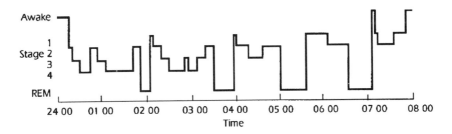

Figure 6.1   Typical patterns of sleep for a young adult

6.4.2 Sleep Patterns

Surveys show that adults sleep an average of 7½ hours, with two thirds of the population sleeping between 6½ and 8½ hours per night. About 16 per cent regularly sleep over 8½ hours and another 16 per cent under 6½ hours (Empson, 1993). Healthy individuals regularly sleeping less than 5 hours or even as little as 2 hours in every 24 hours are rare, but represent a sizeable minority. A laboratory study of two short sleepers found that their sleeping patterns were different from average sleepers. Almost all their time asleep was spent in either stage 4 or REM sleep, giving them a near normal amount of these two stages, and very low levels of light sleep.

    As many people will be aware, sleeping patterns change with age. 20-year-olds sleep with fewer interruptions than 36-year-olds (Feinberg et al., 1967) and increasing fitfulness in sleep continues throughout the lifespan. Whilst there is no difference in REM sleep between 20- and 70-year-olds, there is a reduction of stages 3 and 4 sleep during middle age so that in the over-70s very little stage 3 or 4 is taken. However, some compensation occurs as we tend to stay in bed slightly longer as we get older.

Although most of us regulate our periods of sleep and wakefulness by external events such as changes in light and darkness, going to work, feeding the animals or children, left to its own devices our bodies would still operate on roughly a 24-hour clock. This is part of the **circadian rhythm** which involves daily cyclical changes in body temperature, blood pressure, hormonal secretions and other bodily processes. We normally sleep during the low point of the daily temperature cycle.

Disruption of the circadian rhythm by an extreme change in sleeping patterns may result in a kind of fatigue and disorientation similar to 'jet lag'. We also now know that the neural processes controlling alertness and sleep produce sleepiness and diminished capacity to function during the early morning hours (2.00 a.m. to 7.00 a.m.) and to a lesser degree, during the mid-afternoon. Fatal car accidents, industrial accidents (including the nuclear disasters at Chernobyl and Three Mile Island) and engineering accidents show the same pattern.

6.4.3 Disturbed Sleep

Many people get worried if they are not sleeping as they feel they should and most of us will have experienced disturbed sleep in the course of our lives as a result of work, social or family commitments and pressures. But what effect does lack of sleep have on us?

A common belief is that sleep deprivation can cause temporary psychosis. However numerous studies have shown that although the sleep deprived person may *feel* awful, the only consistent effects of sleep deprivation are drowsiness, the desire to sleep and a tendency to fall asleep readily. The worst thing that happens to people kept awake for more than about 50 hours is that they show 'transient inattentions, confusions, or misperceptions' (Webb, 1975). Although subjects kept awake for eight days did show some disturbed behaviour, interestingly enough, they reported that things got better on the fifth day of being awake and were prepared to continue the experiment providing they were paid for the ninth day (Pasnau et al., 1968). It seems to be the case that hallucinations and other frankly psychiatric symptoms, such as paranoia, are more likely to affect people in solitary conditions or solitary volunteer subjects rather than those selected to be in groups.

Another common belief is that 'dream sleep' (REM sleep) is necessary if sanity is to be maintained. Again, this is something of a myth. Although people do undoubtedly experience longer periods in REM sleep when under stress, being systematically woken at the commencement of REM sleep results only in a 'rebound' effect with an increase in REM sleep of about 50 per cent over baseline measures. So is REM (dream) sleep the body's way of recuperating from stress or is it, as Freud believed, a symptom of stress?

6.4.4 The Effects of Diet and Exercise on Sleep

People often believe that their sleep is affected by what they have eaten during the day. Undoubtedly, indigestion or eating a heavy meal late in the evening will disturb sleep, but what about other effects of food on sleep?

It would seem from clinical observation and the research evidence, that the amount of food intake has some bearing on the amount and quality of sleep. People suffering from anorexia nervosa have been found to sleep little and fitfully (Crisp and Stonehill, 1977). During remission, when these same people were putting on weight, they slept more with fewer intermissions. Another interesting finding was that during remission, there was a massive increase in deep (stage 4) sleep. This is consistent with the restorative theory of sleep mentioned above; that is, that stage 4 sleep is concerned with bodily growth process.

There is not a great deal of research on the effects of specific food substances on sleep. However, it would appear that our mothers (and possibly grandmothers) were right after all! Good old fashioned Horlicks (or any malted milk drink) *does* improve sleep; not so much sleep onset, but it does seem to reduce restlessness during the night.

Most people would claim that they sleep better after taking exercise. However, the effect of exercise on sleep is not simple and the research evidence is somewhat controversial. Horne (1981) concluded from an extensive review of the literature that elevations in deep sleep stages 3 and 4 can occur after increases in the *rate* of energy expenditure, rather than the total amount of energy expended. However, it has also been found that increasing the body temperature can also produce the same effect, so the evidence is difficult to interpret.

So although we may *feel* we sleep better after taking exercise, this may not be always the case. We will see in the next section how those who suffer from insomnia systematically underestimate the time spent sleeping. Could those who feel good from taking exercise do the reverse? That is, overestimate the quality of their sleep.

6.4.5 The Effects of Smoking, Alcohol and Caffeine on Sleep

Studies of smokers who have abruptly given up smoking show an improvement in getting to sleep (from an average of 52 minutes to 18 minutes) and a reduction of time spent awake during the sleeping period. The improvement in sleep quality also appears to be maintained (Empson, 1993).

Although alcohol, like barbiturates, is a sedative drug, unlike barbiturates, it does not suppress REM sleep. The amount of time it takes to get to sleep (sleep onset latency) has been found to be reduced with moderately high doses, but there were no measurable differences with lower doses, although subjects reported that they thought they got to sleep more quickly (Stone, 1980). However, over extended periods of regular drinking sleep patterns may show progressive changes (Empson, 1993).

Caffeine does not just keep you awake. It reduces the amount of stage 4 sleep, increases the number of arousals and at high doses (300 mg, the equivalent of three cups of strong coffee) will cause early waking (Gaillard et al., 1989)

6.4.6 The Effects of Prescribed Drugs on Sleep

Some clients entering counselling will undoubtedly be taking prescribed medicines for conditions or symptoms for which they may be seeking help from a counsellor. The counsellor needs to be aware of the effects on sleep of the drugs most commonly pre-scribed for the alleviation of such symptoms.

Anxiolytics

The benzodiazepines, or minor tranquillizers, are prescribed for both anxiety and sleep problems. The most commonly used drugs in this group for the treatment of anxiety are diazepam (Valium), chlordiazepoxide (Librium) and lorazepam (Ativan). Chlordiazepoxide has been found to reduce the amount of deep slow wave sleep (stage 4) and, over long periods, there is evidence that REM sleep may be reduced. However, there is no strong evidence of REM rebound (a massive increase in REM sleep) on stop-ping the drug. The effects of diazepam seem to be similar (Hartman, 1976).

Hypnotics

Most prescribed hypnotics today are benzodiazepine derivatives such as nitrazepam (Mogadon), flunitrazepam (Rohypnol), flurazepam (Dalmane) and temazepam. Unlike their predecessors, the barbiturates, benzodiazepine derivatives do not appear to sup-press REM sleep when taken in normal clinical doses (Haider and Oswald, 1971), although flunitrazepam (Rohypnol) has been shown with repeated doses to abolish stage 4 sleep. Chloral hydrate (Welldorm) is a different type of hypnotic and, like bar-biturates, suppresses REM sleep initially and causes a massive REM rebound on with-drawal (Hartman, 1978).

Most hypnotics have a long half-life in blood so their effects are not confined to the night and experiments have shown that benzodiazepines can depress performance on simple motor tasks the next day (Walters and Lader, 1970). Benzodiazepines with short half-lives (3–5 hours) such as temazepam are less popular, possibly because they are, by definition, ineffective over a whole night.

None of these drugs are ideal, but the benzodiazepines seem to be the least harmful (Empson, 1993). They are habit forming in some people when taken over long periods. The Committee for the Safety of Medicines in the United Kingdom has warned that as many as 40 per cent of patients regularly taking benzodiazepines may have become physiologically dependent on them. That is, they suffer withdrawal symptoms, includ-ing anxiety attacks and sleeplessness when they stop taking them.

Anti-depressants

The most widely prescribed anti-depressants in Britain are the **tricyclic** anti-depressants, such as amitriptyline. This has been shown to slightly increase sleep time and to slightly reduce REM sleep, but with a relatively short-lived REM rebound on withdrawal.

Another type of anti-depressant, the **monoamine oxidase inhibitor** (MAOIs) actu-ally abolishes REM sleep and virtually abolishes stages 3 and 4 sleep. Surprisingly, patients seem to be able to cope with this, even becoming less depressed (Dunleavy and Oswald, 1973).

More recently the 5-HT uptake inhibitors have been developed. This group of anti-depressants, which include paroxetine (Seroxat) and fluoxetine (Prozac), have also been shown to affect sleep. Fluoxetine, in particular, has been shown to suppress REM sleep and to increase wakefulness (Nicholson and Pasco, 1988).

Beta blockers

These drugs are normally prescribed to reduce blood pressure and heart rate and to reduce the somatic symptoms (such as muscular tremor) of anxiety. Some beta block-ers (the water soluble group, which includes atenolol) do not have any effect on sleep or dreaming but patients on drugs in the lipid soluble group such as propranolol (Inderal) often complain of vivid dreams and nightmares disrupting their sleep (Wood, 1984). In high doses they can also suppress REM sleep, and have been used for the treatment of narcolepsy (see Section 6.4.7).

6.4.7 Sleep Disorders and their Treatment

The most common forms of sleep disorder are related to psychological problems, although there are some rarer syndromes which have medical causes or seem to be innately determined (Empson, 1993). Sleep disturbance is generally related to poor physical health, unhappiness and anxiety. However, although it is common for people suffering from emotional problems to also have problems in sleeping, it is not more likely for people with a history of sleep disorder to have received treatment for a psychiatric disorder (Bixler et al., 1979).

Insomnia

The term insomnia refers to subjective dissatisfaction with the quality or amount of sleep. However, people who complain of insomnia have consistently been shown to overestimate their loss of sleep (Carskadon et al., 1974), although quite why this should be remains something of a mystery. They do, however, take longer to get to sleep, have more frequent wakenings, decreased deep sleep stages (stages 3 and 4) and achieve less overall sleep than normal controls.

Insomnia can occur for a variety of medical, psychiatric, social, psychological and/or drug-related reasons. It can be due to an inherently weak tendency for sleep, perhaps central nervous system (CNS) mediated, perhaps contributed to or main-tained by psychological factors such as bedtime behaviours like keeping irregular hours, worrying, eating or watching television in bed (Dorsey, 1993). It can also be secondary to some other medical or psychiatric cause; for example, pain, depression or mania.

In one major survey (Bixler et al., 1979) almost half of those who reported insomnia had reported **sleep-onset insomnia**, that is, difficulty in falling asleep, stating worry
and anxiety as the main reasons. The relationship between anxiety and sleep disorder,
however, is not simple and subjects selected as being highly anxious generally had no
problem in initiating sleep (although slept less and slept more lightly) (Rosa et al.,
1983). However even if anxiety does not actually cause insomnia, very high levels of
anxiety and worry must be incompatible with good sleep and sleep always suffers in a
psychological crisis. Priest (1983) maintains that it is not so much anxiety that keeps
people awake, but the associated strong emotions of resentment and anger.

Another possible reason for sleep-onset insomnia is disturbance of the circadian
rhythm; going to bed in the early hours of the morning, getting up late, cat-napping during the day. The person may get enough sleep, but at the wrong time.

Almost three quarters of the respondents in the above quoted survey reported difficulty in **sleep maintenance**, with half reporting **early wakening**. These symptoms,
to some extent, are associated with age, but persistent maintenance insomnia in middle age or earlier is associated with depression and mania, drug abuse, alcoholism and
respiratory illnesses. Traditionally in the psychiatry field, early wakenings have been
associated with endogenous depression, and failure to get to sleep with reactive
depression. There is, however, no research evidence for this assertion (Costello and
Selby, 1965).

There have been a number of different cognitive–behavioural methods developed
or adapted for the treatment of insomnia. These methods could readily be incorporated
into counselling by a practitioner with knowledge of, or training in, cognitive–behavioural approaches. **Cognitive therapy** in this context would focus on diminishing
pre-sleep worry and replacing it with thoughts more compatible with relaxation and
sleep. This is often paired with **progressive relaxation training** which concentrates
more on the production of a physiological calm. **Autogenic training** has also been
used to improve sleep. This is a cognitively induced relaxation procedure in which
both self-suggestion and imagery are used to induce relaxation. The images and sensations of warmth and heaviness used in most autogenic training procedures have
been found to be successful in the treatment of insomnia (e.g. Bootzin and Nicassio,
1978).

A somewhat different approach is the **stimulus control** technique developed by
Bootzin (1972). The goal of stimulus control is to strengthen the sleeping environment
as a cue for sleep, rather than other interfering behaviours, such as reading, watching
television, worrying or looking at the clock.

Sleep restriction therapy addresses behaviour at bedtime in a rather different way.
Here the focus is on improvement of sleep quality by regulating bedtime, wakening
time and therefore the duration of time in bed. It is an attempt to consolidate sleep by
systematically restricting the time spent in bed. Although the technique may cause
some discomfort at first, the gains are long-term and include improvement of sleep
quality (Dorsey, 1993).

Finally, probably the most widely used treatment of insomnia is **drug therapy**.
However, as we have seen in the previous section, that is not without its problems.

Whatever the preferred treatment approach of the individual counsellor or therapist, careful assessment of the sleeping patterns and problems is essential as the following example demonstrates.

The client is a 34-year-old woman living on her own. She reported that one of her difficulties was waking and getting up in the morning which frequently meant that she would arrive late for work. She had received a warning from her employers for this. She also suffered from extremely severe acne, a cause of considerable distress to her.

Assessment of her sleeping habits and pattern revealed that she would normally retire late, having spent about half an hour in the bathroom in front of the mirror angrily 'attacking' (her words) her face. She would eventually get to sleep at around 2 a.m. and her sleep was usually interrupted by frequent wakenings. She had her alarm clock set for 7.30 a.m. and would wake at this time. On waking, she would reset her alarm for an hour later. This, she reported, was the best sleep of the night. The problem was that she frequently did not hear the alarm when it went off for the second time, or would turn it off and roll over and go back to sleep again.

In relation to the sleep, there were two main problems. Firstly, she was engaging in arousing behaviours before getting into bed. Attacking her face left her angry and often extremely upset. Secondly, by allowing herself the second sleep having been woken abruptly by the alarm, she may have upset her sleep cycle and been entering deep sleep (stages 3 and 4) usually reserved for the first part of the night. No wonder she found it difficult to get to sleep at night. Of course, this is purely speculative, but it is a reasonable explanation from which to form a hypothesis to guide the treatment approach.

After discussing this hypothesis with the client and giving some information on normal sleep pattern, the counsellor suggested removing the mirror from the bathroom; the client felt avoiding looking in it or covering it would be unsuccessful. She then suggested replacing the 'attacking ritual' with relaxing behaviours such as taking a bath. It was also suggested that the client set her alarm clock for the later time only, which still would give her sufficient time to get to work on time.

Within ten days the client had established a satisfactory sleep pattern, going to sleep at around midnight and getting up at 8.30 a.m. There were, of course, other issues that were addressed in therapy.

Narcolepsy

People with narcolepsy suffer from overwhelming attacks of drowsiness and will fall asleep at totally inappropriate times: whilst carrying on a conversation or driving a car, for example. Episodes may occur several times a day and can last for between 15 and 30 minutes. Narcolepsy is an intrusion of REM episodes into daytime hours. During an attack sufferers go rapidly into REM sleep and may lose muscle control and collapse before they can lie down. Narcolepsy runs in families and there is evidence of a genetic susceptibility.

There is no cure for narcolepsy but it may be controlled by the help of stimulants during the day (Empson, 1993). Beta blockers have also been used (Meier-Ewart et al., 1985).

Sleep apnoea

This is a dangerous and life-threatening condition in which breathing stops until the build up of carbon dioxide in the blood causes sufferers to wake up gasping for air. This can happen as often as 500 times a night. Overweight males are particularly susceptible. The result of sleep apnoea can be that sufferers can spend 12 or more hours in bed each night and still be extremely sleepy the next day. Sleeping pills exacerbate the problem and may prove fatal. Not waking up is probably the main reason why people die in their sleep.

Apnoea can be treated surgically but a less severe treatment is a mechanical aid called a Nasal Continuous Positive Airway Pressure which involves the patient wearing a mask at night.

Sleepwalking and sleep talking

These are specific to stage 4 sleep and are more common in children than in adults. Generally a sleepwalking episode lasts less than 15 minutes, and after some non-purposive activity, the person goes back to sleep, usually in their own bed, or wakes up. The disorder runs in families and there is evidence that somnambulism may be genetically associated.

Night terrors

Again, these are more common in children than in adults. They need to be distinguished from nightmares, which consist of dreams about some frightening or extremely worrying topic, and normally occur during REM sleep.

Night terrors occur during stage 4 sleep and it seems that there is no 'reason' for the fear. Typically, the child wakes its parents with an ear-splitting scream, and remains terrified and inconsolable for 10 to 15 minutes before falling into a deep sleep. In the morning the only people to have any recollection of this will be the parents or carers. Adults can also suffer from night terrors, although usually in a less extreme form.

There is no clear evidence that either psychological therapy or medication will necessarily be helpful in the treatment of night terrors. However, Cushway and Sewell (1991) make some suggestions including information and advice to parents on the management of night terrors.

6.4.8 A Good Night's Sleep

There is reasonable agreement among researchers and clinicians on how to avoid sleep problems. The recommendations below are adapted from Atkinson et al. (1990). Some are based on actual research and some are the best judgements of specialists in the field.

- **Regular sleep schedule**   Establish a regular schedule for going to bed and getting up. Set your alarm for a specific time every morning and get up at that time, no matter how little you have slept. Either take a nap every day or not at all; when you take a nap occasionally, you probably will not sleep as well that night. Waking up late at weekends can also disrupt the sleep cycle.

- **The bedroom**   If you can, organize the bedroom so that it is associated with sleep and not with activities such as studying, watching television etc. Ideally, you should not have your desk or television in the bedroom.

- **Alcohol and caffeine**   Having a stiff drink before going to bed may help put you to sleep, but may disturb the sleep cycle. Avoid caffeinated drinks like coffee or cola for several hours before bedtime. If you have anything to drink, have a milky one such as malted milk.

- **Eating before bedtime**   Don't eat heavily before going to bed, since your digestive system will have to do several hours of work.

- **Exercise**   Regular exercise improves the subjective experience of sleep and may help you sleep better, but it is the rate of energy expenditure rather than the overall amount which seems to be important. But don't engage in a strenuous workout before going to bed.

- **Sleeping pills**   Be careful about taking sleeping pills. All of the various kinds disrupt the sleep cycle, and long-term use can lead to dependency and increase insomnia. A bad night's sleep does not affect performance, whereas a hangover from a sleeping pill might.

- **Relaxation**   Avoid stressful thoughts at bedtime. Try to follow the same routine every night before going to bed and engage in soothing activities such as having a bath, listening to soft music for a few minutes. Find a room temperature at which you are comfortable and, if you can, maintain it throughout the night.

- **When all else fails**   If you are in bed and have trouble falling asleep, don't get up. Stay in bed and try to relax. But if that fails and you become tense, then get up for a brief time and do something restful. Doing pushups or madly cleaning the house is not a good idea.

6.5 DREAMING

Whilst a great deal has been discovered about the physiology of sleep and there are reliable techniques for establishing when people are likely to be dreaming, academic psychology has largely ignored the study of the nature of dreams. There may be a number of reasons for this including disillusionment with the psychoanalytic notion of dream analysis being a cure for psychological ills; dream material being available to only one person and the dreamer and dream data being viewed as perceptual rather than cognitive events and therefore not an appropriate phenomena for 'scientific' research.

Dreams differ from waking consciousness in that dreams happen to us rather than being the product of our conscious control; things happen in dreams and we observe. The content of dreams, as most of us know, varies from the mundane to the fantastic.

We still, however, seem to be somewhat amazed by the bizarre quality of our dreams. How often do we say or hear said, 'I had a very strange dream last night'?

6.5.1 Facts about Dreaming

Does everyone dream?

Although many people say they do not dream, there is no difference in REM sleep between professed non-dreamers and dreamers. In laboratory studies, when non-recallers of dreams are woken from REM sleep, their recall rates are comparable to professed dreamers. It would therefore seem that everyone dreams. Those who say they don't, simply cannot recall them.

How much time do we spend dreaming?

Adults spend about 25 per cent of their sleeping time in REM, or 'dream' sleep in four or five episodes totalling about one and a half to two hours a night.

How long do dreams last?

The idea that dreams are really fleeting impressions formed immediately before waking up is fairly prevalent. The fact is that, when people are awakened from REM sleep and asked to act out their dreams, the length of time it takes to do so is about as long as the REM episode (Dement and Wolpert, 1958). This suggests that incidents commonly last about as long as they would in real life.

Do people know when they are dreaming?

Some people have lucid dreams, when they become aware that they are dreaming whilst they are actually dreaming and are then able to control their dreams by thought. Subjects have been found who are good at lucid dreaming, and experiments have been conducted showing how this level of awareness can be incorporated into dreams (Green, 1968; Hearne, 1990).

   People can also be taught to recognize they are dreaming (Salamy, 1970) and this 'skill' can be used in helping to manage and control nightmares. La Berge (1985) has written extensively on this subject and suggests techniques that will help induce lucid dreams and thereby control, to some extent, the content of dreams. Cushway and Sewell (1992) have adapted and used these techniques with moderate success. They found that where dreamers already have some degree of lucidity, they develop their skills and work creatively with their nightmares in the dreaming state. They caution counsellors and therapists against attempting to induce lucid dreaming in people who have had any kind of psychotic episode or borderline characteristics.

Can people control the content of their dreams?

As discussed above, people can, to some extent become aware that they are dreaming and control the content of the dream by thought. People can also control their dream content to varying degrees by means of pre-sleep suggestions that they will have a particular dream (Cartwright, 1974).

Are dreams related to the events of the previous day?

Dreams occurring in the night's first REM sleep tend to be related to events of the day, whilst those in later REM periods tend to be more vivid, unusual and sometimes anxiety provoking.

Are there any differences between the dreams of men and those of women?

Men's dreams tend to be more active and aggressive than women's. Men use more action terms in describing their dreams, while women use more emotional terms.

Do we dream in colour?

Dreams are frequently reported to be in colour. Colour-blind people dream in the colours they see when awake, and people blind from birth dream in the senses they know, mainly hearing and touch.

Why do we dream what we do?

Psychologists do not have the answer to this question. Investigators do not really understand why we dream at all, let alone why we dream what we do. There are, however, a number of theories about this which will be outlined below.

6.5.2 Cognitive Approaches to Dreaming

The cognitive approach taken by Evans (1984) views sleep as a period when the brain disengages from the external world and uses this time to sort through and re-organize the vast array of information that has been taken in during the day. Evans suggests that dreams have a kind of 'information processing' function whereby the day's events and experiences are organized and stored in long-term memory.

6.5.3 Neurobiological Approach to Dreaming

A rather different view suggests that dreaming is important to our mental functioning not by helping us to remember, but rather by helping us to *forget*. Crick and Michison

(1983, 1986) maintain that if all the information processed during a day were stored permanently in the brain's synaptic connections, the neocortex would soon run out of storage space. They suggest that dreaming is the brain's way of purging itself of unwanted or unimportant material. The implication of this view is that we are operating at cross-purposes with nature when we try to recall our dreams, since they were never intended to be remembered.

6.5.4 Psychotherapeutic Approaches to Dreams

One of the problems with both the cognitive and the neurobiological approaches is that neither of them accounts for the ingenious and creative functions that are evident in so many cultures and that have been documented by so many writers. Nor does either theory assign to dreams the rich symbolism and concealed meanings that typify the psychotherapeutic approaches to the analysis of dream content.

The psychoanalytic approach

Freud saw dreams as the 'royal road to the unconscious' and believed that dreams are a disguised attempt at **wish fulfilment**. That is, that the dream represents wishes, needs or ideas that the person finds unacceptable, and that have accordingly been repressed to the unconscious. In this context dreams tended to be treated as neurotic symptoms rather than an aspect of normal experience.

Clearly all dreams are not wish fulfilment, and Freud explained this by suggesting that these unconscious wishes and ideas appear in symbolic form as the **latent content**, rather than the manifest content of the dream. The manifest dream that we can recall is therefore a compromise in which the wish fulfilments have been disguised. According to Freud, the latent dream, which is only accessible through extensive analysis of the manifest dream, is the 'true' dream. Dreams, as we know them, are the outcome of a process which allows the expression of these unacceptable thoughts and preserves sleep by preventing them from becoming overtly explicit.

Modern psychoanalysts still make use of dream analysis but there is no longer the emphasis on the 'latent' dream. Rather, they tend to use patient's dreams to explore their current preoccupations.

Jung's theory of dreams

In contrast to Freud, Jung saw the dream as a normal creative expression of the unconscious which reflected the workings of an inner drive towards health and maturity. Both Freud and Jung were interested in dream symbolism, but rather than seeing a symbol as a disguise for something else, Jung believed symbols should be seen as having meaning in their own right, and therefore placed more emphasis on the manifest content of the dream than what it may be hiding.

Jung believed that universal themes revealed the existence in each individual of a layer in the mind common to the whole universe. He called this the **collective unconscious**. Archetypes of the collective unconscious are expressions of fundamental and perennial interests which appear as symbolism of many people.

Gestalt theory of dreams

Fritz Perls, who founded the Gestalt school of therapy, developed and extended Jung's theory of dreams. He believed that each object or character in a dream is a part of ourselves, a fragment of our personality that has got projected out of ourselves. He saw the main function of dreams as being to resolve unfinished situations and to integrate these fragments of our personalities. He believed that by working with dreams we can 'reclaim' lost parts of our personality and become more integrated or whole.

Faraday's theory of dreams

Anne Faraday has been very influential in the area of dreaming and has utilized many of the concepts of Jung and Gestalt, but largely rejected Freud's ideas of wish fulfilment and latent content. She proposed that dreams could be interpreted at three different levels. The first level she called 'looking outwards'. At this level she maintains that dreams can provide objective truth about the outside world, often warnings or reminders. At the second level of interpretation, which she calls 'through the looking glass', dreams can act as distorting mirrors which twist external reality according to the dreamer's inner attitudes and conflicts and so can give a picture of the dreamer's internal subjective reality. The third level of interpretation, 'looking inwards' gives access to the internal conflicts and split-off portions of the self (Faraday, 1974).

6.5.5 Common Dream Themes

There appears to be a number of common or, according to Jung, archetypal dream themes which can also, it has been suggested, act as metaphors for underlying content (Faraday, 1974). They may also represent an attempt to make sense out of experiences really occurring in sleep; 'an attempt to make a coherent story out of some pattern of highly active discharges from the hindbrain which are a feature of REM sleep' (Empson, 1993, p. 90).

Common dream themes and their metaphors suggested by Faraday (1994) and Cushway and Sewell (1992) include the following:

- **falling** out of someone's estimation, falling down on a job or falling in love;
- **flying** representing feelings of mastery, being emotionally elevated or trying to escape;
- **teeth falling out** associated traditionally with repression of aggressive wishes but also with growing up or growing old;

- **nudity** often indicating shame and embarrassment; fear of, or wish for exposure, a desire to be more open and honest in one's life;
- **examinations** being put to the test, needing to prove oneself or failing to live up to someone's expectations.

6.5.6 Working with Dreams

Clearly the ways in which counsellors and therapists work with dreams will depend on the theoretical stance taken; and as we have seen, Freud, for example, takes quite a different approach to dreams from Faraday. For Faraday, it is the dreamer's personal meaning that is most relevant, whereas this, for Freud, would represent only the manifest or personally acceptable content.

Cushway and Sewell (1992), drawing on some of the ideas of Faraday and others, have developed a 'dreamwork model' for working with dreams. They classify the techniques of dream interpretation into subjective and objective approaches. In objective approaches, the dreamer is encouraged to step outside any feelings associated with the dream and comment on the dream and its symbols from an outsider's perspective. According to this view, it is only after the symbols have been interpreted as far as possible that emotional aspects are re-integrated.

With subjective approaches, which would include the Gestalt way of working, the dreamer is encouraged to re-enter the dream and work from within it. This may take the dreamer well away from the original dream content and lead to exploration of new and different areas of experience.

6.6 HYPNOSIS

Hypnosis can produce striking changes in consciousness and behaviour. Like dreaming, it is surrounded by an aura of mystery which psychologists, as is their wont, have succeeded in dispelling. Some psychologists see hypnosis as an altered state of consciousness, characterized by narrowed attention and an increased openness to suggestion. Others view it as no more than a mixture of relaxation, imagination, suggestion, obedience, conformity and role-playing (Baker, 1990). Hypnosis is not 'magical'; it can be explained by normal psychological principles. It remains, nevertheless, a fascinating subject.

6.6.1 Hypnotic Susceptibility

People differ considerably in how responsive they are to hypnotic suggestion, and hypnotic susceptibility seems to be a stable trait over time (Piccione et al., 1989). People who are imaginative and prone to fantasy are often highly responsive to hypnosis but those who are not can also be hypnotized (Lynn and Rhue, 1988). It seems that the main factor in hypnotic susceptibility is the willingness to be hypnotized. About 8 people out 10 can be hypnotized, but only about 4 out of 10 will be good hypnotic subjects.

6.6.2 Hypnotic Experience

In all but the deepest hypnosis, people remain aware of what is going on; but when hypnosis is induced a number of changes occur. These have been summarized by Hilgard (1965) and include:

- **Basic suggestion effect**   Hypnotized persons feel that suggested actions or experiences are automatic, they just happen to them. They do not like to initiate any activity for themselves but prefer to take a passive stance and to wait for directions from the hypnotist.
- **Changes in attention**   Attention becomes much more selective and the hypnotized subject, if directed to do so, will ignore everything other than the hypnotist's voice.
- **Dissociation**   In some people hypnosis can cause a 'split' in awareness. For example, when hypnotized subjects were asked to plunge one hand in iced water, subjects told to feel no pain reported none. However, when asked if there was any part of their mind that did feel pain, with their free hands many wrote that it hurt. This part of the mind, termed the **hidden observer**, is aware of the pain, but it remains in the background (Hilgard, 1977).
- **Increase in suggestibility**   There is some evidence for this but less than might be supposed (Ruch et al., 1973).
- **Ability to fantasize**   This is enhanced, so that people can easily put themselves into various scenes or relive old memories.
- **Reduced reality testing**   A hypnotized person may readily accept imagined experiences; for example, talking normally to an imagined person.
- **Post-hypnotic amnesia**   Many people cannot remember what happened when hypnotized and highly responsive subjects can be instructed to forget what happened under hypnosis and memories can be restored when a prearranged signal is given.

6.6.3 Effects of Hypnosis

There have been many claims made for the effects of hypnosis, but what is the evidence for these claims? In some cases it is incomplete or conflicting; but, on the whole, the following conclusions seem to be justified:

- **Memory**   Although there is some evidence that hypnosis can enhance memory, it also frequently increases the number of **false memories**. People's confidence in hypnosis can prompt them unintentionally to distort information and inaccurately reconstruct events (as we discussed in Section 4.8.4 on the Effects of Hypnosis in Memory).
- **Age regression**   Hypnosis has been used to 'regress' patients and subjects to childhood. It has, however, been noted that some age-regressed persons continue

to use knowledge they could only have learned as adults and that this suggests that people are only 'acting' child-like. However, Foenander and Burrows (1980) maintain that subjects only confabulate when memory traces are not available. When memory is available, they claim that there is actual regression.

- **Sensory changes**   Hypnotic suggestions can alter colour vision, hearing sensitivity, time sense, and many other sensory responses (Kihlstrom, 1985).

- **Pain relief**   There are numerous examples of the use of hypnosis for pain relief in, for example, obstetrics, cancer, burns and dentistry. Although many of the studies in this area are methodologically unsatisfactory, it is evident that when appropriately used, hypnosis can be useful as a therapy for pain, either as a supplementary therapy or on its own (Hilgard, 1980).

- **Post-hypnotic suggestion**   There is considerable evidence for the power of post-hypnotic suggestion; that is, a suggestion given to hypnotized people that they will behave in a particular way after they have been wakened. Unfortunately, this effect seems to be strongest for performing behaviours which have little therapeutic value, such as when the subjects are instructed to run their hands through their hair whenever they hear a particular word (Orne et al., 1968). Modifying behaviours such as smoking and over-eating by hypnotic suggestion is far more problematic. The research results are fairly dismal in relation to smoking, although the chances of giving up and maintaining it are higher when motivation is strong (Collinson, 1980). In the case of obesity, the research evidence for the effectiveness of hypnosis is difficult to interpret, as most therapeutic programmes include a variety of techniques in combination.

6.6.4 Hypnosis, Therapy and Counselling

Hypnosis in the treatment of psychological disorders has a long history. Freud believed that the hypnotic relationship, because of its intense emotional involvement, could contribute to the faster removal of defences as well as facilitating the transference relationship (which enables the client to displace feelings and attitudes applicable towards others onto the therapist).

Although Freud himself subsequently abandoned hypnosis in favour of his developing further the techniques of psychoanalysis, the integration of psychotherapy and hypnosis has been continued by others and has taken various forms. In some cases, hypnotic sessions are simply introduced periodically with no other modification of the therapeutic technique; in others, procedures such as age regression, induced dreaming and automatic writing have been employed.

In addition to its use in psychodynamic therapy, hypnosis is used for making direct suggestions and, as discussed above, has been shown to be particularly effective in the treatment of pain. Although employed for controlling smoking, eating, and alcohol intake, it seems to be better at changing subjective experience than at modifying behaviour. It seems to be most effective when combined with behavioural methods.

So where does this leave the counsellor who may be contemplating using hypnosis? Firstly it is important to have some knowledge about what hypnosis can and cannot do.

Secondly, counsellors should be aware of the power of the hypnotic relationship and the issues of transference that this relationship engenders. Is this the kind of relationship you want with your clients? One of the major criticisms coming from psychoanalysis is that positive transference is so powerful in the hypnotic relationship that it interferes with the therapeutic process (particularly the expression of resistances). Counsellors may feel the same, but for rather different reasons.

Thirdly, it is essential to be aware of the possible dangers of hypnosis as well as of those for whom it would be unsuitable or damaging. Crasilneck and Hall (1985) list the dangers as including:

- the possibility of precipitating a psychiatric illness, such as dissociative neurosis and schizophrenia;
- making an existing disorder worse, particularly by the indiscriminate removal of symptoms;
- causing regression;
- prolonging treatment in patients with passive–dependent and hysterical personality disorder;
- masking illness;
- excessive dependence.

Crasilneck also states that there are certain personality types and disorders that should be treated with extreme caution by the hypnotherapist. These include patients with strong paranoid tendencies, persons acutely depressed with a history of suicide attempts, those addicted to hard drugs and pathologically masochistic individuals. To this list should be added those suffering from schizophrenia, from other psychotic disorders and from borderline states.

Even though, with little training, it is relatively easy to induce a hypnotic state in a willing and cooperative subject or client, it should be obvious from the above that hypnosis should not be treated lightly nor embarked upon by counsellors or others without the necessary training in both hypnotherapy and in counselling or psychological therapy.

6.7 MEDITATION

With meditation, a person achieves an altered state of consciousness characterized by a separation of mind and body, a feeling of being divorced from the outside world, of inner peace and tranquillity and of being involved with a wider consciousness, however defined. In this state respiration, heart-rate, muscle tension and oxygen consumption decrease, and there is usually a considerable amount of alpha wave activity, the brain wave pattern commonly found in waking relaxed states. The physiological state is the same as that induced by other relaxation techniques such as biofeedback and deep muscle relaxation.

This state is usually brought about by methods associated with **focusing**, aimed at narrowing the attention to just one thing (which could be a **mantra**) long enough for the meditator to stop thinking about anything else. What is focused on is much less important than doing so with a **passive attitude**.

Meditators frequently report that it helps them to understand themselves better and to decrease stress and anxiety and the associated problems of high blood pressure and insomnia. On personality tests, meditators' scores indicate increases in general mental health, self-esteem and social openness (Shapiro and Giber, 1978). Meditation has also been used in sports psychology to enhance performance (Syer and Connolly, 1984).

Above all, proponents of meditation claim that, even though physiologically it is indistinguishable from relaxation, meditation alone can create the uplifting altered state that they believe leads to true enlightenment (Holmes, 1984). Exactly how meditation produces its effects is unclear.

6.7.1 Meditation and Counselling

Unlike hypnosis, meditation is not generally considered in western societies to be a therapeutic tool. This may be partly for cultural and partly for historical reasons. Traditional forms of meditation follow the practices of **yoga**, a system of thought based on the Hindu religion or **zen**, which is derived from Chinese and Japanese Buddhism. In the west, and very much more recently, a somewhat commercialized and secularized form of meditation known as **transcendental meditation** (**TM**) has been promoted. TM has its own training and organizational structures and although widely practised, has not, to date, been integrated or incorporated into mainstream therapeutic practice. Nevertheless, some clients seeking counselling or therapeutic help use TM as an adjunct to counselling. The precautions given above about suitability of hypnosis for certain clients would also apply to meditation.

6.8 DRUG-INDUCED ALTERED STATES OF CONSCIOUSNESS

For thousands of years people have used drugs to alter their state of consciousness: to enhance their perceptions, to help them relax, to stimulate, to prevent or to induce sleep. Such drugs are usually called **psychoactive**. Most counsellors will experience clients, clients' relatives or friends whose lives have been affected by drugs of one sort or another. The following section outlines the effects of such drugs on consciousness, mood and behaviour. A particular drug, however, may affect different people in unpredictable ways depending on factors such as the dose, frequency of use, the person's size and psychological state. In describing the effects of drugs, we can therefore only speak in generalities.

This section is intended to do no more than inform the counsellor of the more immediate effects on consciousness. The long-term effects, and issues relating to addiction and withdrawal, are beyond the scope of this chapter.

6.8.1 Depressants

Drugs that depress the central nervous system include the **benzodiazepines** (minor tranquillizers such as Valium, Librium and Ativan), barbiturates and alcohol. Of these, **alcohol** is probably the most frequently abused.

Alcohol affects conscious experience initially by increasing energy and sociability. Self-confidence may increase, inhibitions decrease and motor reactions begin to slow down. As the blood alcohol level increases the body begins to react in quite the opposite way. Feelings of fatigue, nausea, unhappiness and depression may occur. Thought process and physical coordination become progressively disorganized and reaction time, hand–eye coordination and decision making are all impaired.

6.8.2 Stimulants

The two most widely used stimulants are **amphetamines** and **cocaine**. In contrast to depressants, stimulants increase arousal. Amphetamines, popularly known as 'speed' or 'uppers', bring about an increase in alertness and confidence and a decrease in feelings of fatigue and boredom. After the stimulating effects wear off, there is often a period of compensatory let down during which the user feels depressed, irritable and fatigued.

Cocaine, or 'coke', and its derivative 'crack' dramatically increases energy and self-confidence, making the user feel witty and hyper-alert. Tolerance develops with repeated use and restless irritability follows the euphoric high. This, with use, becomes depressed anguish which can be alleviated only by more cocaine.

6.8.3 Opiates

Opium and its derivatives which include **morphine** and **codeine** are widely used medically for their pain killing properties. They also produce mood changes, sometimes euphoria.

Heroin, a derivative of morphine, produces a 'thrill' or 'rush' minutes after an intravenous injection. The user feels 'on top of the world' yet peaceful, with no worries or concerns. Once again, tolerance builds up and the user requires stronger and stronger doses to produce the 'high' and to avoid the intense physical discomforts of withdrawal.

6.8.4 Hallucinogens

Hallucinogens or **psychedelics** include **LSD** (lysergic acid diethylamide), **PCP** (phencyclidine), known as 'angel dust', and **mescaline**. These drugs typically alter the person's perception of both internal and external worlds. The effects, however, are heavily influenced by the user's mood, attitude and environment.

Hallucinogens usually distort or intensify sensory experience so that normal environ-mental stimuli are experienced in a completely new way and sounds and colours can seem completely different. Perception of time can become so distorted that minutes seem like hours.

Mystical experiences are reported and users may also experience exhilaration, with-drawal from reality, violent outbursts, self-destruction and panic. The mental effects of hallucinogens are always unpredictable and their effects may recur as **flashbacks** days or even months after the drugs have been taken.

6.8.5 Cannabis

As with that of alcohol, the reaction to cannabis has two stages: a period of stimulation and euphoria, followed by a period of tranquillity and, with higher doses, sleep. There may be some sensory and perceptual changes, distortions in space and time and changes in social perception. Sixteen per cent of regular users report anxiety, fearfulness and confusion as a usual occurrence and about a third report that they occasionally experi-ence such symptoms as acute panic, hallucinations and unpleasant distortions in body image (Halikas et al., 1971; Negrete and Kwan, 1972).

6.9 CONCLUDING COMMENTS

For counsellors, an awareness and some knowledge of the psychology of consciousness, of sleep and of dreams is of direct relevance to their therapeutic practice. All psycholo-gists and most others would agree that a part of our existence is carried out below the level of consciousness. Whether we believe that this is concerned with the sort of information processing that cognitive psychologists study or with unacceptable thoughts and feelings as Freud believed will depend on our own personal and professional orientations and phil-osophy. Whatever they may be, an awareness of alternative theories and explanations can enhance our understanding of our clients and their experience.

All clients sleep and all have dreams. Many experience difficulties in or have con-cerns about sleep and dreaming. Generally speaking, working directly on assessing and improving sleep falls within the domain of cognitive behaviour therapy but these tech-niques can quite readily be integrated into other approaches to therapy and counselling.

In contrast to the psychology of sleep, which is firmly rooted in experimental psy-chology, interest in dreams has developed out of working directly with clients in thera-peutic contexts. Many counsellors accordingly will find themselves quite 'at home' with working with clients' dreams, and that integrating dream-work into their thera-peutic practice comes quite naturally.

The sections of this chapter concerned with hypnosis, meditation and drugs are intended to inform at a very basic level, and to be of more general interest. Some coun-sellors will be trained in hypnosis, some may be considering using it and others merely interested in it. Although psychologists frequently state there is no mystery to hypnosis and that it can all be explained in psychological terms, its use in the control of pain is nevertheless fairly impressive. Unfortunately its track record in other areas such as of treating the behaviours that many people would like to change (smoking, for example) is not so striking.

Although studied by psychologists, meditation is not usually considered to be one of the psychological therapies. As with hypnosis, although some psychologists would deny it, psychology has not entirely accounted for its 'mystical' effects.

A chapter on consciousness would be incomplete without mention of the effects of various drugs on consciousness, cognitions and behaviour. It is only intended to be the briefest of introductions and any counsellor working with clients using drugs will, of course, need to be far better informed than the scope of this chapter allows.

It can thus be seen that the study of consciousness and its altered states covers a wide range of human experience, and includes normal everyday activities, such as sleeping and dreaming, the more esoteric, as with meditation and the frankly bizarre and hopefully uncommon experiences which result from the effects of psychotropic drugs such as LSD. What these rather disparate areas have in common is that they all involve the notion of consciousness.

7

The Social Psychology of Self and Relationships

Jill D. Wilkinson with Adrian Coyle

CONTENTS

7.1 INTRODUCTION

Most people, if they were asked to identify what was the most important thing in their lives, would reply it is their relationship with others: their family, their friends and their partners. If asked what was the cause of most discontent or pain in their lives, many people would similarly report it was their relationships with others. Relationships, as well as being a source of pleasure, contentment and joy, can bring frustration, pain and suffering.

We need relationships. We need them for our genes to survive and we need them in order to establish and maintain an organized society. At an individual level, we need relationships for stimulation (as Robinson Crusoe found), for support in times of crisis (Sarnoff and Zimbardo, 1961) and we need them in order to give meaning to our lives. Sharing our experiences and our lives, caring about others and being cared for are fundamental aspects of human experience.

Clients in counselling often report difficulties in their relationships. These may be primary, and the reason for which the person has sought help, or they may be the result of other factors in the person's life, such as a bereavement or problems at work which may be affecting relationships. Sometimes the difficulty centres around a particular relationship, but for other clients it may be a much more generalized problem which affects the person's ability to make or maintain any satisfactory relationships, or relationships of a particular type, such as intimate relationships.

The study of relationships has mostly been the province of social psychologists. Social psychologists view people not just as individuals who can be explained in terms of their cognitive and psychological processes, but as products of their social environment. They have, accordingly, tended to study people in their natural environments rather than in the laboratory. However, as most researchers are academics, and academics have access to large samples of college-aged subjects, some of this research has its limitations. We know, for example, a great deal about interpersonal attraction (particularly in adolescence); somewhat less about mature relationships.

This chapter is concerned with the social psychology of relationships. It begins at the beginning; with ourselves. The way in which we are aware of, know and understand ourselves plays a vital part in the way in which we relate to others. It then moves on to the area of person perception; how we form impressions of others and how we develop our own understanding of those we relate to. Next it looks at forming relationships before discussing some of the main theories of relationships and relationship breakdown. Finally, the chapter takes a brief look at the research on gay and lesbian relationships and how they may be similar to, and differ from, heterosexual relationships. Throughout, we shall be discussing the implications of this work for the relationship between client and counsellor—the therapeutic relationship.

7.2 THE SELF

Our sense of self forms the very centre of our world and colours the way in which we view and relate to the world around us. If, for example, we consider ourselves as socially timid, we may react and respond very differently from if we see ourselves as bold and adventurous.

The 'self' is the entire person's awareness and representations of themselves. It a unifying phenomenon which provides direction and will to the person; it is the site of consciousness.

For Carl Rogers, the self was a central concept of his theory of personality. This self consists of all the ideas, perceptions and values that characterize 'I' or 'me' and includes the idea of 'what I am' and 'what I can do'.

But the term 'self' as we shall see is used in many ways. It includes both individual characteristics, such as intelligence, as well as social characteristics which relate to us as members of groups. Indeed, it is in the context of our social relationships that we develop our sense of self.

7.2.1 Self-awareness

Some social psychologists maintain that the ability to see oneself as others do, to be able to reflect upon one's actions, thoughts and emotions, is essential for being human. Experience alone does not result in understanding, one has to be able to reflect upon that experience to learn from it. This ability to mentally represent ourselves to ourselves as though to another develops gradually throughout childhood.

To be able to interact with another we need to be able to have some idea about how that other will respond to us; that is, we have to be able to see ourselves from the perspective of others. Of course, the accuracy of these perceptions will vary depending upon both who is the perceiver and who is the perceived.

Extreme self-awareness, however, is very unpleasant, particularly when the person becomes painfully aware of a discrepancy between their behaviour (as perceived by themselves) and what they consider to be appropriate behaviour in the situation, as dictated by the social norms and accepted standards of behaviour.

Extreme self-awareness is often associated with the person expecting others will be evaluating them, and this, in turn, leads to uncertainty about their own abilities. The negative cognitions that result from such expectations (for example, 'I'm making a complete fool of myself, they must think I'm absolutely stupid') play a major part in the development of social anxiety; that is, anxiety in the presence or anticipated presence of other people (Beck et al., 1987). Chronic social anxiety may lead to reduced social contact and withdrawn behaviour when in the presence of others. This may feed back into reduced opportunities to learn social skills and, thus, increased shyness.

Probably everyone has experienced acute social anxiety at some time. However, it is more likely to affect people with low self-esteem than those with moderate to high self-esteem. There are also a number of factors that have been shown to affect how likely any situation is to lead to acute social anxiety. These include how conspicuous the person is, the novelty of the situation, the number of people present in the 'audience', the relative status of the audience, their familiarity to the person, their similarity in other respects to the person, and their behaviour.

When working with clients suffering from extreme self-awareness it is important to assess whether the associated anxiety is the result of 'faulty' beliefs, such as 'no-one will like me unless I am witty and amusing all the time', lack of social skill (performance deficits) or what is probably most likely, a combination of the two. A social skills approach with a strong cognitive component and emphasis on shifting attention onto the other(s) in the situation is one approach which can be taken in counselling with clients who experience very high levels of self-awareness and social anxiety.

Therapist Self-awareness

Repeatedly, throughout this book we have been highlighting the importance of the therapist's self-awareness in connection with the therapeutic relationship. Self-awareness involves the ability to see ourselves as our clients might see us and to understand the possible impact that our personality, beliefs and behaviour might have on them.

7.2.2 Self-monitoring

A related concept to self-awareness is that of **self-monitoring**. Snyder (1987) found that high self-monitors are very aware of how they are behaving and are highly sensitive to social cues and to the social demands of the situation. The problem is, they may spend the time reacting to the demands of the situation and act in ways that are inconsistent with their inner convictions; in other words, they may lose track of themselves.

In contrast, low self-monitors either cannot, or choose not to, act in such chameleon-like ways and tend to express themselves far more consistently with their view of 'true' self. The problem at this end of the self-monitoring dimension is that the person may be, or appear to be, insensitive to the demands of the situation, including the emotional needs of others in the situation.

The implication of these finding for counsellors is fairly clear. If high self-monitoring is causing difficulties for the client, they may need to keep more 'in touch' with their own goals, agendas or needs. If it is low self-monitoring that is causing the problem, then the client can be helped to be more aware of situational and interpersonal demands and to learn to respond with more flexibility in the situation.

Low self-monitoring usually manifests itself only indirectly to the person concerned. It is the people with whom the person is interacting who generally experience the problem directly.

In family therapy it emerged that a father's attempts at what he thought were 'helpful' remarks to either of his adolescent daughters were usually perceived as critical, and would lead to quite violent family rows. Although the step-mother could see why the girls reacted as they did, she felt that she should either stay out of the arguments or support her husband, who was under considerable pressure from work and also under severe emotional strain resulting from his first wife's chronic illness and deteriorating condition.

Both daughters had complained on a number of occasions that they felt they did not spend enough time together as a family (that is, with their father and step-mother). On the occasion in question the family had decided to go out for a meal together but this was cancelled because the girls decided to visit their mother who had been particularly unwell. When the father tried to reschedule the meal for the following evening, one of the girls stated that she had made arrangements to go out with her friends, whereupon her father stated that she really did have to decide where her priorities lay and that he too wanted them to operate as a family. This is fairly typical of how rows in the family started.

When confronted in counselling, the father stated that he had been completely unaware of the effect this could have on his daughter; he had never stopped to consider what impact his behaviour could have on the situation. It was also at odds with what he wanted to achieve in the family.

Role-play with video-feedback following a social skills training approach (see Section 7.5.4) was then employed. The father's aim was to achieve an appropriate level of self-monitoring, concentrating on responding to members of his family with more self-awareness and awareness of the possible outcome of the interaction without losing sight of his own goals in the situation.

Self-monitoring and the counsellor

The process of counselling, as we discussed in Section 5.2.1 (on Attention and the Selection of Information) requires a high level of attention and also a considerable degree of self-monitoring, or switching of attention between client and self. This self-monitoring process alternates, in turn with thinking, or processing information, about the client in relation to implicit or formal theoretical models. This is an extremely complex cognitive process which makes considerable demands on information processing. Counsellors, as do other people particularly in the 'helping professions', need to be aware of the dangers of 'burnout' discussed in Section 10.7.3.

7.2.3 Self-concept and Self-schema

Self-concept is a general term used to describe how we think about or evaluate ourselves; the way in which we know who we are. Frequently clients in counselling will say, 'I don't know who I am any more', 'I thought I knew myself, but now I'm lost'. Psychological theory and research on the subject of self-concept is therefore highly relevant to all counsellors.

The cognitive components of self-concept are referred to as **self-schemas** (Markus, 1977) which contain information, memories and beliefs about oneself. Very often we identify our schema by negative means and will say, 'I couldn't possibly do. . .', or 'I'm not the sort of person who could . . . '. Not only do we have self-schemas for our current selves, we have them about possible selves; the selves we might become (Markus and Nurius, 1986).

Our self-schema influences what we attend to and what we remember, and we will often disregard information if it does not fit or is inconsistent with it. In this way schemas can be self-perpetuating and resistant to change. They can also be 'past their sell-by date'. The circumstances may have changed, the person has moved on but their self-schema remains the same. In spite of the fact that self-schema is relatively resistant to change it may be affected by self-esteem, which may fluctuate, or be 'dented' by negative experiences such as rejection or being made redundant. Many counsellors will work with clients' self-schemas and possible self-schemas in 'identity work' in counselling.

Several sources of information contribute to the development of our self-schema, but as we shall see, reflected appraisals, social comparisons, self-perception and self-efficacy are particularly influential.

One way in which we know who we are is by others' reactions to us. Our perceptions of how others appraise and judge us is referred to as **reflected appraisal.** The way in which others respond to us when we are children is particularly influential, which is why relations with parents, siblings and peers can play such an important role in shaping our self-schema.

A second important process in the development of self-schema is **social comparison** (Suls and Marco, 1991). At a relatively early age, children begin to compare themselves with others, and this process continues throughout life. This may be why siblings of very bright children sometimes view themselves as inadequate in areas where their brothers or sisters excel, even though they may be average or above-average (Fiske and Taylor, 1991).

Thirdly, **self-perception** contributes to the formation of our self-schema. We develop beliefs about ourselves based on how we view ourselves. Sometimes, however, we get it wrong. We may blame ourselves for something that was out of our control and we mistakenly attribute our actions to our own characteristics because we fail to realize the power of external influences which were operating in the situation.

Finally, our feelings of **self-efficacy** affect the way in which we come to view ourselves. Self-efficacy relates to our perceptions of our own ability to cause desired outcomes and avoid undesired ones. It therefore contributes to our sense of control. To act to cause desired outcomes we must believe that we can do so. Self-efficacy is therefore related to motivation, cognition and behaviour. Self-efficacy may be affected by many factors including our past performance, observation of others, our emotional state and factors relating to the situation. We will be discussing self-efficacy in relation to reactions to stress in Section 10.6.3.

7.2.4 Social Roles

We are all members of a number of different groups: the family, departments at work, clubs, church groups, neighbourhood groups, sports teams and the like. All groups influence the behaviour of their members and in each group we occupy a position in the structure of the group. **Roles** are the patterns of behaviour expected of people in their particular position within a particular group.

Some of our roles are under our control or **achieved**, such as the roles of spouse or partner, teacher or counsellor; others are **ascribed** to us, for example, male/female, son/daughter, adolescent, old-age pensioner. These are not under our control.

Our own social roles influence the way in which we see ourselves and also act as a guide to behaving in an expected or acceptable way within a particular group. For example the person who has 'achieved' the role of rebel in a group will be expected to act in a particular way, or live up to this role and others may be quite surprised if the person suddenly starts conforming.

A person will probably occupy a number of roles and it is not unusual for two or more roles to conflict. So the counsellor at his or her sports club might want to say to another club member who has been going on a bit about the break-up with her latest boyfriend, 'For goodness sake, stop wingeing on about it, pull yourself together and do something about it'. He or she may, however, be caught up in a certain amount of **role-conflict** which may prove difficult or frustrating.

7.2.5 Self and Identity

The study of self and identity has a long history but, as with the study of consciousness, went out of favour during the rise of behavourism to re-emerge with force in the subsequent 'cognitive revolution' (Gecas, 1982).

The whole area of self-concept and identity is rather problematic and confusing because different theorists and researchers in the field frequently use the terms somewhat differently, and sometimes the distinction between the two is not at all clear. However, in Britain, identity theory has been tended to be concerned with social identity, that is, the study of the nature of self within the context of social group membership, and a distinction is often made between social and 'personal' identity.

Identity process theory (Breakwell, 1986) abandons this dichotomy (between social and personal identity) and proposes a dynamic model of identity which is particularly concerned with the process of identity change in relation to the impact of events, especially those which may pose 'threats' to identity.

Three 'principles' of identity are seen to be central to this theory and are also included in many other approaches to identity. These are continuity, distinctiveness, self-esteem. More recently self-efficacy (discussed in Section 10.6.3) has been added.

Identity, according to this model, provides **continuity** over time. This does not necessarily mean that a person has to believe that he/she is the same at one time as they were at an earlier time but that any change is explicable in terms of that person's understanding of their own history. Given a perceived discontinuity in the self people will try to reconcile the new self with the old. Sometimes this can pose problems for the individual.

A client, a twenty-year-old woman, was referred for counselling because of obsessive ruminations which took the form of desperate attempts to remember the details of quite ordinary events in her recent past. She would go to great lengths to try to remember exactly what she was wearing on Tuesday of the preceding week, for example, or who was sitting next to her in the canteen at work ten days ago etc.

She was an only child from a very close-knit family and was about to get married to someone from a very different family and social background. She was aware of the fact that her parents (particularly her father to whom she was very close) did not entirely approve, although they had not said it as such.

From the perspective of identity theory, these ruminations could be seen as the client's attempt to keep in touch with her previous 'self', fearing that she might lose her sense of continuity between her old and 'new' married self.

Identity provides a **distinctiveness** which both individuates a person from others and assimilates them into groups, thus providing distinctiveness and similarity. This can be as much a function of the context as of the person. Distinctiveness is not in itself positive or negative although identity process theory implies that we are motivated to seek positive ways of being distinct.

Self-esteem in some form is a fundamental feature of all identity theories. Self-esteem has been defined in a number of ways but it is generally seen as a fundamental motivation to maintain and enhance a positive conception of oneself.

From the above it can be seen that, ideally, one would have a strong sense of continuity, moderate distinctiveness and high self-esteem to be a well-adjusted and reasonably content person. However, people often do not have this profile. People may fail to develop these characteristics or events may occur which change or threaten the established self-image.

Changes in employment, in family situation, and in health may all be perceived as presenting threats to the sense of self. So becoming unemployed may lead to a perception of a loss of continuity in the self, a loss of opportunities to demonstrate skills and self-efficacy, a loss of a sense of distinctiveness and a lowering of self-esteem.

Threats to identity, to one's sense of self, can be extremely distressing.

One particular client was referred for counselling when he reported to his GP that he was in a complete 'turmoil', unable to 'think straight', had lost confidence, could not get up in the morning, function at his job, cope with the tasks of daily life, had lost his appetite and would tremble, sweat, and so forth.

The client had considered himself to be reasonably satisfactorily married (although the relationship did have its 'ups and downs' and he and his wife had rather grown apart) when he met, and fell in love with, a woman on a plane. They continued the relationship by letter, as both lived in separate continents. He enjoyed this and felt very comfortable with the arrangement. After some time the two 'pen-lovers' met up again, and the relationship immediately became intense and passionate. By this time it had emerged that the client's wife was far from happy in the relationship with her husband and had, it transpired, thought of entering into a relationship with a work-colleague. It seemed to be a logical next step for the client and his wife to separate. There were no children involved and, on the face of it, all seemed to be fairly straightforward.

So why was the client so devastated by these events? Was it because he loved his wife more than he had realized? Were there some unresolved issues relating to attachment? Exploration focusing on self-concept and identity revealed that what was so distressing was the fact that what he had done was completely at odds with the sort of person he had always considered himself to be, and the sort of person he felt others had known him as. In fact, he could not face any of his friends or family who 'knew'. He could not accept that something like this (falling in love, leaving his wife) could ever happen to him. This was not the man he thought he knew. He could not integrate into his self-schema the idea of breaking up his marriage. It had shaken the whole foundations of his sense of self.

If the situation was going to be resolved, it would seem that he would either have to change the way in which he thought about himself to make his self-schema compatible with his actions or go back to acting in ways which would be consistent with his view of himself.

According to Breakwell, we attempt to cope with threats to our identity in a variety of ways. **Intrapsychic strategies** may involve some form of deflection such as temporary denial as a way of 'buying time' to adjust to the threat, or we may engage in 'anticipatory restructuring' as a way of gradually altering our identity if a known threat approaches, such as the death of a partner; we may gradually prepare ourselves for a new, albeit unwelcome, identity as widow, widower or single person.

Interpersonal strategies of attempting to cope with threat can include social avoidance or isolation; that is, removing ourselves from others in order to avoid stigma or pity. Some people also engage in social deceit, such as the person who has been made redundant leaving home at the same time as before so that the neighbours or their partner will not realize they are unemployed.

Finally, **intergroup strategies** may be used as a way of coping, such as seeking social support from a different group or joining a pressure group or self-help group.

The work on identity can provide the counsellor with a useful framework in which to explore identity issues generally and threats more specifically. As we have seen, people attempt to cope with threats to identity in a number of ways; some 'healthy', others less so. Here the counsellor could work with the client on replacing maladaptive ways of coping with more positive strategies.

7.2.6 The 'Real' Self?

So far, we have been talking about the process of self-awareness and the concept of self and identity. But is there such a thing as the 'real' self?

The humanistic psychologist Abraham Maslow (1970) certainly believed there was. He assumed that each person has a unique, essential 'inner core of self'. He used the term **self-actualization** to describe the process of recognizing, accepting and expressing that inner core. Psychological difficulties arise, according to Maslow, when this process is thwarted or blocked. As we have discussed elsewhere (Section 2.6 on Humanistic and Phenomenological Approaches to Personality) this idea is central to Carl Rogers' client-centred approach to counselling.

But what is the evidence for the existence of this 'true' self? Research results are mixed. However, much research shows that there are often contradictions between different aspects of the self and that people have less unitary selves than self-actualization theory might predict (Gergen, 1968). This is something of which most counsellors are well aware.

7.3 PERSON PERCEPTION

The way in which we respond to people depends not only on our understanding of who they are, but on why they behave as they do. Firstly, we form impressions of people, often based on incomplete and conflicting information. In doing this, we take into account characteristics of the person, the nature of the situation and the person's behaviour in the situation. We then make inferences, or **attributions**, about the causes of that person's behaviour and employ **implicit personality theories** to explain how particular characteristics or qualities in people are linked.

7.3.1 Impression Formation

Research confirms the conventional view that first impressions are extremely important (Hamilton, 1988). When we meet someone for the first time we do not perceive every aspect of that person. Instead, we take short-cuts and employ **schemas**, generalized views or representations stored in memory. Our schemas about grandmothers may lead us to expect them to be elderly, comfortable and grey-haired. If so, we will be surprised to meet one with purple hair and a ring through her nose.

We use our schemas to infer a great deal about a person on the basis of limited information, often filling in missing information by using knowledge stored in long-term memory. This is how we come to form impressions quickly (Brewer, 1988). It is typical for someone to take a few isolated bits of non-verbal and verbal behaviour and infer all sorts of things about the person's life and personality. Some may be accurate, others not.

In addition to being formed easily, first impressions tend to be lasting and difficult to change. This may be firstly to do with the fact that people, on the whole, tend to be confident, sometimes over-confident, about their judgements. They are sure they are right even when they have very little to go on (Fiske and Ruscher, 1989).

Secondly, we tend to interpret new information in ways that are consistent with the original impression (Park, 1989); so the same behaviour might be conceptualized as confident in someone of whom we have formed a positive impression, and arrogant if the earlier impression was negative.

Thirdly, we tend to remember the general schema better than we remember any 'evidence' that may be contrary to our overall impression. So if a new piece of information about a person does not 'fit', we will tend not to remember it.

Finally, people often act in ways that elicit from another person behaviour that is consistent with their overall impression (Snyder, 1984). An initial impression can therefor become a **self-fulfilling prophecy**. So, for example, if we perceive someone as friendly, we are more likely to behave in ways that will elicit a friendly response than if we perceive them as suspicious.

Cognitive schemas and clients

Although as counsellors and therapists most of us would like to think of ourselves as 'non judgemental' and not 'leaping to conclusions' about our clients, we cannot be immune from applying our own schemas to our clients. We can, and do, form lasting impressions on the basis of first impressions.

If we have some knowledge about the processes which help to maintain what may be, in some instances, erroneous impressions, we may be able to challenge our own rigid schemas. We should not be over-confident about our initial impressions, we need to be careful about interpreting new material in a way that makes it consistent with our earlier conceptualizations and we need to be prepared to adjust our views of the client in the light of new evidence.

7.3.2 Situational Scripts

In the same way in which we have schemas about people, we also have schemas about situations. These are known as **scripts**. We develop scripts, based on **norms**, for a variety of situations. Scripts help us act, hopefully appropriately, in a range of situations without engaging in too much thought. We have scripts for greetings, for partings, for asking for information from a stranger, for parties, dating etc.

As well as guiding our own behaviour, our scripts contribute to our interpretation of the behaviour of others. If someone's behaviour departs in a significant way from our script for a particular situation, we will form a very different impression from if the behaviour conforms to our expectations.

People can develop scripts which may be inappropriate, as the following example demonstrates.

> *One client's script for 'dating behaviour' involved wining and dining his potential girlfriends on the first date. This would be followed up by flowers, romantic cards, little 'surprises', further wining and dining etc. He was following his script for making a relationship, but somehow it never worked. He was a very nice young man, 'all the mothers think I'm wonderful', he said ruefully. The problem was that he was not dating the mothers and the young women in question had very different scripts. He clearly needed to find someone whose script matched his own, or change his script. He worked with the counsellor on the latter.*

Here we can see that scripts not only guide a person's behaviour, but also affect the way in which others perceive us, and the impressions we make on other people.

Scripts in the counselling situation

Most clients also have scripts about the therapeutic situation: what is expected of them, what is appropriate for them to disclose and what it is acceptable for them to do.

Counsellors also have their own situational scripts which may be different from those of their clients. What the client may be expecting from the counselling situation may not match what the counsellor or therapist is offering. Here the counsellor may need to negotiate with the client to arrive at a mutually acceptable way of working.

7.3.3 Attribution Theory

Impressions of others are only one aspect of social perception. We are also constantly attempting to understand why people behave as they do. The process of assigning causes to both our own and the behaviour of others is termed **attribution** (Heider, 1958).

People tend to attribute behaviour in a particular situation either to mainly **internal** causes, which are those that reflect characteristics of the individual, such as personality traits, abilities or attitudes, or to **external** causes, which arise out of the particular situation. Attributions to internal causes are also referred to as **personal attributions**, and attributions to external causes, **situational attributions.** So if we hear of a mother who has gone to work and left her twelve-year-old child alone when she was off sick from school with a cold and high temperature, we may attribute her behaviour either to the fact that she is an irresponsible mother (personal attribution) or to the fact that she is in an impossible situation: her husband has left her, she can't afford child care and she will lose her job if she takes time off to look after the child (situational attribution).

In deciding whether a behaviour is caused by situational or personal factors three factors have been identified as being important (Kelly, 1973). The first is **consistency** of behaviour. Consistency is high if the person always behaves in a similar way. The second factor is **distinctiveness**; does there seem to be anything special about the person's behaviour in this particular situation? If so distinctiveness will be high. Finally there is **consensus**, the extent to which other people might be expected to behave in this way. If it is believed that most people would do the same in the situation, then consensus would be high.

When consistency is high and distinctiveness and consensus are low we are especially likely to attribute behaviour to internal, or personal, causes. Thus if the person who left her child alone does so often (high consistency), if the situation is nothing out of the ordinary (low distinctiveness) and if we would not expect other people to leave their children alone under such circumstances (low consensus), then we are likely to attribute the behaviour to a personal trait of irresponsibility.

On the other hand, if it is unusual for the child to be left alone (low consistency), and if we hear that there were about to be cuts in the workforce where the woman worked (high distinctiveness) and we believe that most mothers under the circumstances would do the same (high consensus), then we would attribute the behaviour to external or situational factors. External attributions are often made to other information patterns as well.

There is considerable evidence that people take consistency, distinctiveness and consensus factors into consideration and often make thoughtful attributions in the way suggested above. But people often also take short-cuts and make snap judgements which can result in attributional biases or errors, the most common of which is the **fundamental attribution error**. This is the tendency to attribute the behaviour of others to internal or personal factors. This may lead people to blame the victims of various unfortunate circumstances (Ryan, 1977): the unemployed as lazy, the homeless as irresponsible, the abused as asking for it.

However, people tend to *avoid* the fundamental attribution error when explaining their own behaviour. (So if it happens to you, it's your fault, but if it happens to me it's force of circumstance.) This is known as the **actor–observer bias**. It serves as a defence, particularly when our behaviour is inappropriate and involves failure: 'I bumped my car into the post because it was a stupid place to put a post (not because I wasn't looking). Actor–observer bias may also occur because we have direct access to the external factors which may influence our own behaviour in a way in which we do not about the behaviour of others. So I may know that the post into which I bumped was sited in a way that was extremely difficult to see from my particular car.

The degree to which people attribute their own behaviour to external factors depends on whether the outcome is positive or negative. There is a marked tendency to take credit for success known as the **self-serving bias**. So if we have done well in an examination, it is because we have worked hard, are clever after all, etc., but if we have done badly, it was a lousy paper (Smith and Ellsworth, 1987). It has also been found that in general, males are more likely to attribute success to internal factors and failure to external ones while the reverse is true of females.

7.3.4 Attributional Style and Depression

In addition to the distinction between internal and external attributions, psychologists have argued that attributions may reflect some other dimensions. The main ones are a **stable/unstable** dimension; that is, how stable the characteristic is over time and a **global/specific** dimension; that is, whether the cause is believed to apply to a large number of things or just one particular one.

Attributions can therefore be internal or external and also reflect the above dimensions. If I think I failed an exam because I did not work hard enough, this attribution would be internal, unstable and specific. But if I believe it was because I am unintelligent, the attribution would similarly be internal, but this time stable and global. Alternatively, I might attribute failure to a belief that multiple choice exams are unfair. This would be an example of an external attribution which is stable and global.

It has been argued that the way in which people explain failure to themselves determines its subsequent effects. Global attributions should increase the generalizability of the effects of failure. So that if I attribute my failure to lack of intelligence (global) rather than I'm not very good at maths (specific) my belief is likely to be applied to other areas of my life. Attributions that are stable are likely to make the belief long-term. So attributing failure to lack of intelligence, which is stable as well as global, will produce a longer-term belief than if I attribute failure to being overtired.

People become depressed, it has been suggested, when they attribute negative life events to stable, global characteristics. Whether self-esteem is adversely affected depends whether or not the attributes are internal or external. If the attributes are internal and the person blames him or herself, then self-esteem will be adversely affected.

(It would therefore seem to be that the person who always blames everything or every-one else for their misfortunes may not be particularly likeable, but they may be pro-tected from depression.)

The 'depression-prone' individual, according to this model, has this particular type of **attribution style**, which means that when they experience a bad event, they will believe that it is caused by them (internal), that the cause is long-lasting (stable) and that the cause will make other things bad too (global).

There is something intuitively appealing about this theory, but what about the evi-dence? Sweeney et al. (1989) conducted a survey of more than 100 studies looking at the relationship between attributional style and depression and found that the correla-tional evidence is supportive. However, all this says is that depressed people have this particular attributional style, not that the attributional style *causes* the depression.

In order to test the 'vulnerability' model, that is, that the attributional style makes you 'teeter on the brink', but you need a bad event to push you over studies would have to be prospective; they would need to be conducted before you had been pushed over. This is clearly very difficult, costly and time-consuming to do and the most that can be claimed at the present time is that there is evidence of a relationship between attribu-tional style and depression.

The work on attribution has had considerable impact on cognitive therapy. However, even if the counsellor or therapist is not trained or does not choose to work in this way with clients, attribution theory and research can add to both the client's and the coun-sellor's understanding of the way in which the client's world is conceptualized and how they come to the conclusions they do.

7.3.5 Implicit Personality Theory

Our own **implicit personality theories** (which we discussed in Chapter 1), will also influence our impressions of people we meet. We use our implicit theories to help to explain why someone may think, feel or act as they do and we also make assumptions about how particular characteristics or qualities of people are linked. For instance, some people assume that 'intelligence' is linked with 'coldness', that fat people are more gen-erous than thin people, or that women are more intuitive than men.

The contents of implicit personality theories develop through social interaction, i.e. they are not just the products of purely individual processes of information processing, which is what a purely cognitive approach would imply. The social origin of many implicit personality theories explains their commonality across social groups.

The accuracy of people's implicit personality theories has been debated vigorously. As these theories assume some consistency of personality, the debate overlaps with that on the stability of personality traits discussed in Section 2.4.1 on Trait Approaches to Personality. Mischel (1968) found that most personality traits, measured using scales devised by psychologists, showed only low correlations with behaviour across time and contexts. This suggests, at the least, that people over-estimate the degree of personality consistency and, thus, their implicit personality theories are sometimes inaccurate.

Implicit theory and counselling

This subject was covered in some detail in Chapter 1.

7.4 FORMING RELATIONSHIPS

Social perception clearly plays an important part in how we think and react to other people; but what determines whom we like and dislike, how do we form and maintain social and intimate relationships and why do relationships fail? These are just some of the questions social psychologists working in the area of interpersonal relationships have addressed.

In looking at factors that promote liking or interpersonal attraction, psychologists have focused their attention on three main variables: physical attractiveness, proximity and similarity. It should however be noted that much of this research has been conducted on samples of US heterosexual college students.

7.4.1 Physical attractiveness

Research has shown that even though people say otherwise, physical attractiveness plays a central role in liking; at least in the early stages of relationships (Tesser and Brodie, 1971; Walster et al., 1966; Mahes, 1975). Physical attractiveness has also been found to be related to how popular children are at school.

Physical attractiveness, however, does not appear to be the key to happiness. Firstly, physical attractiveness during college years is unrelated to life satisfaction in middle age (Berscheid, 1984). Secondly, physically attractive people do not necessarily have the highest levels of self-esteem (Major et al., 1984). Indeed very attractive people can be beset by great self-doubt and insecurity, possibly because others relate only to their 'surface' characteristics, not to their inner personal qualities.

Although people are attracted to attractive people, what seems to happen is that we are most likely to end up in close relationships with someone similar to ourselves in attractiveness (Baron and Byrne, 1991). This is known as the **matching hypothesis**.

7.4.2 Proximity

Do we actively choose our friends and/or partners or do circumstances where people are 'thrown together' exert a strong influence on the formation of relationships? Research shows that physical proximity between two people strongly affects the likelihood that they will form a relationship. Although familiarity can breed contempt, overall physical proximity has a positive influence on attraction (Festinger et al., 1950).

This clearly has implications for making friends and meeting potential partners. The workplace or an activity which brings people into close contact for sustained periods may be a better place for making relationships than a social club or a dating agency. A person who is in, or creates a situation of, close proximity is probably better placed for making relationships than a person who goes along to a club or bar with the hope of meeting someone. (Advice to friends who want to form relationships might be to get a job which brings you into close contact with others, or, alternatively, take up round-the-world sailing!)

Of course, close proximity does not determine the quality of the relationship. This may be why, in the workplace, we sometimes see the most unlikely people getting together to form an attachment. If we are thinking about quality of relationships we need to look further, possibly at similarities between potential partners.

7.4.3 Similarities

On the one hand we hear that 'birds of a feather flock together', and on the other 'opposites attract'. Popular thinking is clearly rather contradictory on this issue.

Attention in the research has focused on similarities of dimensions such as age, education, social class, attitudes and interests and personality. The evidence from this research suggests that it is perceived similarity, not dissimilarity, that increases attraction in both short-term and long-term relationships (Neimeyer and Mitchell, 1988). This is one of the strongest and most consistent findings in the literature.

The strongest effects of similarity occur in relation to **attitudes, beliefs and values**, particularly in relation to such things as religion, music and politics (Byrne et al., 1986). However, once you begin to develop a close bond with someone, your attitudes might become more similar to those of the other person, or you might change your perceptions of the other person's attitudes to make them appear more similar to your own. Clearly though, one could only go so far in this direction without feeling that the compromise was too great.

If relationships are going to develop and partners remain attractive to each other, it might be expedient to explore attitudes and beliefs at an early stage in the relationship. This requires a certain level of social skill and awareness. Some people may lack the necessary skills of self-disclosure, appropriate questioning and responding, others may 'kid' themselves that similarity exists where there is, in fact, very little. These are areas which can be addressed in counselling or therapy.

There is also a good deal of support for the claim that people with similar **personalities** are attracted to each other. It has also been found that the personalities of partners in stable marriages are more similar to each other than those in unstable marriages (Cattell and Nesselrode, 1967).

It has also been suggested that the similarity principle extends to the way in which we 'tell our stories' about our relationships and the nature of these stories (Weber et al., 1987). It can be distressing towards the end of a relationship for the partners to realize they have developed very different accounts of the nature and meaning of the relationship. This must be a situation with which most couples counsellors will be familiar.

Client–therapist similarities

We have seen how similarities have been found to be an important factor in forming potentially close relationships; but what about in the therapeutic relationship? Are such similarities between therapist and client beneficial to the client and related to positive therapeutic outcomes?

The results of a large number of studies suggests that both similarities and differences in client–therapist values are related to outcome (Beutler et al., 1994). Similarities in the relative value placed on such qualities as wisdom, honesty, knowledge and intellectual pursuits are associated with more positive therapeutic outcomes, as indeed are *discrepancies* between client and therapist in the value placed on social status and friendships (Arizmendi et al., 1985) and interpersonal goals of treatment (Charone, 1981).

It has been suggested that the values held in common by therapist and client that are associated with improvement (wisdom, honesty etc.) reflect humanistic values that are important for maintaining social order. In contrast, discrepant values that are associated with improvement (e.g. social status) may be more closely associated with the issues for which the client may be seeking help (Beutler and Clarkin, 1990)

Although similarity of personality has been found to be an important dimension in interpersonal attraction and in forming close personal relationships, the research does not support the view that similarities between client and therapist personalities is related to therapeutic benefit. On the contrary, one study found the opposite; that it was contrasting personality styles (of dependency and autonomy) that were associated with positive outcome (Berzins, 1977).

A number of other areas of client–therapist similarities and differences have been investigated. These include the effects of differences in age, sex and ethnicity on therapeutic outcome.

Although one study found that therapists who were more than 10 years younger than their clients obtained poorer outcomes when compared to those whose age was either similar or older than their clients (Beck, 1988), many other studies in this area have been inconclusive (Atkinson and Schein, 1986). As far as sex of the therapist is concerned most research on the topic has failed to find significant differences in outcome that are attributable either to the sex of therapist or to therapist–client matching in this respect.

Research on therapist ethnicity parallels that on therapist sex (Beutler et al., 1994). Results are, at best, mixed and are difficult to interpret.

In conclusion, it would seem that although similarities in terms of values and personality might be important in forming close personal relationships, the only client–therapist similarity that has been shown to be consistently influential in relation to outcome in therapy is similarity in values.

7.5 MODELS AND THEORIES OF RELATIONSHIP DEVELOPMENT

Some relationships go no further than initial attraction, others develop to a deeper level of intimacy and commitment. How do close relations progress and what determines their development?

7.5.1 Stages of Relationship Development

As relationships develop, they often go through a number of stages. These stages are not necessarily discrete nor are they followed rigidly. It should also be noted that the models discussed below were developed to understand romantic relationships where a degree of exclusivity is often expected. People obviously form a range of relationships in different circumstances and for different reasons.

- **Stage 1—Sampling**   This involves a filtering of those with whom interaction is desired and likely, from those with whom it is not desired. This filtering is gradual and most people are excluded at an early stage on the basis of superficial information. The desire for different types of relationships may lead to people being excluded from one group but included in another. For instance, friends may be selected on a different basis from romantic partners.
- **Stage 2—Bargaining**   This involves the formation of acquaintanceship and the assessment of expected rewards and costs (see 'Social exchange theory' below). This is a complex on-going process.
- **Stage 3—Commitment**   This involves the expression of some form of public or private bond. Commitment involves the mutual recognition of the relationship.
- **Stage 4—Institutionalization**   This involves the expression of the relationship in terms of a socially recognized institution, such as marriage. The relationship has more formal elements and may become legally constrained in some respects.

Walster et al. (1978) propose that as relationships develop there is an increase in the following:

- **Intensity of liking and/or loving.**
- **Depth and breadth of information exchanged**   Those who are intimate know much more about each others' idiosyncrasies, personal histories, vulnerabilities, etc. (see Section 7.5.3).
- **Actual and expected length of relationship**   Each person will be making estimates about the expected progress of the relationship—whether it will yield positive outcomes, how long it will last, etc.
- **Value of resources exchanged**   As the relationship develops, partners are more ready to invest significant resources in the relationship but also gain an ability to

punish more severely through termination of the relationship. Each person will carry out an analysis of his/her inputs to and outputs from the relationship. Comparisons will also be made with other possible relationships (see below).

- **Interchangeability of resources**   For example, a person may repay a partner's cooking with verbal and non-verbal praise.
- **'We-ness'**   This is the tendency for partners to define themselves as a unit in interaction with the external world.

7.5.2 Social Exchange Theory

Social exchange theory (Thibault and Kelley, 1967) suggests that the move towards closeness is governed by the balance of **rewards** and **costs** encountered in the relationship. While there are a number of slightly different versions of social exchange theory they all emphasize the exchange of resources of one kind or another.

Rewards in relationships might include companionship, emotional support in times of stress and satisfaction of other needs. Costs can include time, money, effort spent to maintain the relationship, suffering in times of conflict and the passing up of other relationship opportunities (Kelly, 1979).

This theory suggests that people evaluate the ratio of their costs and benefits (or **outcome**) in several ways. These include:

- **Own costs against own benefits**   Do the costs (the time, effort, etc. put into the relationship) exceed the benefits (emotional rewards, social support, etc.) gained from the relationship?
- **Own costs/benefits against other's costs/benefits**   This involves asking who is putting more into the relationship and who is getting most out of it. Of course, one may be satisfied to get less out of a relationship if one is putting less into it.
- **Expected balance of costs/benefits**   This is known as the **comparison level** and is based on personal experiences and observation of other people's relationships. According to Thibault and Kelly, outcomes that meet or exceed the comparison level are satisfying; those that fall below are dissatisfying.
- **Current relationship against other relationships**   Could one get more or would one get less out of another relationship, i.e. what alternatives are there? This question is more abstract than the preceding three, which ask about the actual relationship. Instead, here the person has to imagine possible other relationships that they might have. The failure of many people to imagine realistic, better alternatives to their current state may explain why some people stay in unsatisfactory relationships. This evaluation has been called the **comparison level for alternatives**.

7.5.3 Self-disclosure and Social Penetration

The process of getting to know another person means that people must reveal more and more of themselves as the relationship develops. One of the most important aspects of a close or intimate relationship is the sharing of our innermost thoughts and feelings, or **self-disclosure** (Jourard, 1971). **Social penetration theory** (Altman and Taylor, 1973) suggests that relationships progress from superficial exchanges to more intimate ones as people begin to give more of themselves to each other.

As the relationship becomes more intimate, the disclosures by one person are 'matched' by the other in term of both the breadth of the disclosure and the depth (Altman and Taylor, 1973). That is, each partner reciprocates the other's disclosure in terms of level of intimacy. Matching has been found to be more important in the early stages of developing a relationship. Well-established relationships are more tolerant in expectations of immediate reciprocation of disclosures.

Regulating self-disclosure is one way in which we can control the level of intimacy in a relationship. Many of our relationships involve fairly low levels of self-disclosure and that is as far as we want to go with them. Social norms will also affect the degree and type of self-disclosure. Negotiating an agreed level of disclosure is therefore an important skill in many different kinds of relationships.

Problems with self-disclosure can take many forms but the most common difficulties encountered by clients attending counselling include over-disclosure, under-disclosure, mismatching of disclosure and 'pseudo-disclosure'.

Over-disclosure is when the person discloses all: the 'I'm an open book' syndrome, 'What you see is what you get'. The problem with this is that firstly, the person leaves themselves undefended and open to criticism, ridicule etc. Secondly it places the other person in a very uncomfortable position. What are they supposed to do? They may feel under pressure to reciprocate, but be nowhere near ready to do so.

Under-disclosure results in the relationship failing to develop. It may also leave the other person in an uncertain position. They may have engaged in a certain level of self-disclosure, and be left feeling rather vulnerable as a result of there being no reciprocity.

Mismatching of disclosure content may occur if a person has undergone some trauma or experienced a high level of distress or symptomatology which is outside the experience of the other. If this is the case it is going to be inherently difficult to 'manage' reciprocal self-disclosure.

Some people will unfortunately have experienced traumatic experiences, such as rape or child sexual abuse, about which they may feel deeply ashamed. It may take a considerable time before they can trust another person sufficiently to disclose this sort of information. Some people, of course, never feel safe enough disclose such deeply painful experiences. In the mean time, the other person may have interpreted the 'holding back' as a reluctance to engage and may have withdrawn from the relationship.

People who are disfigured by nature, accident or by surgery may also have difficulties with self disclosure, but of a different kind. If the disfigurement does not show, the stage in a potential relationship at which the person should disclose such information becomes a major concern.

One twenty-one-year-old female client with an ileostomy pouch agonized over when to disclose this highly personal information to her new boyfriend. After discussing it and 'rehearsing' the situation with her counsellor, she finally plucked up the courage to tell him. She was immensely relieved at his response, 'I'm so glad it's just that. I'd been imagining all sorts of dreadful things. I even thought you might be frigid . . .' etc. He had obviously been acutely aware of her reticence and was relieved she felt she could now trust him sufficiently to tell him.

Most counsellors will be familiar with the client who engages in **pseudo-disclosure**: the person who *describes* feelings rather than self-discloses at an emotional level. Here the counsellor may want to assess whether this is the result of the demands of the situation; is the client reluctant to disclose because it is in some way expected and subsequently resists it? Is it because the client does not trust the therapist? Does the client trust anyone? or does he or she lack the basic skill of self-disclosure and have no idea of what is expected or how to behave in this respect in this or any other situation?

Social exchange and self-disclosure in the counselling relationship

The counsellor–client relationship, like other relationships, forms through the exchange of various resources (e.g. information, expertise, time, respect, status, money, services, energy and trust), the assessment of costs and rewards and the expectations about future outcomes. All these processes occur within the constraints of social norms, such as norms of equity, and of equality.

One of the inequalities in the exchange process in the therapeutic relationship is self-disclosure. The counselling situation is one in which information, often of a very personal and intimate nature, is disclosed by the client to the counsellor. Usually in close relationships where information about the self is revealed it happens reciprocally, i.e. both people disclose information of roughly the same degree of intimacy about themselves. Gradually, as the relationship develops (and a cause of its development), the amount of information increases (i.e. greater breadth of information) and the information becomes more intimate (i.e. greater depth of information).

However, the counselling situation does not involve a reciprocal relationship between the two people. The client is expected to reveal more and deeper information about his/her self than is the counsellor. While norms of behaviour vary depending upon the context so that reciprocity is not expected in all interactions, this inequality of disclosure does present both counsellor and client with an imbalance in the exchange.

Sometimes clients will attempt to redress this imbalance by seeking personal information from the counsellor. This happens particularly when the client, for some reason, senses an inequality or feels a lack of trust in the relationship. A careful assessment of the reasons underlying this tendency needs to be made before the counsellor decides how to act in this situation.

The counsellor can also redress the imbalance in the relationship by consciously using self-disclosure. This was advocated strongly by the psychologist Sidney Jourard (1971) who proposed that disclosing therapists precipitated client self-disclosure. The assertion that therapist self-disclosure is beneficial has some experimental support and one study (Barrett and Berman, 1991) found that when therapists disclosed personal information, their clients experienced a greater improvement in their symptoms than when they did not disclose. Clearly, however, self-disclosure on the part of the therapist or counsellor needs to be done with awareness and handled carefully.

7.5.4 Social Skill and Relationships

Making and maintaining satisfactory and rewarding social and intimate relationships requires considerable social skill. For example, establishing a new friendship involves the successful negotiation of several stages. As well as the skills involved in gradual and reciprocated self-disclosure, skills are required to arrange meetings, to deal with misunderstandings, to be sufficiently rewarding to each other and to relate to others in the other person's social group. In order to maintain the relationship, it is necessary to keep up the level of rewards and to avoid, or deal with, sources of conflict (Argyle, 1988).

In long-term intimate relationships self-disclosure continues to be important. Both men and women report the highest levels of satisfaction when self-disclosure is high. In fact, mutual sharing of interests, beliefs and opinions is often more important than sex (Sternberg and Grajek, 1984).

Conflict and anger are a part of all marriages and close relationships, but dealing with them effectively is the hallmark of the most satisfying marriages (Repetti, 1989). Skill is needed at negotiating points of disagreement and in diverting interaction sequences which have led to conflict in the past.

Argyle and Kendon (1967) proposed an information processing model of social skill which provides us with a cognitive behavioural explanation of the process of 'normal' social behaviour. They saw the process in terms of a cycle consisting of the person's goals, perceptions, the translation of perceptions into action, motor responses (verbal and non-verbal) and observation of feedback from the interpersonal partner. Wilkinson (1985) later expanded the model to include cognitive schemas (of self, other and the situation) and social knowledge (of norms). Other workers in the field have emphasized the importance of self-monitoring to social skill.

Social skills training was devised by Argyle and Kendon (1967) as a therapeutic approach to treating skill deficits. Although it was conceived as a group approach to training more generic skills, such as opening and maintaining conversation, a number of psychologists and others have adapted the methods for working therapeutically with a variety of populations and problems (e.g. Trower et al., 1978; Wilkinson and Canter, 1984). Social skills training can also be adapted for working with individual clients with specific problems, as the following example demonstrates.

The clients are a couple who have been having some difficulties in their relationship. After seeing them both together for two sessions, it has been decided that, because both partners have their own specific difficulties, particularly in their styles of communication, the counsellor will work with them individually for a few sessions before continuing the joint sessions.

One area of concern that the husband voiced is that his wife was 'fiercely independent'. By this, he means that she will never accept any offers of help from him (or anyone else, for that matter), nor does she respond in any way other than negatively to compliments or when he buys her presents, even Christmas and birthday presents. He finds this particularly difficult because he has always thought of himself as a genuinely generous person who has always enjoyed giving. One of the effects his wife's negative responses have on him is to make him feel redundant in the relationship. He feels his wife does not need or value him.

On exploring this with his wife, it became apparent that she had developed this so called 'independent' behaviour as a way of coping as a child with a chaotic environment and an alcoholic mother. 'You ought to be grateful' was a frequent saying of her mother's.

She was aware that, as well as causing difficulties for her husband, this behaviour alienated her colleagues at work and annoyed her friends. She decided that she no longer wanted or needed to respond in this way but found it almost impossible to change. She did not know how to respond in this sort of situation.

*After some discussion with the client, the counsellor decided to work directly with the behaviour concerned using a social skills training approach within the session. This involved identifying the 'target situations', identifying the client's **goals** in those situations, doing an **assessment role-play** to identify 'target behaviours', 'training' the target behaviours using **instruction** and **behavioural rehearsal** and **shaping** the behaviours by the use of **feedback** expressed in such a way as to provide **reinforcement**.*

Social skill and the therapeutic relationship

Therapeutic skills are a particular type of social skill. The cognitive components of therapeutic skill such as self-monitoring and social perception which we have discussed above are probably very similar to those required in social situations. The behavioural components, however, are somewhat different.

Although therapeutic skills are influenced by the theoretical orientation and the personal style of the counsellor or therapist, there are an number of skills which are common to most approaches and most therapists. These are the skills which most counsellors and therapists learn during training. Learning is necessary because, for the most part, these skills are not in our existing behavioural repertoire.

The most common behavioural therapeutic skills (verbal and non-verbal) are probably those involved in communication attention and understanding, and facilitating exploration of the client's thoughts, feelings, motives etc. This involves very different 'talker–listener' sequences from those found in social conversation, with the client talking very much more than the listener. This is facilitated by the therapist's use of statements reflecting the manifest, the latent or the emotional content of the client's responses and by the use of 'process questions'. These are questions that are couched in terms that require the client to think further or more deeply on a particular topic.

7.6 INTIMACY AND LOVE

Social psychologists have only fairly recently turned their attention to studying what must surely be the richest and most complex of area of human experience—love.

Love is an emotion (see Chapter 3). As such it is something that happens to you. You do not choose to 'fall in love'; nor can you can you make yourself love another person.

Most people, including social psychologists, would agree that there are different types of love. One widely accepted distinction is that between passionate and companionate love (Hatfield, 1988).

Passionate love is an intensely emotional and absorbing love that involves a high level of physiological arousal and intense yearning for the partner. Sexual feelings are very strong and thoughts of the other frequently intrude on the person's awareness.

Companionate love, on the other hand, involves an affectionate relationship marked by deep caring about the partner's well-being and happiness combined with a commitment to being there for the other (Caspi and Herbener, 1990). It is more stable than passionate love, which sometimes evolves into companionate love over time (Metts et al., 1989).

Part of the difficulty with this approach is that the concepts of passionate love an companionate love are treated as categories rather than dimensions of a relationship. This is not the case in Sternberg's (1988) **triangular model of love**. The three components of this model are

- **passion**—including feelings of romance as well as physical and sexual attraction;
- **intimacy**—the closeness the two people feel for each other and the extent to which they count on each other and share themselves and their possessions with each other;
- **commitment**—the decision to remain in the relationship and the labelling of the relationship as a 'love' relationship.

Variations in the strength of each component gives rise to qualitatively different types of relationship. According to this model, liking that occurs in a close friendship is high in intimacy but low in passion and commitment; passionate or romantic love would involve passion and intimacy, but may lack a meaningful degree of commitment, and what Sternberg refers to as 'fatuous love' (the type of love when two people meet and fall madly in love and marry after a short whirlwind romance) is based on passion and commitment. When passion dies, all that is left is commitment, which is unlikely to survive in the absence of intimacy. Thus fatuous love is often short-lived.

According to Sternberg's model, the most complete and satisfying love is 'consummate love', which involves a high level of all three components (passion, intimacy and commitment). Consummate love is difficult to attain, even harder to maintain but, according to Sternberg, is the ideal basis for long-term intimate relationships.

The models of love presented above are all essentially descriptive. They do not *explain* why different people love in different ways. The **attachment approach** (Shaver et al., 1988) has attempted to do this. There is growing evidence that early attachment to parents or care-givers can have a lasting impact on how we relate to others. A large-scale study has shown that three primary attachment patterns: secure, avoidant and anxious–ambivalent, seen in early child development, manifest themselves in adult relationships.

It seems clear from this study that a pattern of secure early attachments in which the child felt loved and accepted is related to the most positive outcomes in terms of adult relationships. A **secure attachment style** in adulthood was marked by caring, intimacy, supportiveness and understanding. Secure people regarded themselves as friendly, good-natured and likeable and they tended to think of others as generally well-intentioned, reliable and trustworthy. Unfortunately, in this study, this included only 56 per cent of a sample of over 600 adults.

The rest of the sample were divided between the two categories of avoidant and anxious–ambivalent attachment. Those who reported **avoidant attachment** with their parents (feelings of rejection) were uncomfortable with closeness in relationships as adults, feared intimacy, were suspicious, aloof and sceptical about love and tended to pull back when things went wrong in a relationship. The person with an avoidant attachment style tended to see others as either unreliable or overly eager to commit themselves to a relationship.

Finally, the **anxious–ambivalent attachment style** was marked by mixed emotions about relationships. Conflicting feelings of affection, anger, emotional turmoil, physical attraction and doubt often left the person in an unsettled, ambivalent state. People with anxious–ambivalent attachment styles tended to regard themselves as misunderstood and unappreciated. Whilst they wanted to be close to their partners, they were likely to be preoccupied with doubts about their partner's trustworthiness and dependability and beset with worries that their partners did not really love them. They reported a tendency to want to merge completely with their partners, whilst at the same time fearing abandonment by them.

Whilst these findings are intuitively satisfying, the relationship between early attachment and later development is not quite as clear-cut as this study might suggest. The reader is referred to Section 8.4.1 on Attachment and its Consequences for Later Life for a critical discussion of this topic. Nevertheless, the attachment approach to relationships has considerable implications for the counsellor, although this is not to suggest that clients should be pigeon-holed into the various categories. It highlights the importance of early experience on subsequent development; this theme is enlarged upon in the next chapter. The central issue in relation to counselling and therapy though is the extent to which the client who engages in avoidant or anxious–ambivalent relationships can change. Chapter 2 deals with this issue in more detail.

7.7 RELATIONSHIP DECLINE AND BREAKDOWN

There is considerably more written in social psychology about making relationships than about breaking them. Yet many relationships diminish in closeness and some disintegrate entirely.

The reason for, and management of, the disengagement varies with the type of relationship. A friendship may not stand up to reduced frequency of contact due to geographical separation. Other reasons for the decline of friendship are related to friendship 'rules': rewardingness, keeping confidences, standing up for each other and being jealous of other relationships (Argyle and Henderson, 1984).

As we have discussed, there is usually a high level of conflict in close relationships, and couples may not have the skills for resolving conflict peacefully. In both happy and unhappy marriages it has been found that men tend to respond to anger from their spouse with anger of their own. But in happy marriages the cycle of angry reactions is broken, usually by the wife, allowing the couple to deal with the problem more calmly at a later stage. In contrast, in unhappy marriages, both husband and wife fall into a cycle of trading increasingly angry and hurtful remarks, minor irritations escalate, blame is attributed to the other and communication breaks down (Gottman, 1979). Typical sources of conflict are money, unfaithfulness, in-laws and drink. Often in the breakdown of the relationship there is a precipitating event, such as violence, drunkenness or infidelity. This is followed by a period of separation, which may become permanent (Argyle and Henderson, 1985).

Depression is a common response to relationship breakdown and may be associated with loneliness, apathy, sadness and regret. A person's role in the separation will affect the likelihood of depression. The person who wants to end the relationship is less likely to be depressed when it does end than the one on the receiving end. This may be the result of feelings of helplessness and impotence which are often associated with depression. Here the counsellor may be able to help the client take more control over their situation, thereby increasing their sense of self-efficacy.

An obsessive mental recapitulation of events may occur in which scenes are replayed repeatedly. From this the person develops an account of the breakdown that becomes incorporated into their self-concept. This account can present a version of events that supports and protects that person's self. It may enable the person to feel stronger and more in control in the short-term, but may not be helpful in the longer-term.

In traditional relationships and contexts, a man may to some extent be protected by maintaining self-esteem through his work-role. This may also serve as an important source of distraction and routine. However, men may have fewer opportunities than women for emotional expression, and be left with unresolved feelings of conflict and grief. Repression of these feelings may give the man a short-term sense of being in control but may result in a new set of problems and difficulties.

Women, on the other hand, are more likely to have a network of women friends to whom they can unburden themselves, but may not have the work-role to bolster their self-esteem. Professional women could come off worst of all. Although they have their work-role and identity, they may find it difficult to repress painful feelings; as a result their work becomes a source of stress and they may additionally, be reluctant to admit to needing professional help.

Finally, both ex-partners' life-style may change. Financial resources may be reduced, especially for women, and both may have to relinquish old roles, take on new ones and possibly develop new personal and social identities.

7.8 LESBIAN AND GAY RELATIONSHIPS

Whilst there are many similarities between heterosexual and lesbian and gay relationships, there are also some significant differences.

These relationships are often portrayed as intrinsically unstable and short-lived. However, the difficulties involved in establishing and maintaining any relationship are multiplied if the relationship is unacknowledged, devalued and unsupported by significant others in the partners' social network. This lack of support from heterosexual significant others often characterizes lesbian and gay relationships (Kurdek and Schmitt, 1987) and may make them harder to sustain. Thus the belief that gay and lesbian relationships are short-lived may become a self-fulfilling prophecy.

Peplau and Cochran (1990) reviewed research on lesbian and gay relationships and reported that between 45 and 80 per cent of lesbians and between 40 and 60 per cent of gay men are involved in steady relationships. The factors that influence the success and longevity of heterosexual relationships also tend to be important in lesbian and gay relationships. For example, lesbian and gay relationships tend to last if the partners are from similar backgrounds and have a similar level of commitment to the relationship (Peplau, 1991). The processes that influence relationship satisfaction have also been found to be similar across lesbian, gay and heterosexual relationships (Kurdek, 1994).

However, the nature and structure of lesbian and gay relationships may differ considerably from heterosexual relationships (Kitzinger and Coyle, 1995). One potential area of difference concerns 'rules' about sexual exclusivity (Davies et al., 1993). However, the process of negotiating sexual non-exclusivity may be difficult as there is no social 'script' to guide the process.

There may also be differences between heterosexual and lesbian and gay relationships in terms of how power is distributed between partners. Research has suggested that in lesbian relationships, power tends to be fairly equally distributed, whereas in gay male relationships, as in heterosexual relationships, the partner with the higher income tends to have more power (Blumstein and Schwartz, 1983).

The end of lesbian and gay relationships may present particular difficulties for those involved. For example, the tendency to equate attractiveness with youthfulness is particularly noticeable in gay male social contexts and publications. For older gay men who have experienced a relationship break-down, fears about being unable to secure another partner may therefore be particularly acute. Also, if a lesbian or gay man is concerned about the potential negative effects of disclosing their sexual identity to others, relatively few people in their social network may be aware that they were involved in a relationship. Hence, if that relationship ends, there may be little support offered by members of the individual's social network.

If the partners in the relationship have chosen to make the relationship known to only a small number of people, this may also limit the provision of social support in the event of the death of one partner. The family of the person who has died may exclude or marginalize the bereaved partner in funeral arrangements and mourning rituals. This denial of the nature and/or significance of the relationship that has been lost may exacerbate the distress of the surviving partner. The bereavement experiences of gay men who have lost partners to AIDS are further complicated by the social stigma associated with this condition. This further reduces the chances of the bereaved individual receiving adequate social support. This factor, together with the possibility of gay men experiencing multiple bereavement as members of their social network succumb to AIDS, renders AIDS bereavement a particularly traumatic experience for gay men who are affected by it (Wright, 1993).

Counsellors and therapists working with lesbians and gay men who have lost partners therefore need to assess the level of social support and to explore possible new sources. If counsellors are informed about and comfortable with lesbian and gay issues, they themselves can provide effective social support through the counselling sessions.

Finally, counsellors working more generally on relationship issues should be aware of the implications of the research which highlights the differences between lesbian, gay and heterosexual relationships and should avoid generalizing from heterosexual relationships to lesbian and gay relationships and indeed from gay male relationships to lesbian relationships.

7.9 CONCLUDING COMMENTS

This chapter has presented some of the main areas of theory and research into making, maintaining and ending relationships. In conducting much of their research, social psychologists have moved out of the laboratory and into the supposedly real world. It is, however, a somewhat restricted world. Many of the existing models of relationships take for granted a traditional marital and family paradigm and fail to take into account the context of the relationship. For example, feminists assert that by defining marital problems in purely relational terms, power relationships, which can be particularly problematic in situations of violence, are omitted from many analyses of marital patterns (Alexander et al., 1994)

There are of course a number of different treatment philosophies, models and techniques for working with marital and relationship difficulties. These include marital behaviour therapy, cognitive-behavioural marital therapy, emotionally focused marital therapy and insight-oriented marital therapy. It is beyond the scope of this chapter to review these approaches. Rather, we have presented an outline of the theory and research on which some of these therapeutic approaches are based or on which they draw.

The counselling relationship is a particular type of relationship; one which probably has no parallel in the lives of most clients. Although this chapter has mainly been concerned with the development of close social and intimate relationships, as we have demonstrated, much of the work in this field is of relevance to the counselling relationship.

However, in extrapolating from the social–psychological literature on self and relationships there are an number of factors which counsellors and therapists need to take into consideration.

Firstly, in working on relationships, it is important to avoid **reductionism** which leads to a focus on individuals rather than on the unit (the couple or the family) or on the interaction. So, for instance, when looking at the communication within a relationship the sequencing of messages and the pattern of sequential interaction is as important as what any one person might say.

Secondly, **cognitive, affective and behavioural aspects** should all be taken into account when exploring relationship issues. Behavioural aspects of course include both **verbal and non-verbal** elements. It is possible that different messages are being transmitted by different channels, thus resulting in an inconsistent message.

Thirdly, we need to keep in mind the **dynamic** nature of relationships. Processes such as attraction, attribution and exchange interact with each other and may be differentially salient at different times throughout the course of a relationship. So what may be good for a relationship at one time may not be so later and vice versa. Thus, we need to focus on the integration and interaction of these different processes in a dynamic model which highlights the constantly fluctuating and evolving nature of human relationships.

Finally, as it is all too clear, it has not been possible to capture the richness, depth and diversity of human relationships in psychological theory and research. For that, one has probably to turn to literature, to dance, art or philosophy—and to real life.

8

Lifespan Development: Infancy and Childhood

Alyson Davis

CONTENTS

8.1 INTRODUCTION

The first aim of this chapter is to present a select summary of the issues currently being explored by **developmental psychologists** in their attempts to describe and explain development in childhood. A good deal is known about the abilities of children at different ages and how children develop; but providing a summary of such developmental milestones would barely meet the aims of this volume and would do little more than replicate what is already available in developmental text books.

Instead, 'themes' will be presented which have relevance to those involved in counselling and therapy where the evidence is particularly compelling or intriguing. This has the added advantage of bypassing the traditional sections on cognitive, social, linguistic and motor development which provide rather artificial distinctions in our understanding of early life.

Although written with the particular interests of counsellors in mind, the content of this chapter is not based on psychopathology. In other words it does not concentrate on development which 'goes wrong'. Rather it looks at normal development and what is known about that, instead of focusing on gross deviations from development.

There are good reasons for taking this stance. Firstly, many people who seek counselling in life either as children, adolescents or adults have undergone 'normal' rather than abnormal development. Secondly, even where development is exceptional to the norm, the explanation of such development is often better understood in terms of its deviation from the norm rather than being treated as a totally independent account of abnormality.

The second aim concerns an overarching issue about the status of childhood. Most of us attribute to childhood unique qualities. We assume it has a privileged position in the lifespan regarding the role our early experiences play in later adult life. We marvel at those who have emotionally and materially successful adult lives despite having deprived or unhappy childhoods. Yet at the same time we are tempted to interpret failure or deviancy in later life in terms of 'difficult' childhood experiences. In other words, we interpret the world assuming a good deal of continuity between stages of development and are surprised by instances of discontinuity. Are we right to do so? This question is addressed most directly in the section on early relationships but it pervades the whole of the chapter.

8.2 WHERE DOES PSYCHOLOGICAL DEVELOPMENT BEGIN?

Development is characterized by age-related changes which are progressive and result in behavioural change and in many cases psychological advance. The abilities of, say, the three year old are not only different from the three month old, they are also an advance on earlier skills. This principle is most clearly demonstrated in motor development. The motor skills of the toddler who can run, skip and hop are not only different from the young baby, they also incorporate and build on those earlier abilities. But where should the study of development begin?

Psychologists, understandably have began with birth; the point when the infant literally enters the world. However, more recently, changes in theoretical standpoints coupled with changes in technology have shifted our starting point for studying psychological development. 'Real-time' ultrasound scanners allow us to observe the baby *in utero*, giving us privileged access to behaviour before birth. Likewise sensory development in the latter stages of foetal development are well documented, including thumb-sucking and startle responses. Thus while birth represents a crucial point in life (the newborn must breathe for the first time, experience a totally new sensory and psychological environment) it is not necessarily the starting point for psychological development.

For example, research has provided good evidence for *in utero* learning. During the last month of foetal development hearing is well developed such that external sounds like the mother's voice or music can be heard above the considerable noise of intrauterine life. This sensory capacity has been shown to have psychological significance too. Spence and DeCasper (1982) have shown that newborns exposed to a particular piece of prose their mothers repeated to them *in utero* showed a preference for that piece over another and even prefer the familiar piece spoken by the mother rather than another person. The significance of this type of finding lies not just in terms of its confirmation of the sensory capacities of the foetus, but it suggests that the foetus is capable of learning—the newborn actually recognizes the prose and the speaker as in some way being familiar.

There are two points to be made in the face of this kind of evidence. First it shows that developmental psychology must literally take a step back and seriously consider development before birth. The second is more controversial. This kind of evidence of psychological life before birth may in the longer term give scientific credence to psychoanalytic accounts of early development which propose that the very earliest of experiences are of real psychological relevance.

8.3 MODELS OF THE 'COMPETENT' CHILD

If one were asked to identify a single change in developmental psychology over the last 30 years then the one which most developmentalists would offer is the general shift in our attitudes to infant and child competence. We have moved from a distinctly negative view of early life towards a much more positive one.

Piaget, the scientist who almost single handedly put developmental psychology on the map, characterized development as a rather gradual (although highly successful) process. In doing so he inevitably focused on those abilities lacking at earlier stages of development which then constituted the achievements of later development. Thus, perhaps almost by default, he drew attention to what babies and young children could *not* do rather than what they can do.

This trend has in recent years has been reversed. Today, developmental psychologists paint a rather different picture by concentrating more on the achievements and competencies of early development rather than their deficits. There are endless examples to chose from so it has been necessary to be selective.

8.3.1 Achievements of Early Infancy

Our characterization of the competence (both cognitive and social) of infants has shown the most dramatic shift. William James (1890) described the world of the newborn as one of 'a blooming buzzing confusion' and the newborn as a 'lowly piece of unformed protoplasm'. If this were the case then the young baby could not even merit psychological enquiry.

However, we now know that this attitude to early infancy is quite simply wrong. The neonate has remarkably well-developed sensory capacities, particularly vision and even the ability for complex learning (Papousek, 1967). Of all the evidence on neonatal skill two areas of research will be discussed which illustrate the general point particularly well while at the same time having profound implications for later social life.

During the first two years of life the infant learns about the world of objects and people and even how to talk about that world. This mastery is quite remarkable. Many of the prerequisite skills for this development are either innate or learned very rapidly and therefore provide something of an explanation for the achievements of infancy. But precisely how does development take place? Why is it that infants take so little time in coming to terms with the world and become active participants in it?

It is tempting to suppose that we must appeal to nativist arguments, in other words that these skills are pre-wired genetically and unfold in much the same way as motor development does as a sequence of inevitable ordered events relatively unaffected by environmental influence. Alternatively, we might be tempted to argue that early development is so successful because of the extraordinary expertise with which adults structure and impact on the baby's first few months thus literally creating development on behalf of the child.

Both these viewpoints are reflected in psychological theory to a greater or lesser extent and the problem for developmental psychologists is not to choose between the two but to specify the nature of their interaction. Two quite contrasting examples illustrate this point.

The first example comes from work on early face recognition. There is currently an ongoing debate in the scientific literature concerning the age at which infants recognize faces and the mechanisms involved in doing so. It is a classic example of the nature/nurture debate. Is the ability to recognize the human face inborn—pre-wired in some way or is the ability to recognize faces learned more gradually over time?

This kind of question has obvious interest to those interested in early cognition, but there are more than cognitive skills at stake here. Recognition of the mother's face has enormous implications for those who want to propose early social, as well as cognitive, competence to the young baby. Some recent work in this area has fuelled both the specific debate and contributed to our recasting of early social competence.

Work by Ian Bushnell and colleagues (Bushnell et al., 1989; Sai and Bushnell, 1988) has shown that within the first few days (and in some cases hours) of life the neonate can distinguish her/his mother from that of a stranger of similar appearance. Moreover, these newborns do so on the basis of visual rather than olfactory, auditory or other cues. The finding is quite staggering as a measure of visual competence and so are its implications for social development. This finding of a skill within the first few weeks of life is usually taken as evidence of innate capacity.

However, in this instance it would be ridiculous to propose infants are born knowing what their mothers look like! Furthermore, Bushnell's evidence from a further study shows that some learning is clearly involved since he found that infants recognize their mothers in full face and half-profile some time before they recognize the profile view. Here is early knowledge which can be measured in the very first weeks of life but which clearly involves environmental experience. Before looking at a possible explanation of these findings we move on to consider another example which challenges the conceptualization of nature versus nurture as a dichotomy.

This second example concerns the theoretical claims about imitation. The debate here again centres on the question about the role of imitation in general as an explanation of developmental change, and the issue concerning the age of onset, i.e. when can babies first imitate?

Learning theorists such as Skinner proposed that imitation is fundamental to human learning. He even went as far as arguing that language development could be accounted for by appeal to these principles. The young infant vocalizes, and parents, Skinner argued, selectively reinforce those vocalizations which best approximate the words of their native language, thus increasing the frequency of their production by the baby.

Unfortunately, however, the argument simply does not hold. Chomsky pointed out that as an explanation of language development, this theory suffered from fatal flaws. Firstly, language development is far too rapid to explain it in terms of imitation. Secondly (and more seriously) children make systematic errors in their language which quite simply cannot be imitated from adults, since adults do not make these types of mistakes. For example, children make errors of over-regularization—'he goed' instead of 'he went' or 'she's house' instead of 'her house'. Chomsky argued that these creative errors can only be explained by an innate sensitivity to the regularity of language rather than appeal to imitation. Thus imitation cannot be the sole or primary mechanism of language development.

This said, it would be ridiculous to dismiss the role of imitation altogether. The fact that children acquire their native language (be it English, French or Japanese) rather than some developmental form of Esperanto, indicates that imitation does occur. Beyond the example of language learning, most of us would accept it is bizarre to assume that imitation is psychologically irrelevant. Many skills acquired throughout the lifespan stem from the simple but powerful fact that human skills and behaviour are directly displayed by others and by the simple act of copying many of these are available to the less knowledgeable or able individual.

Piaget, like Chomsky, was at pains to marginalize the role of imitation for fear that his account might seem compatible with learning theory and thus undermine the significant role played by the child in development. Piaget avoided this dilemma by proposing that imitation needed prerequisite cognitive skills and therefore true imitation comes relatively late in infancy when the child has already established the very bases of mental representation.

However, recent evidence by Meltzoff and Moore (1983) has shown that soon after birth infants have the capacity for deferred imitation, a capacity which Piaget denied them until well into the second year of life. Meltzoff has shown that certain gestures (such as tongue protrusion) displayed by an adult will be reliably copied by newborn babies, demonstrating the capacity to imitate others from the very beginnings of life.

These two examples, neonatal recognition of the mother, and early imitation, present a powerful challenge to our conception of early life. Both demonstrate the remarkable competence of infants and yet neither forces us to appeal to innate mechanisms or environmental influence alone. Both Bushnell and Meltzoff account for their findings in terms of a capacity known as **cross-modal mapping**, which refers to the infant's ability to treat sensory input from the different modalities as equivalent.

This explanation means that we need neither appeal to innate devices nor resort to the primacy of environmental influence. Instead, it supposes we acknowledge the rapidity of learning made possible by a cognitive mechanism which ensures that the newborn is maximally sensitive to the environment, especially the social world.

The impact of this type of research in changing the way we think about infancy has been matched by research on development in childhood. Again, there has been a marked shift towards describing and explaining the impressive abilities of the young child rather than simply describing their cognitive and social deficits relative to older children. In almost every aspect of development children below the age of 6 or 7 have been shown to have remarkable abilities which are denied them under Piagetian theory.

8.3.2 Cognitive Competence in Childhood

The young child has been shown to be a competent thinker (Donaldson, 1978), to be capable of inferential and deductive reasoning (Bryant, 1972), to have adult-like memory capacity (Chi, 1978) and even to be mathematically able (Gelman and Gallistel, 1978). The list is apparently endless. So, are there no differences between the 5-year-old and adults in terms of cognitive ability?

The research, which suggests extraordinary competence in children, also reveals that children can only operate 'like adults' under rather specific conditions—their ability is highly **contextually sensitive** or **domain-specific**. In other words their ability to succeed on the various cognitive tasks used to test them depends on the way the task is presented, their familiarity with the area and the context of the task itself, particularly the social context and interaction between adult and child. In short it shows that children can reason properly and perform (simple) mathematics when the task is presented in a way which is meaningful to them, when they understand the adult's intentions and when they understand the nature of the task. Without this kind of contextual support, young children make just the kinds of mistakes that we might expect from them taking a traditional Piagetian perspective.

The important point about our characterization of the child (as opposed to the infant) as being cognitively able in specific contexts is that it highlights the social sensitivity of the young child by showing that even thinking itself cannot be understood without reference to a consideration of social aspects.

The social world is as important to the young child's understanding as it is to the young infant and social development cannot really be easily separated from cognitive development nor vice versa. Furthermore, we know that adults, like children, are susceptible to similar kinds of contextual influence. The gap between adult and child is far less than previously thought.

Typically then the model of the competent child is represented as having impressive cognitive skill but this should be considered in a social context. From an applied perspective there are clearly important educational implications at stake about the way that children are taught in schools. But there is also a wider implication that lies at the centre of those who become involved with children in any kind of counselling context—namely that we must take children and what they say more seriously.

We cannot automatically dismiss their claims or behaviour as being a result of their failure to understand (although this will of course sometimes be the case) because of 'their age'. Instead, we are obliged, given the weight of the psychological evidence about precocious cognitive capacity, to take a closer look at the precise context of the behaviour. An example should illustrate this point.

There has long been a debate as to the validity of children as witnesses in legal cases. It used to be thought that children, before their teens, made unreliable witnesses because they lacked the memory capacity of adults, or they were more prone to distort their evidence. The most recent research evidence suggests, similarly to the general research on cognitive skills, that this need not be so. Rather it seems that children, like adults, are vulnerable to the passage of time in terms of their accuracy of recall but that they are no more prone to make outlandish claims about what they have seen or what has happened to them than adults (Dent and Flin, 1992). While this research has been concerned specifically with addressing questions about eye witness testimony, it has broader implications for those of us who deal with children and have little else to go on except what they literally tell us.

So far in this section, a rather general view of development has been taken without specific reference to individual differences in children or adults. Before moving on to looking at questions about the nature of relationships it is appropriate to take a step back and consider some of the striking differences which are known to exist between children, and between the way that different adults relate to their children even at the most basic level.

8.3.3 Individual Differences and Temperament

Many students of psychology express their disappointment that psychology seems to spend so little time explaining the difference between people, since this is what, for many of them, the very role of psychology should be—why some people act in one way while others act in another. Developmental psychology has found itself particularly focused on questions of universals—those developments which occur without cultural or individual variation. But there are some notable exceptions.

An obvious exception is in the field of developmental behaviour genetics, the area which attempts to describe biological constraints on behaviour. For example, how far is hyperactivity or autism explained in terms of genetic predisposition? But there are also examples from within mainstream developmental psychology which point quite distinctly to aspects of development which seem to be sensitive to differences between individual children or differences between the way that adults respond to children. I shall take an example of each of these to illustrate the importance of variation in development. The first relates to infant temperament.

A colleague once described temperament as something you believe in if you have more than one child. Books on child care and infant behaviour are full of rhetoric about the well-managed baby who sleeps for four-hour stretches and then feeds before entering a further four-hour sleep. It is true that some infants do precisely just this (although who has ever met one?) but most do not. How can we explain why within a family one child will always sleep through the night while another with equal consistency will never do so? Similar differences in behaviour can be found for eating and crying patterns as well as differing reactions to psychological stimuli.

Interestingly, many explanations such as learning theory rely on appeal to environmental influences, particularly parental (especially mother's) behaviour, and there is good research evidence to show how child care practices do influence infant behaviour. The most striking evidence can be found in cross-cultural studies; for example Super and Harkness, (1982) found that in the Kipsigis people in Kenya where infants spend most of their time day and night with their mothers, there is no tendency toward a pattern of day-time waking and night-time sleeping. In fact in their study, the longest period of time which these young infants slept was 4.5 hours compared with 8 hours in the western sample of infants.

At some level then, behaviour is controlled and adapted to social patterns and influence and provides an explanation of cultural differences. But what of individual differences between children within a given culture or family?

The pioneering work on this question was carried out by Thomas and Chess (1977), whose original longitudinal study, following children over time, showed that from birth, infants show marked temperamental differences. They identified three main clusters of temperament: easy, difficult and slow to warm up.

- **The easy child** is one who is generally in a positive mood, quickly adapts to routines and new experiences.
- **The difficult child** on the other hand tends to cry frequently, reacts negatively and is irregular in routines.
- **The slow to warm up child** is characterized by a low activity level and is less adaptable.

In terms of frequency the figures are approximately 40 per cent, 10 per cent and 15 per cent respectively for the three groups and the claim is that these basic temperamental characteristics remain reasonably stable across childhood.

This suggests a powerful genetic link with temperament which has some support from the various twin studies which have been carried out. Nevertheless, there is also an important link between the infant's temperament and parental behaviour and it seems that the critical factor is the match between infant temperament and various parental attributes (Plomin and Thompson, 1987).

While an easy infant literally makes the job of parenting easier, characteristics of parental temperament and behaviour can have a significant outcome on the child as well. In other words infants can influence their parents as well as parents influencing their children. Even the most dedicated behaviour geneticists focus as much on these gene–environment interactions as they do on trying to pursue a heritability index alone. Indeed, intelligence itself is now couched in these terms and hence shifted the debate from the original argument of nature versus nurture.

These pronounced interactions between biological constraints and environmental factors lie at the heart of much research in developmental psychology today and frequently add to the debate about cause and effect in development. The point is that we have reached a position where the debate is an appropriate one, but it is an extremely difficult task to specify the nature of the interaction.

8.4 EARLY RELATIONSHIPS AND THEIR IMPACT ON DEVELOPMENT

The question of the role of early experience in determining later development is central to this chapter but as indicated already in the preceding sections, there are no easy answers. However, in this section the problem will be tackled head on as we move to consider early emotional relationships and their later impact. Before looking at the available evidence and associated theories some key issues will be outlined which psychologists must deal with, and which act as qualifying statements on what is probably a widely held belief in the special nature of childhood.

The first is evidential. What evidence do we have that childhood exerts an influence on later life? Are there scientific grounds for believing in the potency of childhood? Secondly, is there reason to believe that early experiences are more important than later ones in determining psychological well being? That is, should we credit childhood with a privileged position over adolescent or adult experiences? Thirdly, are there some experiences which are critical in their influence? This supposes that some early experiences will leave such a pronounced long-term mark that no later compensatory ones will erase the early damage or early benefit. Finally, are there periods of development within childhood itself which are peculiarly psychologically sensitive which need to be recognized as such?

Good answers to these questions would indeed provide a remarkable spring-board to anyone involved in counselling others, be they adults or children. If such answers could be given they would carry with them prescriptions about how to deal with adults experiencing difficulties as well as providing hard and fast rules about parenting and child care. Furthermore, we might make informed guesses as to how to compensate those whose early lives were in some way lacking, and even make decisions as to who would or would not benefit from counselling or some such psychological intervention.

The questions as outlined above have all been addressed by psychological theory and research to a greater or lesser extent. The ways in which these questions have been tackled will be discussed, even where the answers turn out to be less than clear cut.

8.4.1 Attachment and its Consequences for Later Life

Attachment refers to a close emotional relationship between the infant and primary care-giver. Developmental psychologists have been exploring the nature of this relationship and its consequences since it was argued by Freud and later by John Bowlby to be so critical to normal emotional development. Freud (as we discussed in Chapter 2) argued that infants become attached to the person (usually the mother) who provides oral satisfaction. However, in a renowned series of studies by Harlow (e.g. Harlow and Zimmerman, 1959) it was found that food and oral gratification were not the prime source of infant attachment. Harlow's results found that when monkeys were separated from their mothers at birth and 'raised' by two surrogate mothers one made of wire which supplied food and one made of cloth, they spent more time with the cloth surrogate than the wire mother even though it was the latter who provided the food. Furthermore, the monkeys used the cloth mother as a source of comfort when faced with novel and threatening events in preference to the wire mother. These findings suggested, that for infant monkeys at least, it is contact comfort which the infant seeks rather than food *per se*.

In terms of human relationships the most influential figure in the field has been John Bowlby (e.g. Bowlby, 1953, 1980) who emphasized the central nature of early mother–child attachment and took psychoanalytic claims about its impact on later development much further than Freud had done. Bowlby's early claims (Bowlby, 1953) about mother infant attachment centred on his belief that the mental health of infants depended on having a 'warm, intimate and continuous relationship with his mother' (p. 13).

There are two key aspects of this claim which need exploring. Firstly, Bowlby's argument was concerned with a 'monotropic' relationship—i.e. a single attachment with the mother. Secondly, he argued that the attachment must be continuous and not disrupted. Following from these criteria Bowlby supposed that the damage which would result from either failure to form a satisfactory attachment very early in life or for an attachment to be broken due to mother–infant separation was inevitable and irreversible. In addition, Bowlby was influenced by ethological theory which supposed that there are critical periods of development during which attachments must be made.

These claims have far reaching implications about the type of early relationships and the proposed disasters which will ensue for the infant in later life if these are not satisfactory. In support of his claim, Bowlby appealed to evidence from Goldfarb (1945) on the effects of institutional rearing of infants. Goldfarb had shown that children separated from their mothers and raised in institutions were at significant risk of developing profound personality disorders in later life compared to children raised in normal family units.

Yet, the original argument went beyond claims of negative effects of childhoods spent in institutions, since even the briefest separation from the mother (such as hospitalization) would have profound effects. A whole area of research developed concerning the effects of 'maternal deprivation' based on Bowlby's claims.

Much of the most recent research has taken a highly critical stance to Bowlby's extreme position and does so on the basis of good evidence. Before considering this evidence it is worth putting Bowlby's work in perspective. Like any major figure in psychology who has written over a long period of time, history tends to report a rather static view of his work. In doing so the fact that Bowlby altered his views quite dramatically in his later writing (e.g. Bowlby, 1988) is often overlooked.

Secondly, it is somewhat ironic that it was the most extreme and most criticized aspects of Bowlby's work which has had the most impact on social policy. For example, Bowlby was instrumental in changing existing hospital policy about allowing parents to stay with their children in hospital. Rudolph Shaffer, who worked with Bowlby in the 1950s, talked of his dread of Sunday afternoons when parents made their weekly visits to see their sick children. He spoke of the sounds of children crying on their parents' departure knowing that another week must pass until their next visit. Today parents can visit their children freely and even stay with them throughout periods of hospitalization as a result of Bowlby's work. He successfully put emotional life on the agenda of policy makers and furthermore was even more successful than Freud theoretically in so far as attachment has remained a key issue in developmental research to this day.

The argument which has raged more recently then is less about whether we should explore early relationships or ignore them, and more about the particular emphases of Bowlby's work. The first aspect to be discussed concerns Bowlby's claim of the primacy of the mother–child relationship and its monotropic nature. Is it the case that infants only form relationships with a single person and does this have to be the biological mother?

The evidence is clear cut. There is now overwhelming evidence to show that by the age of 18 months infants can form multiple attachments (to mothers, fathers, siblings and other care-givers) (Schaeffer and Emerson, 1964). Furthermore, it is also evident that the quality of attachment is not diluted in any sense by having multiple attachments. In short, this aspect of Bowlby's argument has not stood up to the empirical test.

The second aspect of Bowlby's theory under dispute is the claim that the attachment relationships need to be continuous—in other words that the attachment bond cannot withstand even minor disruptions. Again, the evidence forces us to be highly sceptical of this. In a review of the evidence, Rutter (1981) demonstrates the resilience of children, and the attachment relationship, to withstand temporary and even long-term breakdowns of the primary attachment. Rutter shows that the key factors in determining the effects of short- and long-term separation include: the reasons for the separation taking place, the quality of 'substitute' attachments available during the separation phase and the quality of the relationship on reunion. In addition Rutter points out that there are multiple reasons for disruption of any relationship and that these have differential effects on outcome.

The third claim which needs unpacking relates to the suggestion from Bowlby that disruption of the attachment bond has **irreversible** consequences. Within the literature there are some documented cases (thankfully very few) of children whose early lives have been deprived of the most basic of human relationships (see Skuse, 1984 for a review) alongside other deprivations; where children have been given only the minimum of food to keep them alive but deprived of human interaction altogether. These tragic cases are testimony to the resilience of development and provide evidence against Bowlby's claim by showing that the effects of early deprivation are reversible. The psychological outcome of these children following their eventual discovery is varied but some common patterns emerge.

Firstly, recovery from the deprivation is typically extremely rapid indeed. Secondly, the key predictor in determining the long-term outcome is the *quality* of care following discovery. In other words, where children are removed from their deprived environments and placed in the context of loving, caring relationships the prognosis for near normal development is extremely good indeed. In fact Thompson (1986) cites the case of a toddler having experienced no interpersonal relationships in his early life, on being adopted by a family, going on to excel academically at school and being emotionally indistinguishable from his peers. The evidence suggests quite clearly that negative early experiences can be compensated for by good quality later emotional experiences.

So far then, in this section it has been argued that we must be sceptical about general principles which suppose that early relationships must be singular, with the biological mother and continuous. In its place we have support for the resilience of human infants to form multiple attachments and recover from either failure to form initial relationships or from the disruption of those early bonds. From this it is clear that counsellors and therapists should not 'jump to conclusions' about the possible effects of early separation.

But throughout this discussion the issue of the way in which early attachments are assessed by psychologists and the role of individual differences in attachment behaviour has been avoided. In order to understand the way attachment theory has developed over the last few decades it is essential to consider the measurement of attachment, since this provides the very basis from which attachment theory has maintained its claims over the importance of early experience on later development.

8.4.2 The Assessment of Attachment

At the heart of attachment theory lies the notion of individual differences between children and their relationships with their care-givers. It is only in psychologists' ability to classify attachments differently that they can make claims about the outcome of having 'good' or 'bad' attachments. So how do we assess the quality of these early relationships? The vast majority of studies rely on what is known as the **strange situation paradigm** which is usually (but not always) carried out in a laboratory setting.

The strange situation was pioneered by Ainsworth et al., (1978) and involves a series of short episodes in which infants (between 6 and 24 months) are observed. In the typical situation the mother and baby are left for about 3 minutes together, at which point an unfamiliar adult (the stranger) enters the room. After a further three minutes the mother departs, leaving the baby alone with the stranger before returning again after a further three-minute interval at which point the stranger departs. The infant's response during all the episodes is observed with particular attention being paid to his or her reaction to the mother's departure and the subsequent reunion. The evidence from large numbers of studies employing this paradigm suggests that there are three main categories of attachment.

- **Group A: anxious–avoidant** (approximately 15–20 per cent). This group of infants actively avoid reunion with their mothers on her return despite not having been particularly happy when left with the stranger.
- **Group B: secure** (approximately 60 per cent). Securely attached infants are content with the strange situation as long as the mother is present but show distress on her departure. However, they soon settle when she returns.
- **Group C: anxious–ambivalent** (approximately 15–20 per cent). These infants show ambivalent relationships towards their mothers. Prior to separation they may seek such close proximity to her that they avoid exploration and yet on reunion (following the separation period) they may actively avoid her.

Attachment measures in infancy have been used as predictors of later developmental outcome. A review by Thompson and Lamb (1986) found that secure attachment is associated with good social functioning in the pre-school years and other studies (as discussed in Section 7.6 on Intimacy and Love) have found links much later in life (Shaver et al., 1988). Moreover, securely attached infants have been found to out-perform insecurely attached groups on various cognitive measures which suggests that adequate relationships early in life may impact on all round psychological well-being in later development. These findings must be taken with caution, however, since they rely on the reliability and validity of the strange situation as a measure of quality of attachment.

The strange situation does show reasonable retest reliability in so far as children classified as securely attached during one testing session are likely to be classified in the same way at some subsequent testing but there are some worrying exceptions to this general trend. For example Thompson et al. (1982) found that approximately 50 per cent of infants actually changed their attachment classification during their second year of life. Even if we accept that the strange situation is a reliable measure this still leaves us with the larger problem of its validity. To what extent does the strange situation really assess the quality of mother–infant relationships?

Some researchers such as Kagan (1989) have questioned the role of temperament in determining the infant's response to the strange situation irrespective of the attachment itself. In a similar vein, Clarke-Stewart (1989) has argued that the strange situation is an invalid test for children of working mothers since the paradigm itself involves a situation which is 'strange' for children of non-working mothers but which is, in fact, very familiar to those of working mothers. Given the large and increasing numbers of children who are cared for by friends, relatives and other carers while the mother works, this criticism of the attachment literature needs to be taken very seriously indeed.

The general claim that emanated from Bowlby's writings that early relationships, particularly the mother–child relationship, are the *key* to explaining later difficulties does not hold. The fact that infants form multiple relationships from early on, coupled with Rutter's repeated claims that it is the quality of the relationship following any period of separation which determines psychological prognosis, forces us to take on board a more sophisticated analysis of the relationship between early and later development.

The exclusive focus on *mother–child* relationships has seriously disadvantaged our understanding of the value of social support networks throughout the lifespan in determining psychological well-being. This mother-centrism exists as a commonly held lay-belief as much as it does in psychological research. Fortunately more recent researchers have begun to acknowledge this and the shift towards broader social networks involving other family members and peers is discussed in the following sections.

8.5 BEYOND THE MOTHER

When Bowlby and others talked about primary attachments, they were generally referring to traditional families in which the mother is the primary care-giver. Here we look at the influence of other family members on the development of the child.

8.5.1 Father Influence

Developmental psychologists began to show an interest in father–child relationships in the 1960s. At around that time it was becoming clear from research that many young children were attached equally to both parents, and in some cases showed preference for their fathers (e.g. Schaeffer and Emerson, 1964). But, to a large extent this early interest mirrored work that had been carried out earlier on mother–child relationships. Questions were asked about whether infants could in fact form attachments to their fathers and whether fathers could interact with their infants in the same way as mothers.

The answers were clear cut and affirmative. Studies from the delivery room to the school room showed that mutually warm relationships existed between fathers and their children. Initially, then, the psychologists' interest in fathers was to establish the similarity between both parents in terms of their psychological impact. Prior concern about 'maternal deprivation' was matched by equally emotive concern about 'father absence' and this research (perhaps not surprisingly) was met with the same types of evidential and theoretical criticism.

By the end of the 1970s the focus had shifted towards acknowledging the different roles of both parents as a result of two types of emerging evidence. Firstly, with regard to child care, there was overwhelming evidence that fathers, while perfectly competent at caring for their offspring, in practice did so very rarely! (see for example Lewis, 1986). Secondly, another set of questions was being asked about the father's long-term effect on children's psychological development.

The results of this research showed that fathers interacted quite differently with their children than did mothers, with correspondingly differential effects on development. Fathers tend to engage in direct physical 'rough and tumble' play and direct tutoring of objects. In contrast, mothers tend to interact more calmly and in a way which promoted their children's linguistic development. The stage was set for an explanation of complementary parental roles which while being quite distinct are both equally essential for development.

This rather rosy picture of family life in which mother and father contribute in different but equally valuable ways has been disturbed by social reality and by the emerging research evidence. The problem is that for many children life does not consist of two parents (a working father and mother at home). Many families consist of single parents and even the most stable of middle class homes often have mothers who are working.

Similarly, research on professional working mothers (Brannen and Moss, 1987) showed that despite widely held beliefs by both parents that child care and responsibility for children should be shared equally, in the vast majority of the cases it was the mothers who took prime responsibility for both the day-to-day provision of child care and wider issues about children's schooling and general welfare. This suggests we need to take a much broader perspective when we consider family influences on child development.

8.5.2 Sibling Influence

Over the last 20 years psychologists' concern with the family has extended from a focus on mothers and then fathers to an acknowledgment of the potential impact of siblings. Siblings are a normal part of family life—around 80 per cent of children share their childhoods with brothers or sisters and they do so irrespective of whether they are raised in two-parent, in single-parent or other non-standard family units. Early research was founded on psychoanalytic traditions, which placed a negative emphasis on sibling relationships by concentrating on sibling rivalry, or was concerned with factors such as birth order. More recently, however, the sibling relationship has been studied directly in terms of its impact on development with considerable theoretical consequence.

A key worker in this area is Judy Dunn, whose observational studies of siblings and their relationships has dramatically altered the way developmental psychologists conceptualize the nature of social development and relationships within the family. It may seem obvious that being raised in a family unit comprising other children as well as adults should affect the child's social understanding and indeed it does. But Dunn's work (e.g. Dunn, 1988; Dunn and Kendrick, 1982) has used this to reframe the way that we consider children's cognition.

Piaget's account of how children come to understand the social world is for the most part clear cut. He argued that social understanding is essentially driven by cognitive development. Dunn presents a totally contrasting and a rather more convincing view. She suggests that children's early involvement in family life leads to an early understanding about the behaviour, goals and intentions of other people.

Family life is ridden with emotion. Sharing, negotiating, pleasing, teasing and arguing are an integral part of family life and children must learn from a very early age how to share in this level of social activity. Dunn's research evidence shows that in the first three years of life children learn to do just this. However, this social competence is not to be separated from cognitive competence by supposing that the former simply develops earlier than the latter. Rather, Dunn's thesis is that these most fundamental of social achievements actually drive cognitive development. In other words Piaget's account is turned on its head.

In a series of longitudinal studies (studies over time), young siblings from infancy to the pre-school period were studied in their homes in the course of everyday life. The findings are really quite striking when compared to laboratory findings. Dunn looked at questions of sibling rivalry and sibling cooperation and found that there were high levels of conflict between young children. For example, in one study pre-school siblings were found to average around 8 quarrels an hour! (Dunn and Munn, 1985), but these results were matched by findings of very high levels of concern and co-operation between siblings. The children were sensitive to each other's needs and emotions (even when these were in direct conflict to their own) and behaved in very non-egocentric ways towards each other. The ability to recognize and cooperate with another's goal was apparent as early as 14 months of age and indications of sensitivity to moods of others comes even earlier, at around 8 months.

Another point which arises from this research concerns the complex nature of the patterns of behaviour. For example Dunn and Kendrick (1982) studied toddlers' reactions to the birth of a new sibling and, as might be predicted, some children responded dramatically to this event. Some of the toddlers showed behavioural signs of being disturbed such as sleep disturbances and increased clingingness to the mother. In short, they had what appears to be a clear negative reaction to the new baby.

But what impact does this have on the later relationship between the siblings? In fact, the results showed that some toddlers who had the most negative reaction to the baby's arrival went on to develop very positive sibling relationships with the baby in subsequent months. Similarly, some of the most 'disturbed' toddlers were also those who showed the most interest in the baby. Taken together the evidence supported a very complex chain of patterns of behaviour and disputed the notion common in child'care books about the primacy of early relationships on later ones. The work on siblings contributes to an increasingly held view of the need to look at family influence within a wider framework. In attempting to understand current psychological functioning, the counsellor therefore needs to explore this very important area of influence.

8.5.3 The Effects of Birth Order

It so often seems to be the case that one can attribute certain characteristics or behaviour to birth order. For example, we commonly think of the oldest child as being responsible and the youngest as being more relaxed, possibly because they may have been left to 'occur' rather than having their parents' child-rearing ideas imposed upon them. However, the evidence suggests that birth order only plays a role in the more extreme family circumstances such as very large families or single child families. Families with over six children tend (not surprisingly) to restructure child care and have less time to spend in individual interaction with their children. In some circumstances this makes these children more at risk in terms of academic achievement and antisocial behaviour (Wagner et al., 1985). This said, these effects should be taken alongside the fact that large families are also often severely economically disadvantaged, and so the 'effects' of family size may simply reflect well-established effects of poverty (Rutter and Madge, 1976). At the other extreme, first-borns and only children have been found to have both short- and long-term advantages in academic achievement and personal characteristics due to their 'privileged' relationship with their parents (Sutton-Smith and Rosenberg, 1970).

Despite these findings, birth order effects need to be kept in perspective since there are profound individual differences due to temperament and family circumstances. Moreover, the theoretical focus towards studying positive aspects of sibling interaction, for example, has displaced traditional approaches that tended to see birth order as a 'risk' variable.

8.5.4 Influences outside the Family

The previous sections have concentrated on family issues. It is hardly surprising that this should be so given that most children develop within the context of a family in some form or other. However, development is not exclusively family-based and it is necessary to consider development in a wider context. There are major issues about race, schooling and other social variables which impact on children's lives but in this section we focus on the role of peer relations.

Peer relations, including friendships, are important because of their truly developmental significance throughout the lifespan. Furthermore, they represent an influence outside the family which is, at least to some extent, under the influence of the individual child, in a way which race or ethnicity for example are not.

Do peers have any real impact to make on children's lives? Within developmental psychology peer influence takes on two quite different guises. The first is peer influence on cognitive development and the second is peer influence as general social support. The fact that these two quite distinct areas are covered under the same umbrella should highlight the significance of peer relationships.

Peer influence on cognitive development

Even in the most cognitive of accounts of development, such as that offered by Piaget, the role of peers and friendships was given a central place. In his early work Piaget argued that peers are actually causal in the child's development since they provide the possibility for cognitive conflict necessary for development itself to take place. Adults, Piaget argued, are too far removed (both intellectually and socially) from children to play a significant role. Instead, the mixing of young children with their age mates is viewed as necessary for children to appreciate the limitations of their understanding of the world.

By interacting with peers young children at least would be confronted with the fact that their view of the world (being extremely ego-centric and logically deficient) was simply not viable. Neo-Piagetian studies of peer interaction (e.g. Doise and Mugny, 1984) showed the benefits to individual children of working for a period of time in pairs or groups on problem-solving tasks. A given child working with another child is more likely to succeed on a similar subsequent task presented individually than a child not given the benefit of peer interaction (e.g. Blaye et al., 1991). More recent work has shown that children do not even have to interact with each other to benefit in this way—the mere presence of another child can be enough to improve performance. Given the strength of the evidence of peer influence on cognition it is then not surprising that peers are known to have a significant contribution in children's social development.

Peers as social support

From the initial work on attachment, peers have been identified as being important. Ainsworth (1989) has argued that, even for young children, peers can represent crucial attachment figures and carry the enduring qualities of parental attachment, a claim which is backed up by findings using 'the strange situation' described above. It was found that infants were comforted by siblings as well as their primary care-giver. Peer relationships can also play an important protective role for the most vulnerable children. Research on divorce, for example, has shown that a single close friendship can offer 'protection' even to the most vulnerable child (e.g. Hetherington, 1989).

Early Peer Relationships and Adult Functioning

More generally Asher et al. (1993), have looked at the relationship between peer relations and later functioning in adult life. They present strong evidence that mental health in adults is associated with earlier peer relationships. It has been found that in particular, early poor peer relationships are linked with later risk of disorder. A case in point is the tentative association between peer rejection in childhood and adult depression. But again, these patterns are not clear cut. Many people experience poor early peer relationships but do not go on to have difficulties as adults. It would be a mistake to assume too great a continuity.

However, this kind of link highlights the importance of looking outside the family for background factors which impinge on later adult functioning. For counsellors involved with adults experiencing difficulty there may be far more to be gained by adopting an approach which looks at social support networks as a whole in childhood rather than merely family relationships (see Champion and Goodall (1993), for a wider discussion of social support throughout the lifespan).

8.6 FAMILY BREAKDOWN AND DISRUPTION

Everyday conflict between family members (who has the first turn on a new toy, what food should be had for lunch, whether to go to the park or to the shops) is a normal part of family life and development. But at what point does conflict become abnormal and have serious effects on children? One problem in dealing with this question is in deciding what is meant by 'abnormal'? Should a negative effect in itself define the cause as abnormal? If so then many parental separations and divorce might need to come into this category. But divorce, in social terms, can almost be considered as normal in that around 30 per cent of marriages end in divorce; the figure for re-marriages is higher still.

Most divorces involve children; up to 40 per cent of children will experience their parents' divorce and so it is not surprising that concern is expressed about its impact on children's psychological well-being. In this section some of the available evidence on the effects of family breakdown on children will be discussed.

It is important to have an understanding of both the short- and long-term effects of disruptions brought about by divorce as well as the continuity of effects. As it turns out the evidence (like that considered in previous sections) is complex but reasonably consistent. Divorce does cause short-term psychological trauma to children but the long-term effects are mediated and even eliminated by other variables. Furthermore, some children are more vulnerable than others, and social factors can interact to intensify or reduce this vulnerability. Acknowledging these facts is essential for those involved in giving support to adults and children alike.

Early evidence on the effects of parental separation was incredibly pessimistic, and assumed a host of psychological and behavioural problems which followed. However, this early work was beset with methodological weaknesses; few studies were longitudinal in nature, many lacked control groups from 'intact' families and worse, many were retrospective, taking clinical referrals only from individuals who had already displayed profound personal difficulties. Such evidence was not very revealing about the effects of divorce on the substantial group of 'normal' children whose parents separate during their childhood.

More recent work, however, has gone some way in rectifying these initial research weaknesses to the point that we can now sketch out the main variables which we ought to be aware of. First there are a number of child factors which are clearly influential of which the two key ones are the age and sex of the child at the point of the parental separation.

8.6.1 The Effects of Age and Sex of the Child

Several studies have shown that younger children (pre-school) are most affected initially by their parents' separation, showing signs of disturbance at home and in their school lives (e.g. Wallerstein et al., 1988). But for children of all ages these effects become much less marked within two or three years.

Interestingly age appears to be much less crucial than sex of the child. Boys, in line with other areas involving stress, are much more vulnerable than girls to the process of divorce. Thus while Wallerstein et al., found that girls had made an almost complete psychological recovery within two years, for some of the boys in the sample, the initial negative effects were still apparent on some of the measures many years after the initial separation. Furthermore, boys seem to take not only longer to 'recover' but also show overall lower levels of recovery compared to their female counterparts.

However, there are two reasons why even these findings should be treated with caution. Firstly, a large scale study by Allison and Faustenberg (1989) did not replicate this female advantage even on a very large sample of children. Secondly, even where girls seem to be less sensitive to the negative emotional impact there are other factors which mediate outcome irrespective of sex.

8.6.2 Post-divorce Relationships and Family Arrangements

The quality of the post-divorce relationship is a much more central predictor of outcome than individual variables such as age and sex. Here the evidence is quite clear. In cases where the post-divorce arrangements are stable and involve little family conflict the prognosis for the children's well-being is good. It seems particularly important that the separated parents do not continue hostilities following separation and that the children remain in contact with the (typically) absent father (Richards 1988). In fact, this finding has led some courts (particularly in the USA) to recommend shared parenting where children divide their time with each parent. At least the practice of joint access is well founded in research evidence.

A further finding relates to a complicated interaction between sex of child and post-divorce family arrangements. In the majority of divorce cases mothers are given custody of their children and many of these mothers go on to remarry. Thus, many children acquire step-families, especially step-fathers. A close analysis of the findings shows that the benefit of girls in the post-divorce period up can be reversed in a step-father situation. Girls are more likely to be adversely affected by their mother's remarriage than boys, who have been shown to benefit.

These subtle interactions along with other findings have drastically altered the way that developmental psychologists consider divorce. Divorce is no longer conceived of as an *event* with a series of adverse consequences which can be assumed and measured. In contrast, divorce is considered as a *process* which involves a series of complex and changing family relationships which begin long before the legal act of parental separation and which continue long after it. Early work on the effects of divorce was couched theoretically in terms of attachment theory and therefore treated divorce as an event involving undesirable separation of the child from a key attachment figure. The effects were interpreted in terms of 'loss' and therefore pinpointed the problem and its effects at the point of parent separation. We now know that this approach is misleading and unhelpful.

8.6.3 Family Conflict

While divorce does have negative psychological effects on children, they are not primarily a result of the separation. Instead it seems that it is the family *conflict* which is present both before and after legal separation which is disturbing to children.

The most convincing evidence of this comes from a study by Block et al. (1986). This study followed a group of children longitudinally from the ages of 3 to 14 years. Of the 128 children studied some 41 experienced parental separation. The results showed that many of the behavioural characteristics found in previous studies following children after divorce were to be seen in the 'divorced' group several years before the divorce took place. Thus many of the so-called 'effects' are not effects of the divorce since they were measured beforehand. So what are they? Block et al. conclude that the atmosphere of parental conflict was a key factor and such conflict could be measured as much as ten years before parents actually divorce.

This finding is much more than an academic clarification. It shifts our focus of attention from a single event of separation between parents and therefore between departing parent and child towards acknowledging that severe levels of parental dispute will have adverse effects on children's psychological adjustment irrespective of whether parents separate or not. The evidence on the effects of divorce has many parallels with that considered in relation to more extreme forms of deprivation. We cannot undergo a simplistic analysis and there are no simple answers. Yet, the complexity is beginning to be unravelled so that the scale of the task of explaining these complex social acts is at least outlined despite there being no clear immediate answers.

8.7 CONCLUDING COMMENTS

The themes which have been outlined in this chapter should at least offer a taste of the research areas currently explored by developmental psychologists, whose work, either intentionally or otherwise, has relevance for those involved in counselling.

As an academic group developmentalists are typically very reluctant to be prescriptive about the way their research may impact on individual cases for a variety of reasons—some better than others. One reason is certainly due to the fact that researchers in this area are aware of the huge gaps in our knowledge which prevent the kind of clear cut messages about the psychological world which physical and medical science can offer; but this reason is by no means the most important one.

The last 20 years or so have seen enormous gains in our knowledge base and this very increase in our knowledge of development has paradoxically increased the developmental psychologists reluctance to come forward in some instances. We now know just how complex development is—single factor explanations are unlikely to explain anything other than the very simplest developmental phenomenon. But acknowledging the complexity has paid off. In all areas of psychology, including developmental, there is an expectation that answers to identified questions and problems will be complex and multivariate; but the jigsaw is starting to take shape.

So if we take the recurring theme of the effects of early experience on later functioning, the problem has been redefined. We have moved from the earlier question 'what are the long-term effects of early trauma?' towards asking 'what are the factors that mediate any effects and therefore enhance recovery?' and 'which children are the most vulnerable and why?' This new perspective need not be seen as complicating matters but as a recasting of the problem more appropriately. As such the answers to identified 'problems' become more, rather than less, answerable. It is hoped that this kind of optimism rings true for those professionally involved with children and adults experiencing psychological difficulties.

9

Lifespan Development: Transitions from Adolescence to Old Age

Adrian Coyle

CONTENTS

9.1 INTRODUCTION

Although all clients are unique in the way they experience their particular difficulties, there are nevertheless undoubted similarities in the problems that clients present. Each stage of life carries with it certain 'tasks' and demands which must be negotiated with some degree of success if we are to attain a reasonable level of psychological well-being.

A developmental task has been defined as 'a task which arises at or about a certain period in the life of the individual, successful achievement of which leads to his happiness and to success with later tasks, while failure leads to unhappiness in the individual, disapproval by the society, and difficulty with later tasks' (Havighurst, 1972, p. 2).

The developmental tasks of adolescence and adulthood include the negotiation of independence from parents; the development of identity, including sexual identity; the establishment, maintenance and termination of sexual and emotional relationships; coping with employment and unemployment; parenting; managing the so-called midlife 'crisis'; coming to terms with ageing and retirement; loss and bereavement; and of course, preparation for death. Clearly, these represent many of the major issues which clients raise in counselling contexts. In this chapter, some of the major transitions associated with the broad life stages of adolescence and early, middle and late adulthood will be discussed, sometimes in outline and sometimes in detail.

9.2 ADOLESCENCE

One of the problems in dividing the lifespan into particular stages is the question of how to determine where these stages begin and end. There are many ways of defining adolescence but for the purposes of this chapter, we have adopted Bee's (1994) definition of adolescence as 'the period that lies psychologically and culturally between childhood and adulthood rather than as a specific age range' (p. 253).

Adolescence is commonly thought of as a particularly stressful life stage because of the series of major developmental tasks that arise during this period. These include negotiating changes in relationships with parents; establishing and maintaining relationships with peers; developing identity in a range of contexts, including sexual identity; establishing sexual and emotional relationships; and beginning the process of making occupational choices. Some of these tasks will already have been encountered during childhood but changed social norms and expectations will mean that the nature of these tasks is quite different in adolescence.

The tasks outlined are the most common ones encountered by adolescents. However, some adolescents have additional issues to address. For example, some adolescents may also find themselves having to negotiate developmental tasks that are thought of as more usually occurring in early adulthood, such as marriage and parenting; gay and lesbian adolescents may face problems in negotiating the meaning, management and expression of a socially devalued sexual identity; and adolescents who were adopted in childhood and who do not have information about the circumstances of their adoption may feel that they lack important elements for a satisfying 'reworking' of their identity. Some writers have addressed the issue of identity formation in adolescence among different ethnic groups (Phinney and Rosenthal, 1992). Membership of particular ethnic groups obviously carries with it differential status and value in society. Adolescents who belong to those ethnic groups that have been discriminated against may have particular problems in negotiating their adult identities. In general, how the developmental tasks of adolescence are negotiated may have far-reaching implications for the young person's future and an awareness of this may increase the stress associated with this life stage.

The psychosocial context of the adolescent's life has also changed. Adolescents are no longer seen as children but are not yet viewed as adults. Although social expectations concerning their behaviour will have changed as they left childhood, they may still be unclear about what exactly is expected of them. However, despite the tendency to represent adolescence as a time of acute 'storm and stress', research has suggested that it is no more stormy than other periods of transition during the lifespan (Powers et al., 1989).

9.2.1 Physical and Cognitive Changes in Adolescence

The developmental tasks of adolescence arise at a time of major physical and cognitive change. With the hormonal changes of puberty, the young person matures sexually and their body also alters in terms of height, shape, muscle development and fat distribution.

Within Piaget's framework of cognitive development, the young person enters the stage of formal operations during adolescence. This allows them to think about possible occurrences rather than real events, to search systematically for an answer to a problem, and to understand logical relationships.

The development of formal operational thought has implications for the ways in which counsellors may frame interventions with adolescent clients. However, it should be remembered that the timing and extent of the development of formal operational thought (the ability to think and reason about possibilities in the abstract) varies considerably from one person to another. This can itself be a source of psychological difficulties. In a school context, within the same class, those who have attained the stage of formal operations may excel while others who have not reached this stage of cognitive development may struggle. This may give rise to such problems as low self-esteem and challenging behaviours.

9.2.2 The Development of Identity in Adolescence

One of the major dimensions of transition during adolescence is the development of identity. We have discussed in Section 7.2.5 above Breakwell's theory of identity process. Another very influential model of identity is that of Erikson (1959). His eight-stage model of psychosocial development was, in fact, conceived as a 'lifespan' model. The developmental tasks he described are present to some extent throughout the lifespan but become focal tasks at particular life stages.

Erikson saw the person as subject to demands from the social context throughout the lifespan. These demands provoke emotional crises which, if successfully resolved, lead

Table 9.1   Erikson's model of psychosocial development

Approximate age	Crisis
0–1	Basic trust versus basic mistrust
1–6	Autonomy versus shame and doubt
6–10	Initiative versus guilt
10–14	Industry versus Inferiority
14–20	Identity versus role confusion
20–35	Intimacy versus isolation
35–65	Generativity versus Stagnation
over 65	Ego integrity versus despair and disgust

to the development of what Sugarman (1986) has called 'a new "virtue" or "vital strength"' (p. 84). If the crisis is not resolved, the person is left in a state of psychological disequilibrium.

Possible positive and negative outcome states are described in the names given to the particular crisis associated with each stage. For example, during adolescence, the person is said to enter the fifth stage of development in which they have to negotiate a period of 'identity versus role confusion'. However, the developmental outcome of each stage need not be either of those specified. Instead, the outcome may lie somewhere between the two.

During the adolescent stage of identity versus role confusion, the young person is subject to new social demands and expectations as they move beyond childhood. In response to these demands, they try to discover 'who they are', where their skills or talents lie and what roles might be appropriate for them in adult life. Although these questions can be partly answered by making suitable career choices, many young people may find that their social circumstances allow them little scope for choosing social roles generally, and occupational roles in particular.

Erikson's model, however, extends beyond career choice. He saw the young person experiencing a fundamental need to establish a new sense of self and a personal value system and world view at this point. The young person also seeks to construct some continuity in their identity while negotiating the physical and psychosocial changes of adolescence that may have disrupted their sense of continuity.

In childhood, we gain our sense of self primarily through identifying with significant others, usually our parents. Some adolescents resolve identity conflicts by continuing to adopt wholesale the values of significant others. Marcia (1980), who has expanded Erikson's ideas, has called this **identity foreclosure**. Those who follow this identity path have been described as conventional, authoritarian and inflexible in their ideas about what is right.

Other young people select from, retain and discard aspects of their childhood identifications to create a new identity. They seek roles that will allow them to construct a new synthesis of some of their former identifications. Marcia has referred to the outcome of this process as **identity achievement**. Identity achievers have been described as psychologically strong but flexible, open to new experience and capable of sustaining intimate relationships. The achievement of an appropriate and psychologically healthy synthesis takes time. The young person needs to develop an ability to deal with periods of uncertainty when their identity is in flux. During the identity transition, the young person is described as being in a **moratorium**. An example of a young person at this particular stage is the client described below.

This is an eighteen-year-old woman who was referred to the counsellor following termination of a pregnancy. She was in her final year at school and lived with both parents. Her elder brother was at university. From the age of fourteen or so she has been involved in a number of 'incidents' at school when she was identified as the 'ringleader'. She was asked to leave her last school.

She reported that she was extremely fond of her parents and had enormous respect for both. However, she found it very difficult to live up to their high standards and to conform to the type of person they expected her to be. She reported that they did not appreciate how 'good' she was, compared to her friends. She goes to church every Sunday with them, stays in most Saturday evenings for meals, is usually home after going out by midnight, and is generally obedient to their wishes and has never challenged or confronted them openly.

However, every so often she 'breaks out' and does, in her own words, 'something totally daft', often risking getting caught. Examples of this are driving without insurance, playing truant from school and becoming pregnant. She desperately wants to be 'her own person', but equally desperately, she wants to be a 'good girl' and please her parents, whom she admires and respects.

Here it would seem that the client was experiencing some conflict between identity foreclosure and identity achievement. Here the counsellor might help the client to identify ways in which she differed from her parents with respect to, for example, attitudes, values and beliefs and work out ways of appropriately confronting them with the person she feels she is, rather than going through the motions of being the 'ideal daughter'.

If the young person fails to resolve the identity crisis of this stage, this may result in **role confusion** (also discussed in Section 7.2.4 on Social Roles) and a lack of stable identity. This has also been referred to as **identity diffusion**, i.e. an uncertainty about who you are and what you will become. This may manifest itself as low self-esteem, low autonomy and an inability to form intimate relationships. The young person may try to boost a fragile sense of identity by identifying closely with particular peer groups or individuals. If these peer groups or individuals are engaged in socially undesirable behaviours, the young person may also adopt these behaviours. Such behaviour patterns may bring them or their parents into contact with a counsellor.

Of course, the individual may purposefully choose to identify with others who engage in socially undesirable behaviours. If this is not continuous with their upbringing, it may represent an attempt to construct identity anew rather than to create a new synthesis from existing identity elements.

One problem with Erikson's model of development that is relevant here is that psychological health is defined within existing social norms. What might to one person appear to be socially undesirable behaviour resulting from over-identification with certain peers might, to another person, be radically different ways of behaving that rightly challenge the repressive social status quo. This question of who and what defines behaviours as problematic and appropriate for therapeutic interventions is a major consideration within the mental health field and is beyond the scope of this chapter.

Also, the idea that adolescence is characterized by an identity crisis locates his model within the 'storm and stress' view of adolescence, which has not always been supported by research evidence. Siddique and D'Arcy (1984) found that only a quarter of the large sample of adolescents whom they studied experienced psychological distress during adolescence: the majority seemed to progress to adulthood fairly smoothly. Undoubtedly, major change occurs in the roles that people play as they move from childhood to adolescence to adulthood but these changes may not be so overwhelming that they spark an identity crisis. Perhaps Erikson's description of the identity transitions in adolescence is simply too dramatic or perhaps it applies only to some adolescents.

Nevertheless, if the more problematic aspects of Erikson's model are omitted or amended, it remains a useful way of conceptualizing the identity-related developmental tasks that some adolescents may face. It also provides pointers for the counsellor who is trying to understand the difficulties that may be faced by some adolescent clients and to frame appropriate interventions.

9.2.3 Adolescent Identity Issues and Counselling

Kroger (1989) has collected together recommendations on therapeutic interventions with young people experiencing various difficulties in the identity versus role confusion stage. Those in the identity moratorium may benefit from exploring elements that could potentially be incorporated into an identity synthesis. The young person may be encouraged to try out different identity options. Until the person attains a workable identity synthesis, the outcomes of this testing process should be seen as exploratory rather than as identity commitments.

Those who have foreclosed on identity development may only present for counselling if something has occurred which has shaken the borrowed certainties upon which their world view is based. Counsellors working with those who have foreclosed need to recognize the security that the person's rigid identity structure has provided, while also opening up new identity possibilities for them. This must be undertaken with sensitivity because a direct challenge to the foreclosure identity commitments may lead the person to adhere even more rigidly to these commitments and avoid exploring new possibilities.

The person who has experienced identity diffusion will require interventions that address the particular developmental conflict that gave rise to their diffusion. This may involve working back through the person's experiences of previous Eriksonian developmental stages. For example, the person may have been positioned at the negative pole of the developmental continuum of the first stage, i.e., they may have developed mistrust rather than trust. They may need to develop trust in themselves and in others before developing autonomy and initiative, which are the positive outcomes of the second and third developmental stages. Without these qualities, the processes of identification and identity synthesis are impossible.

Identity problems are not, of course, confined to adolescence. As Erikson (1956) himself noted: 'a sense of identity is never gained nor maintained once and for all . . . instead . . . it is constantly lost and regained' (p. 74). Counsellors may find themselves having to address identity issues with clients of all ages. It may be that clients never attained successful resolutions of identity crises during adolescence. Alternatively, former resolutions may need to be revisited and reworked because of changed circumstances. The case study below offers an example of a client who is in the stage of early adulthood with whom a counsellor might usefully explore adolescent identity issues.

> *The client is a 30-year-old man who qualified as a psychiatric nurse six months ago. His career path has been somewhat erratic. At school, he was a good student and achieved sufficient A-level grades to study architecture at university. He explains his choice of subject saying 'I thought it would be creative and would allow me to leave my mark on my surroundings—make an impact, you know.' After doing well early in the course, his performance deteriorated and he ended up with a lower second class degree. 'It just got so boring,' he says. 'It was all technical, so soulless. It had nothing to do with people at all.'*
>
> *Not knowing what to do next, he began a postgraduate diploma in architecture but left the course shortly before his exams. Feeling that he wanted to do 'something useful with people' and always having had an interest in complementary medicine, he took a short course as a massage practitioner. After qualifying, he tried to establish himself in private practice but with no success. 'To be honest,' he says, 'I just didn't have the drive needed to set up my own business.' Pursuing his desire to work in the health field, he began a nurse training course, intending to train in adult nursing. Half-way through the course, after some enjoyable mental health placements, he switched to mental health nursing.*
>
> *Since qualifying as a psychiatric nurse, he has found it difficult to secure a job. He is uncertain about what to do next and about what career path he really wishes to pursue. As he says himself, 'I just can't seem to be able to settle to anything but I don't want to end up never having done anything worthwhile with my life'. The arrival of his 30th birthday three months ago made him aware that 'time is moving on' and left him fearful that 'I'll never achieve anything. I'll never amount to anything.'*

The counsellor here might understand the client's difficulties as ones of identity diffusion or role confusion. We have noted above how this might be associated with low self-esteem and a poor sense of personal autonomy. The counsellor might therefore help this client to explore his underlying feelings related to his lack of self-worth and feelings of power or 'mastery' in work settings.

9.3 EARLY ADULTHOOD

By convention, the period of early adulthood is seen as encompassing the decades of the twenties and thirties.

9.3.1 Physical and Cognitive Functioning in Early Adulthood

Physically, the body is at its peak at the end of adolescence. Young adults perform better than those in middle or late adulthood on virtually every physical measure. Compared with those in older age groups, young adults have more muscle tissue, better eyesight and hearing and a more efficient immune system. Most people do not become aware of a significant decline in physical functioning until middle age, although the rate and extent of physical decline are dependent upon lifestyle factors such as diet and exercise.

Cognitive functioning is also at its peak in early adulthood. It has been suggested that adults do not routinely employ formal operational thought to solve the problems associated with the roles they fulfil. Instead, they tend to adopt a pragmatic form of thought (Labouvie-Vief, 1980). While the consideration of endless possibilities may be beneficial when making significant life choices in adolescence, it becomes an unwieldy means of dealing with the less momentous challenges that regularly confront most adults.

Adults also shift away from an analytic mode of thinking in which the emphasis is on arriving at definite answers through a consideration of facts and move towards a more imaginative mode of thinking which can tolerate uncertainty (Labouvie-Vief, 1990). The adult becomes less certain about some of the choices they make and can also accept that it is not always possible to arrive at definite and certain solutions to some of the problems of adult life. A client who has adopted this form of thinking and who enters counselling or therapy may find it relatively easy to relate to the process. They may be open to the idea that counselling may not produce definite, clearcut solutions to their problems. Although there is as yet little empirical evidence for these ideas about cognitive development in adulthood, they make intuitive sense.

9.3.2 Models of Early Adulthood

Turning to psychological and social aspects of adult development, we have already outlined Erikson's (1959) model that describes development in psychosocial terms throughout the lifespan and we will return to this in our discussion about relationships in early adulthood. Another influential model of adult development is that of Levinson et al. (1978). This is rather more descriptive than Erikson's more psychological model, outlining the tasks to be confronted in coping with the adult world.

The period that we have defined as early adulthood encompasses the first five of what Levinson et al. termed the 'seasons' of adulthood (see Table 9.2). According to this model, adult development proceeds through alternating periods or 'phases' of transition and stability.

Table 9.2　Levinson et al.'s Model of adult development

Approximate Age	Stage
17–22	Early adult transition
22–28	Entering the adult world
28–33	Age thirty transition
33–40	Settling down
40–45	Midlife transition
45–50	Entering middle adulthood
50–55	Age fifty transition
55–60	Culmination of middle adulthood
60–65	Late adult transition
over 65	Late adulthood

- The model begins with the early adult transition, which occurs between the ages of about 17 and 22. During this period, the person reappraises and modifies their sense of self that has been created in childhood and adolescence. They may move from the family home both physically and psychologically, fulfil more autonomous and responsible roles and make some tentative choices about their adult life.
- During the second period of **entering the adult world** (ages 22–28), the young adult continues to test and also to refine and consolidate the tentative commitments to the adult world made during the early adult transition. This involves a delicate balancing act between exploring possibilities and creating a stable life structure by making choices and commitments about, for example, careers and relationships.
- The third period, termed the **age thirty transition** (ages 28–33), sees the person establishing the pattern of their adult life. The 'transition' in the title of this phase refers to the way in which choices that have been made earlier may be reconsidered at this point. Here, the person may feel that the time for them to establish a stable life structure is running out and that they must arrive at a workable life pattern soon. Such feelings of time pressure can make this a stressful period.
- In the fourth phase of '**settling down**' (ages 33–40), the person aims to settle for a few key life choices in such areas as work, family and friendships. They consolidate their key commitments to career, relationships or whatever, and progress within these commitments. The later part of this stage may be marked by a struggle for increased independence and self-sufficiency. Note how the emphasis on decision-making throughout adulthood, making life commitments and establishing stable life patterns echoes Erikson's conceptualization of development. These emphases are typical of models of adult development.

The close of the 'age thirty transition' sees the end of what Levinson et al. regarded as the **novice** phase of adulthood. Throughout this novice period, the person is seen as working on five particular developmental tasks. These are: forming and living out a sense of the role one might play in the adult world (what Levinson et al. termed 'the

Dream'); forming mentor relationships with others who will support and nurture the person in their development; forming an occupation (note how the use of the term 'forming' emphasises the development of occupational ideas); forming love relationships, a partnership and possibly a family; and forming mutual friendships. Although these tasks are particularly to the fore in early adulthood, they may continue to be addressed in later life.

Levinson et al.'s model is based on in-depth life history interviews with 40 males in professional jobs. It is therefore only a partial account of adult development as it excludes the experiences of women (the book in which the model is presented is entitled *The Seasons of a Man's Life*) and those from lower socioeconomic groups. For example, the conflict that women may experience between advancing their career and becoming a parent is missing. Also, women who have had children early in their adult life may experience their thirties not as a 'settling down' period but as a time of exploring new opportunities. Women do feature in the description of the developmental task of forming love relationships, a marriage and a family. However, their role is to support the attainment of their husbands' Dream. When their husbands and children no longer require them, they can then form their own identities. Such a conceptualization of the role of women is clearly most unsatisfactory. The model is also applicable only to heterosexual couples.

Another worker in this field, Gould (1978), took a rather more cognitive approach to adult development than either Erikson or Levinson et al.. His four-stage model of adult development covers the period from the age of 18 to the age of 50 and so fits almost entirely within the age range that we have designated as early adulthood. However, the content of the final stage belongs more appropriately in a discussion of middle adulthood.

In Gould's model, the main trend within adult development involves movement away from the assumption that our lives are determined by the rules we have learned in childhood and towards the idea of ourselves as creators of our own lives. His four stages represent the challenging of four major assumptions or beliefs which he maintains are internalized during childhood and which serve to create feelings of safety and security.

From our overview of these models, we can conclude that it is a mistake to assume that models of psychosocial development can be universally applied. Indeed, it is debatable whether any model of psychosocial development could ever apply to all people in all situations because psychosocial development is potentially so variable and so greatly influenced by factors such as gender and culture. A model which did try to represent the experiences of all people would probably be so abstract and so general as to be worthless. This does not mean that psychological models cannot be useful for counsellors. It means that the counsellors need to be aware of the background to the development of the model and to adapt it to the needs of other populations and contexts.

9.3.3 Sexual and Emotional Relationships in Early Adulthood

The specific psychosocial developmental tasks commonly negotiated during early adulthood include the establishment, maintenance and termination of sexual and emotional relationships, parenting, and the development of occupational roles. The focus here will be on the developmental task of negotiating sexual and emotional relationships. Difficulties with this task constitute or contribute to the presenting problems of many clients who seek counselling.

Within Erikson's (1959) model of development, the adolescent stage of **identity versus role confusion** is followed by the stages of **intimacy versus isolation** and **generativity versus stagnation**. Both are said to occur in early adulthood but the stage of intimacy versus isolation is of greater relevance to the establishment of relationships. The intimacy that marks the successful resolution of this stage refers to the ability to commit oneself to affiliations and partnerships and to adhere to these commitments. Having established an identity separate from others in one's family, at this stage the young person returns to fusing identity with others, but this time in the context of sexual and emotional relationships.

This process involves placing at risk the hard-won individual sense of identity achieved during adolescence. Unless this identity is sufficiently strong to avoid being submerged in the identity of a partner, the person may avoid intimate relationships and may experience isolation. In Boldero and Moore's (1990) research, those who had not achieved intimacy often reported loneliness. This emphasizes how developmental work undertaken at earlier stages (in this case, work on identity) will influence an individual's ability to form and maintain relationships in adulthood.

Another suboptimal outcome involves the person over-identifying with their partner, borrowing excessively from their partner's identity rather than fashioning an identity of their own. This simply returns the person to the childhood stage of identification with parents. It also means that the relationship is inherently unequal and that one partner ends up carrying the identity work of two.

For the young adult who can construct a partnership in which there is an intimate, secure attachment, this relationship can act as a secure base from which they can explore the adult world. The person can take psychosocial risks and can risk failure in the knowledge that there is a 'safe place' to which they can return. In this sense, a secure adult relationship serves the same function as the relationship with the mother in early childhood. At that stage (as we have discussed in Section 7.6 on Intimacy and Love and Section 8.4.1 on Attachment and its Consequences for Later Life) if the attachment between mother and child is secure, the child can move out from this place of safety to explore their world, knowing that they can return to the mother for comfort and consolation if things go wrong.

The young adult who is unable to create secure relationships and who therefore cannot construct this secure base may experience isolation and, having to rely on their own resources, may be inclined to avoid risks and exploration. Much of the literature attributes the creation of a secure base to the formation of sexual and emotional relationships but this function can also be fulfilled by close emotional relationships, i.e., by close friendships.

For further discussion on relationships, see Sections 7.4–7.8.

9.4 MIDDLE ADULTHOOD

The mid-life years are seen as extending from about the age of 40 to about the age of 60. These years of middle adulthood are often viewed as marking the beginning of physical and cognitive deterioration. Nevertheless, it should be remembered that chronological age is a less reliable guide to the physical and mental abilities of the middle-aged adult than of the young or old adult. The mid-life stage presents the person with new transitions to negotiate, which are sometimes represented as a 'mid-life crisis'. Let us consider some of the changes of middle adulthood, beginning with physical changes.

9.4.1 Physical and Cognitive Changes in Middle Adulthood

Some physical functions start to decline in the forties and fifties but do so very gradually. Other functions, such as reproductive capacity, vision and hearing, will already have deteriorated significantly by middle adulthood. Health begins to deteriorate too. About half of all adults aged between 40 and 60 have some diagnosed or undiagnosed disease or disability, which is often chronic. Cognitive functioning also deteriorates in the mid-life years. Declining memory functioning is less noticeable when middle-aged adults are dealing with familiar material than with unfamiliar material, especially when they are in their forties and early fifties. There is evidence that although memory for surface detail declines among middle-aged adults, memory for meaning and for broad themes is good (Adams, 1991).

9.4.2 Models of Middle Adulthood

Erikson, Levinson et al. and Gould all have something to say about this period of life. All have somewhat different perspectives and emphasize different developmental aspects.

Erikson's model

Erikson's (1959) stage of **generativity versus stagnation** is said to begin in early adulthood but continues to be a developmental focus throughout middle adulthood. Generativity is defined as a concern with establishing and guiding the next generation. Although it is often manifested through parenting, it can also be expressed through various forms of altruism and creativity, for example, by acting as a mentor to younger colleagues. If the person fails to achieve generativity, this is said to lead to stagnation and personal impoverishment. The energy that has to be directed in some way towards nurturing the next generation in order for personal growth to occur is instead directed inwards. The person thus becomes their own child and focuses all their nurturing capacities upon themselves in a self-centred way.

Levinson et al.'s model

Around the age of 40, according to this model, the person is said to enter the mid-life transition when they have to relinquish the life structures of early adulthood and begin establishing life structures for middle adulthood. They work towards forming a stronger sense of who they are and what they want and towards developing a more realistic, sophisticated view of the world—what it is like, what it offers them and what it demands from them. This is believed to result in increased independence.

However, the more sharply defined sense of self is also said to give the person the confidence to form more intense attachments. Around the age of 45, the individual enters the stage of middle adulthood and may make certain major changes as a result of having reappraised their life. This may involve changes in relationships, career and place of residence. In essence, Levinson et al.'s model ends here. Although it identifies an age fifty transition, a culmination of middle adulthood and a late adult transition leading into late adulthood, these are not discussed in detail.

Gould's model

According to Gould's (1978) model of adult development, between the ages of 35 and 50, various social events may occur which emphasize to the person that they are no longer young. For example, their career has peaked, their parents become more dependent on them and their children have left home. The person realizes that they are mortal and a sense of time urgency develops for the resolution of life questions.

As in Levinson et al.'s 'age thirty' transition, the individual revisits life questions that they had resolved in the past and these resolutions are re-examined. For example, in the past the person may have regarded success at work as a solution to all their problems. At this stage, they may realize that career success will not protect them from death and so may seek to strike a new balance between their work and other aspects of their life.

9.4.3 Challenges of Middle Adulthood

Despite the transitions and developmental tasks outlined by these writers, Bee (1994) has noted that during middle adulthood 'the social clock is ticking much less loudly' because '(m)any of the same roles that dominate early adult life continue' (p. 390). In terms of functioning in the workplace, research has indicated that adults may be at their most productive during middle adulthood and that the quality of their work is high (Horner et al., 1986; Simonton, 1988; Streufert et al., 1990). In middle age, many adults continue to be involved in relationships, continue to be parents and continue to work. However, the nature of these roles may change and sometimes radically, for example, when divorce or redundancy occurs in middle adulthood.

Divorce is a prime example of a 'life event' that can set in motion a process of dealing with transition, a moving through to the next stage. The act of divorce, however, is not a discrete event to be adjusted to. It is more likely to be a process which takes place over time and which requires frequent adjustments and accommodations over a long period, maybe for the rest of the person's life. This is why models of adjustment (such as Hopson's, 1981) which describe various stages of adjustment, are often not appropriate when thinking about and working with real-life clients in real-life settings.

Research on the psychological effects of divorce has suggested that those who have recently divorced may experience feelings of failure and low self-esteem and are at increased risk of physical illness, depression and suicide. For some people, divorce can have an adverse effect on psychological well-being for many years. For others, however, divorce represents a developmental milestone. It presents them with opportunities to take their lives in new directions, with positive outcomes in terms of psychological well-being. Although divorce is more likely to occur during early adulthood than middle adulthood, there is evidence that older adults experience it as more emotionally disruptive (Bloom et al., 1979).

The adverse psychological effects of redundancy and unemployment have been well documented and include anxiety, depression, loss of self-esteem and self-confidence, self-blame, anger, reduced life satisfaction, and feelings of helplessness and loss of control (Daniels and Coyle, 1993). These have been attributed to the loss of the practical and psychosocial benefits of having a job which include income; the social status of being employed; opportunities to engage in meaningful activity, to practise existing skills and develop new skills and to receive positive feedback on one's competence; scope for significant decision-making; interpersonal contact; and the temporal structure of one's day.

Unemployment is often equated with laziness and lack of motivation. Unemployed people are represented as 'social miscreants who have failed in some way to comply with society's requirements and are being legitimately chastised through the loss of paid work' (Breakwell, 1986, p. 57). It is hardly surprising then that their self-esteem and identity are often adversely affected.

Those aged between 30 and 60 appear to show the greatest increase in physical illness and the greatest deterioration in mental health following unemployment (Warr et al., 1988). It may be that older adults will have more economic responsibilities to shoulder than younger people. Job loss may therefore hit them harder. Another factor which may influence the severity of a person's reaction to job loss is the meaning which they invested in their job. If their identity was focused around their occupational role, the loss of that role may affect them very severely. This is especially likely if they experience difficulties in filling the void left by their occupational role and finding another role that provides them with the main psychosocial benefits previously derived from their job.

While there are undoubtedly psychological challenges to be faced by the individual during the mid-life years, some popular notions about the difficulties of this life stage are not supported by research. Foremost among these is the concept of the mid-life crisis, which features in some of the major theories of adult development. Levinson et al. (1978) saw the adult in the mid-life years as having to confront a cluster of developmental tasks such as accepting one's mortality, declining health and physical functioning and changes in social roles. These are held to be of such significance that they often exceed the person's ability to cope, thus precipitating a crisis.

However, most research has failed to find any evidence for the occurrence of a crisis in the mid-life years. One exception has been a study of 1000 men aged 25–69 by Tamir (1982), who found that college-educated men aged 45–49 reported more drinking problems, greater use of prescribed drugs, less 'zest' and more 'psychological immobilization' than other men. However, these features may be particular to this group, perhaps because of the group-specific social demands and expectations that they encounter in middle age.

After summarizing research on the mid-life crisis, Bee (1994) concluded that 'there are stresses and tasks that are unique to this period, but there is little sign that these stresses and tasks are more likely to overwhelm an adult's coping resources at this age than at any other' (p. 381).

9.5 LATE ADULTHOOD

The final decades of the lifespan are characterized by specific developmental tasks such as managing retirement from work and the increased leisure time that this brings, dealing with the death of an increasing number of one's peers and perhaps one's partner, coping with the loss of unfulfilled hopes and wishes and coming to terms with one's own mortality. The nature and management of these tasks and transitions may be significantly affected by an increasing decline in physical and cognitive abilities. For example, with increasing age, parents may come to rely on their children to meet some of their basic needs.

This may herald yet another change in the parental identity of older adults. As their children matured and forged independent lives, their parental identity may have undergone a series of changes. The precise nature of these changes will depend upon a host of factors such as parenting styles and the nature of the family situation. However, most parents begin their parenting career by fulfilling the role of main provider of material and psychosocial care to their child. Thereafter, their parenting identity may involve aspects of advising, counselling, warning, protecting and helping practically.

Although the power base of the parent–child relationship may have become more equal over time, the shift that can occur when parents become physically dependent on their children and its effects on the parental identity may be particularly hard to deal with. Parents and children may find their earlier roles reversed, as the role of parent-as-carer evolves into the role of parent-as-cared-for.

9.5.1 Physical and Cognitive Changes in Late Adulthood

The rate of deterioration in physical and cognitive functioning during late adulthood varies greatly from person to person and increases significantly after the age of 75. Care needs to be taken therefore not to treat all those in the stage of late adulthood (or indeed in any life stage) as a homogeneous group but to recognize that individuals will have particular skills and abilities.

Let us consider some of the principal physical and cognitive changes that often occur in late adulthood. The loss of visual and auditory acuity that begins in middle adulthood continues in late adulthood and can become problematic. For example, the person may experience tinnitus (a ringing in the ears) and have difficulties in hearing high frequency sounds, hearing when there is background noise and discriminating individual words.

If uncorrected, such hearing loss creates communication problems for the older adult. Visual impairment may mean simply the need for glasses, but severe disorders such as glaucoma and cataracts are likely to bring about much greater distress. Although with the sort of blindness which can come with cataracts, the older person has considerable warning, it is still a frightening transition to make.

The risk of back pain increases as shock-absorbing cartilage in the spine becomes compressed with age. Changes in joints may cause arthritis. Immune functioning deteriorates with age, leaving the person vulnerable to conditions that a younger person could combat. Also, the body's ability to repair damage, for example, to bones and muscles, diminishes as does its ability to control cellular growth, which increases the risk of cancer occurring. Sexual function, although variable in older years, may be impaired or lost as a result of ill-health, surgical trauma or by anxiety related to fears of failure.

A range of cognitive abilities has also been found to diminish with age, including memory, reasoning, decision-making, speed of information processing and the ability to comprehend new information. In studies of the components of problem-solving (including organization, creativity, flexibility and the skills of identifying relevant information and abstracting it from concrete situations), older adults (especially those aged over 70) have fared less well than younger adults (Salthouse, 1982). Given these potential changes in physical and cognitive functioning, older adults may be fearful that their activities will be curtailed or that they will lose control of their lives and have to become dependent upon others.

The physical health of older adults appears to be linked to their mental health. Research on psychological well-being among older adults has found that those whose physical health is good score highly on measures of mental health (Gerson et al., 1987). In their review of the literature on mental health among older adults, Hayslip and Panek (1993) concluded that positive mental health in old age is often related to individual characteristics and patterns of coping that have been present throughout life. Positive mental health at any age is said to be related to high levels of self-confidence and self-reliance, realistic perceptions of one's strengths and weaknesses, learning and maintaining effective coping skills and an active approach to one's social environment. Preparation for successful adaptation to ageing involves fostering these skills and qualities throughout the lifespan.

9.5.2 Models of Late Adulthood

Of the developmental models that we have been tracing, only Erikson's (1959) addresses development in late adulthood in a detailed way. His final developmental stage of **ego integrity versus despair** is said to be the prime psychosocial issue for those aged over 65. The ego integrity that arises from the successful resolution of this stage is characterized by an acceptance of how one's life has been, a lack of regret that it could have been different and an acceptance of responsibility for one's life. The despair that is seen as the negative possibility of this stage may be expressed as a fear of death and a belief that there is not enough time left to alter one's life in a more satisfactory direction.

9.5.3 Retirement

It is generally assumed that retirement adversely affects psychological well-being. A person's occupation is often seen as underpinning their identity and as providing them with many opportunities for meaningful and socially valued achievement and for social interaction. After retirement, it is therefore assumed that the person may experience a sense of meaninglessness and depression. The problem with this line of reasoning is that it presumes that everyone who retires derived fulfilment and satisfaction from their job. The person who finds their job tedious and unfulfilling and who sees it simply as a means of 'putting bread on the table' may welcome the release from this situation that retirement brings. Their identity may be focused around domains outside the workplace to which they can devote more time after retirement.

Bee (1994) reviewed evidence from longitudinal studies of adults before and after retirement and concluded that retirement has essentially no impact on life satisfaction or feelings of well-being. Generally, it is not associated with increased depression nor is it experienced as stressful. However, it has been found that those who have little control over the decision to retire (because of ill-health, for example) are more likely to experience lower life satisfaction and higher levels of stress than those who choose to retire (Herzog et al., 1991). A lack of control over retirement renders it similar to redundancy, with the same adverse effects on psychological well-being. From their review of the literature on retirement, Hayslip and Panek (1993) have also pointed to the person's occupational level, the importance they attach to work and the extent of their psychological and financial preparation as influencing the likelihood of successful adjustment to retirement. The scenarios below present two very different reactions to retirement, with the different reactions shaped by the influential variables that have been outlined.

Ben Davies is a 62-year-old man who has recently been forced to retire from his job as managing director of his own company because of ill-health. He describes himself as 'hard-driven and ambitious'. Throughout his life, he devoted all his energies to building his company into a successful enterprise. As a result, his relationship with his first wife suffered and they divorced after ten years of marriage, when Ben was in his late thirties. He remarried soon after but this marriage also ended in divorce after 12 years. He seldom sees his two sons from his first marriage, neither of whom were interested in pursuing a career in business. Since his retirement, Ben has been finding life difficult. He says he feels empty and useless and does not know how to fill his days. He has little involvement with his company because, in the scramble for the directorship following his retirement, he backed an unsuccessful candidate. He has few friends or interests outside his former workplace and does not want 'just to fritter my time away'.

George Green is a 62-year-old man who has recently taken early retirement from his job in a hosiery factory. Although he had worked at the factory in various capacities for 27 years, he never found the work very interesting. 'I work to live,' he used to say, 'I don't live to work.' George's real interests lay outside work, where he pursued various hobbies and sporting interests, sometimes with his workmates but more often with other friends and members of his family. George first married at the age of 25 but this relationship ended after 10 years. He remarried at the age of 40 and is still living with his second wife. He is close to his two sons from his first marriage and enjoys spending time with his three grandchildren. When the opportunity for early retirement was offered to him, he eagerly seized it. He now devotes much of his time to organizing various activities at his local football club and tending his garden (and those of his elderly neighbours). George professes himself to be 'quite content to live out my days like this'. His only regret is that 'I didn't do this years ago'.

9.5.4 Reactions to Bereavement

One task that can impact significantly upon psychological well-being in late adulthood is the management of bereavement. Older adults will experience the death of friends who are of the same age and thus will be made acutely aware of their own mortality.

Inevitably during late adulthood, one partner in a couple will die. In heterosexual couples, given the longer female lifespan, it is more likely to be the female partner who is left to cope with this bereavement. The death of a spouse has been rated as the most stressful life event that most people encounter (Holmes and Rahe, 1967). It is a standard finding in research on widowhood that the first six months after the death represent the most difficult period of adjustment. Studies have generally found no differences in mental health between widowed and non-widowed groups two years after the death of the widowed participants' spouses (for example, see McCrae and Costa, 1988).

The psychological effects of the death of a partner tend to be greater if the death has occurred suddenly. In this case, the surviving partner will not have had the opportunity to prepare for the death or to have engaged in what has been termed 'anticipatory grieving'. This refers to the situation where a death is expected and so the grieving process can begin before the death occurs. This, however, presumes that the surviving partner had acknowledged the likelihood of their partner dying. It ignores people's ability to deny what seems obvious to those around them or to maintain hope in the face of an imminent and inevitable personal disaster.

Also, the predictability of the loss may not prevent adverse grief reactions among older adults who were involved in caring for their partner during their final illness. During this period, they may have neglected their own physical and psychological well-being. This, combined with the many social and psychological losses associated with the death of a partner (including the loss of the role of carer), may render the grief experience extremely painful. Women tend to fare better during widowhood than men (Stroebe and Stroebe, 1986). This has been attributed to the tendency for men to rely heavily on their spouses for emotional support, while women generally obtain such support from a wider circle. Without his partner's support to protect him from life stresses, a man's mental and physical health may suffer badly after her death.

A complicating factor in bereavement in late adulthood is the possibility of 'bereavement overload'. This may be experienced by older adults who have undergone the deaths of many friends over a relatively short period of time. These individuals may find that they have insufficient time to come to terms with one death before another death occurs. Thus, each grieving process is compounded by the one preceding it.

There have been attempts to outline stage models of grieving (for example, see Bowlby, 1980, and Sanders, 1989) but these have been problematic. The experience of grief does not easily fit into fixed stages and not everyone appears to experience the stages that have been outlined. Counsellors therefore need to take care not to use these models in a prescriptive way when working with people who have been bereaved, otherwise they may end up waiting for the person to exhibit the second stage of a particular model of bereavement and may not be aware that the person has skipped that stage and moved from the first stage to the third. It has been known for counsellors to try to squeeze every bereavement reaction within their chosen model or to ignore responses to bereavement that do not fit within the model.

Bereavement counselling has been recognized as a potentially effective means of alleviating some of the distress that the bereaved individual may experience (Barry, 1993). Parkes (1980) has reviewed a number of evaluative studies of counselling services designed to promote psychological well-being among people experiencing bereavement. He concluded that professional and voluntary counselling services and self-help groups can reduce the risk of psychiatric and psychosomatic problems arising from bereavement. However, he emphasized that voluntary and self-help services require professional support. Counselling services may be most beneficial to those who experience severe bereavement reactions because of the circumstances of the death or because of their personal circumstances, for example, those who lack social support to help them through their bereavement and those who have experienced many losses (not necessarily deaths) within a short period of time.

Outside the counselling context, friends and relatives of bereaved individuals are often unsure what they should say or how they should support them in their grief. Lehman et al. (1986) found that what is rated as most helpful is contact with others who have had similar bereavement experiences and who can listen and allow the person to talk about their feelings. Platitudes that minimize the loss or deny its uniqueness—such as 'he'd had a good innings' or 'I know how you feel'—tend to be rated as most unhelpful.

9.5.5 Death of the 'Self'

As life draws to a close, the ageing person faces another death; his or her own death, the death of the 'self' (Raphael, 1984). The awareness that one's life is finite takes on a new reality and the person may go through a process of 'anticipatory grief' as described by Kubler-Ross (1969) and Aldrich (1963) in their work on terminal illness. Sometimes they may want to talk about it, sometimes they will deny that it will come. Some individuals may calculate their life expectancy based on a number of variables such as the age at which their parents died, their own health etc. (Marshall, 1975).

Many elderly people reminisce and this can turn into a 'life-review'; a time for reworking old conflicts and coming to terms with past life (Butler, 1963). And so, according to Erikson, and as we have discussed above, rather than experiencing the pain of personal despair indicated by 'a sense that the time is now too short for an attempt to start life anew', the individual tries out alternate roads to achieving a state of **ego integrity.** If elders have integrity enough not to fear death, then 'healthy children will not fear life' (pp. 28–29).

9.6 CONCLUDING COMMENTS

This chapter has attempted to describe conceptualizations of psychosocial development from adolescence to late adulthood, interwoven with relevant information on physical and cognitive development. Within each life stage, particular developmental tasks and transitions were selected for consideration on the grounds that they may feature among the problems presented by clients who seek counselling. Although lifespan developmental psychology focuses on those developmental issues that are encountered by most or all people, the particular difficulties faced by specific social and cultural groups should not be overlooked within a counselling context. Indeed, it should be remembered that individual patterns of development can vary greatly from the general trends that have been described.

Some writers on lifespan developmental psychology have offered suggestions for interventions that might promote psychological development among clients experiencing problems with developmental tasks (for example, see Sugarman, 1986). Although some general points about counselling practice on certain issues have been included in the present chapter, a programme of specific therapeutic interventions has been deliberately omitted.

Instead, it is hoped that counsellors will use the conceptualizations of development that have been outlined and the discussions of various developmental tasks to inform their counselling practice, to heighten their understanding of clients who are grappling with the issues raised and to develop appropriate and effective interventions for these clients.

10

Stress, Coping, Health and Illness

CONTENTS

10.1 INTRODUCTION

Life, most people would agree, is inherently stressful. There are the day-to-day frustrations of home, family and working life and there are the more major events that most people, at some time in their lives, have to cope with: the break-up of a relationship, illness, moving home, the death of someone close. Some people are also unfortunate enough to experience events which would normally be considered to fall outside the range of 'normal' life experiences, such as rape or the death of a child.

But as well as using the term stress to refer to a broad range of events that may happen to a person, we also use it to describe the individual's reactions—physical, behavioural and psychological—to such events. Accordingly, if the person is not coping with such events, they may be said to be 'suffering' from stress; that is, if they are middle class, professional and possibly male. But if it happens to be a woman of a certain age, 'forty something', who is not coping, they may well be seen to be reacting as they do because they are menopausal; and if they happen to be unmarried with two children, living in a council flat, they would probably be described as plainly inadequate! The concept of stress, as we can see, is not particularly straightforward.

We also sometimes impose stress on ourselves. We decide to apply for a new job or to go walking in the Himalayas (although, at some stages of the journey, we may wonder why on earth we did). In this way, stress can be an internal state that is self-generated, rather than triggered by some incident.

So whilst everyone knows what it means to feel 'stressed' and the word 'stress' is used frequently in everyday language, it would sometimes be difficult to spell out exactly what we mean by the term.

Psychologists and researchers have had similar problems with the definition and in this chapter we will be looking at the various ways they have conceptualized stress. We will be examining the different types of 'stressors' and the various ways in which we react to such events and situations.

The psychophysiological work in this area is particularly intriguing. Our physiological responses are integrally linked to the way in which we perceive and cope with stressful situations. Having some knowledge of this area of theory and research can add to our own understanding (and possibly that of our clients) of the experience of stress. It can also help us to begin to understand the relationship between stress and ill-health.

Another area of the stress literature which is of particular relevance to counsellors is concerned with 'protective' and 'vulnerability' factors. We will be examining what makes some people more 'stress-resistant' than others and exploring ways in which the counsellor or therapist can enhance the protective mechanisms and decrease the tendency towards vulnerability to stress.

Throughout the chapter, we will be giving examples of the way in which work in this area can inform the counsellor and be used therapeutically. The chapter finishes with a brief section on 'stress management programmes'.

10.2 THE CONCEPT OF STRESS

Researchers have tried to study stress in a very wide variety of settings and using many different models of stress. Some have concentrated on the biological or physiological aspects, others have emphasized the meaning of particular events to an individual while yet others have examined community wide stress such as that caused by natural disasters or war.

Given the wide ranging nature of this activity, it is not surprising that many models or concepts of stress are employed by theorists and researchers. Often researchers have failed to make explicit the model of stress that they are operating from and/or have assumed that there is an agreed or 'commonsense' model which is obvious and uncontroversial. Thus it has become a part of our cultural belief system that stress causes heart disease, depression, ulcers and many other conditions. However, such a model, which assumes that any stress can cause any disorder, is not a very helpful one since it is too general to lead to any concrete applications.

The dominance of this generalist or non-specific model of stress can be traced back to one of the earliest theorists in this area: Hans Selye. Selye's (1956, 1982) model is known as the **general adaptation theory of stress**. He suggested that stress produces a typical physiological response in the body which could be thought of as having three stages of adaptation: alarm, resistance and exhaustion. The first stage, the alarm stage, consists of general physiological arousal and activity in which the body's defences are activated. If the stressor persists then, in the second stage, the body attempts to resist whatever the assault on it is. If this resistance is unsuccessful and the stress continues, then the body can exhaust its resources and this is the final stage. This three-stage reaction is known as the **general adaptation syndrome**.

Although this model was originally devised to account for the body's reaction to physiological or biological stress, it has been very influential in thinking about psychological and social stress also. However, the legacy of this model is that we have tended to think of stress as being something essentially undesirable and to be avoided, i.e. it proposes a pathological model and assumes that stress produces a non-specific vulnerability to ill-health.

For example, Holmes and Rahe (1967) assumed a general adaptation of stress when they devised their **social readjustment rating scale.** This scale listed a number of events which would entail some adaptation or readjustment on the part of the individual. Each event on this scale was given a weighting to represent the degree of adaptation that might be expected. For example, death of a spouse had a very high weighting whereas birth of child had a lower weighting. The total sum of the weightings was then taken as an index of the degree of stress to which the person had been exposed.

Numerous research studies have used this or similar checklist measures to examine the relationship between stress and illness. Overall, such studies have claimed to find statistical associations between degree of life change and a variety of physical and psychological symptoms or disorders. However, there are significant conceptual and methodological problems in such research which mean that the results from these studies should be treated with caution.

One way of overcoming some of these conceptual problems is to draw the distinctions between **stressors, stress** and **distress**. It is too simplistic to see 'stressors' as good or bad. Everyone is exposed to a number of stressors at any point in time. Some of these may be independent external events or circumstances, such as noise, traffic jams or housing problems. Others, as mentioned above, may be internally or personally generated, such as going for promotion or sailing round the world. Stressors may be either threatening or challenging or even both at the same time. For example, being made redundant (or even the death of a partner) may be seen as a source of considerable stress at the time, but it may prove to be liberating and a challenge for a particular individual over time.

Clearly there is no simple way of seeing such stressors as undesirable or negative and then adding the number of events together to get a 'stressor score'. Even a person who appears to have a large number of external stressors may not subjectively experience 'stress' as an internal state. Yet each of us knows some individual for whom even the most insignificant stressor can be the source of considerable subjective stress. Therefore we need to have a model of stress which is more sophisticated or complex to do justice to these wide individual variations.

The nature of the link between subjective feelings of stress and any distress is also not entirely straightforward. While some individuals may be said to thrive under stress and appear to find the experience of stress an enabling and energizing one, for others it is quite the opposite. Individuals with a low tolerance of stress may find that they become **distressed,** either psychologically or physiologically.

A comprehensive model of stress will therefore need to be able to encompass individual differences in tolerance for, and reactivity to, internal states of stress. It will also have to be able to be more specific about why in some instances distress is manifested in the form of gastrointestinal or other physical health problems, whereas in others the manifestation may be in the form of agoraphobia, depression or some other psychological condition.

One model of stress which has attempted to do justice to the complexity of the issues involved is the **diathesis–stress model**. Diathesis means predisposition. In this model, external events, or stressors, are assumed to interact with predispositions, vulnerabilities or constitutional factors within the individual person. The interaction of these external and internal factors is what then determines whether distress, disease or disorder comes about and, if so, what particular form it takes.

The adoption of this model of stress obviously calls for much more sophisticated research strategies than simply administering life change checklists and correlating the score on such measures with the number of 'symptoms' a person reports. Such ambitious and more complex research has recently grown considerably after the impetus of the model of life stress suggested by Brown and Harris (1978, 1989).

In their model, the role of life stress in bringing about disorder is seen as being crucially mediated by the 'meaning' of the event in the context of the individual person's biography and current circumstances. This is something which is, of course, recognized by most counsellors and therapists. What we may assume to be to be a source of stress or distress may not necessarily be so, and what, on the face of it, may appear to be insignificant can, to the client, be a considerable source of stress. For example, the acne on the client's face may be hardly visible to the naked eye, but the distress it causes that particular person can only be understood in relation to the meaning it has for them. This may be associated with feelings of worth, how they think others see them and their role and position in their peer group.

10.3 STRESSORS

Although in this section we will be identifying some of life's stressors, these should not, as we have discussed above, be viewed out of the context of the personal factors we shall be discussing in Sections 10.5 and 10.6.

10.3.1 Life Events

Stressful life events vary considerably in severity from minor daily hassles through major life events to catastrophic life events.

Minor frustrations

Often it is not the major life events that produce the greatest stress, but the minor frustrations and annoyances such as driving in the rush hour, dealing with rude or unpleasant customers, queueing at the supermarket, not being able to find a clean mug *yet again* because they are all growing mould in the teenagers' bedrooms. Indeed, one researcher (DeLongis et al., 1982) found that accumulation of daily hassles was an even greater predictor of emotional and physical health than were major life events in peoples' lives.

Major life events

Events that can have a strong impact and long-term consequences such as the birth of a baby, the death of someone close, marriage, failure to get into university, being the victim of a serious crime are considered to be major life events. As noted above, scales have been developed which purport to measure the impact of such events, based on the idea that all change is of necessity stressful and negative. However, as we have seen, this tends to be an oversimplification and more recently scales have been developed which allow for the individual to judge each event as good or bad and estimate its impact on their lives.

However, in spite of the criticisms of life-events studies, there does seem to be some relationship between life changes and health. The majority of people, however, manage to cope with change without becoming ill and clearly other factors are involved. These will be discussed in Section 10.6 below.

Catastrophic life events

Finally, some events that have such a profound impact, and are thankfully outside the range of usual human experience, are usually referred to as catastrophic life events. These include natural disasters, such as earthquakes and floods; man-made disasters, such as wars and nuclear disasters; traumatic accidents, such as car or plane crashes and physical assaults, such as rape or attempted murder. The impact of such events will be discussed in Section 11.6 .

10.3.2 Common Psychological Stressors

Excessive demands

Increasingly we are expected to do more and more in less and less time; increasing our productivity, meeting ever tightening deadlines. Additionally, many of us are required to demonstrate our proficiency and competence. We have to fill in appraisal forms, time sheets, documents for quality control and audit. Professionals fear being sued, many fear redundancy. In some occupations, such as medicine, nursing, air traffic control, people may have to face constant and long-lasting pressure and be required to make decisions under heavy time pressure which involve life and death. People under such pressure day after day can begin to perform poorly, and develop stress-related physical and psychological symptoms which can then become an additional source of stress.

Most counsellors will have experienced clients under this type of pressure and working with such clients can sometimes pose ethical dilemmas for counsellors. What do you do, for example, if your client wants to return to a situation in which the demands are so unreasonable that there is little chance of him/her, or anyone else, being able to function in that environment? Even if the client wishes it, should counsellors or therapists give first-aid 'stress management' which may ultimately lead to more serious distress?

Boredom

This is the opposite of pressure, but boredom, or understimulation, can be a significant stressor, especially if it continues a long time. Boredom often occurs when people feel trapped in situations, metaphorically or literally. An extreme example is the agony of solitary confinement.

Frustration

When some obstacle stands in the way of our personal goals or wishes, it is inherently frustrating. The closer the person is to achieving their goal, the more frustrating it is when they encounter an obstacle which prevents them achieving it. So the situation of almost making the summit when bad weather forced a retreat may be more frustrating than having to give up half way up the mountain. The person who is shortlisted for the job may, although not necessarily, find it more frustrating not to be selected than if he or she had not made it that far.

Frustration can also result from personal factors. For example, if someone desperately wants to become a doctor but clearly does not have the intellectual capability to get into medical school, then it is personal limitations, rather than external forces, that hinder the achievement of the goal. The implications for counselling are different depending on whether the frustration is external or personal.

Conflict

This also can be external or internal and is almost always stressful. The most obvious examples of external conflicts are disputes with family, friends or colleagues. Internal conflicts can be equally, if not more, distressing and occur when a person must choose between incompatible or contradictory needs, desires, motives or external demands.

Common sources of internal conflict include being one of the 'gang' yet wanting to keep out of trouble, choosing between the competing demands of work and family life, the need for relaxation and playing with the children, the need for personal solitude and the desire to maintain a relationship. Exploring and working through such conflicts is often one of the tasks of counselling and therapy. The situation described below provides a good example of internal conflict as a source of stress.

A client was referred for psychological therapy by her GP because she had experienced a number of stress-related physical symptoms over the past four years. Five years ago she was delighted to achieve her ambition by becoming head teacher of a junior school. She had always had a very clear idea of the sort of headmistress she would like to be: someone who was approachable, firm but caring, available to her staff, pupils, parents and governors alike; a 'hands-on' traditional headmistress. Unfortunately she found herself caught up in a changing world: a world of performance-related pay, of budgets, appraisals, league-tables and audits—the world of the head teacher/manager. Nevertheless, she took this on board and indeed became quite committed to the ideas embodied in this new philosophy of educational management. Accordingly, she conscientiously applied herself to all the necessary extra administration—in addition, that is, to the roles, tasks and duties of the traditional headmistress.

Her health began to suffer as she found it harder and harder to cope. She also developed symptoms of depression: she had difficulty sleeping, found it increasingly hard to make decisions, her confidence, never particularly robust, plummeted and she would frequently become tearful. When she was first referred to the counsellor she was on sick leave and unsure when she would return to work.

Therapy centred around the conflict. The client found it extremely difficult to relinquish her traditional role by, for example putting a 'DO NOT DISTURB', notice on her door when working on the administrative tasks (this being inconsistent with her view of herself as a traditional headmistress). Nor did she feel she could delegate any more than she had been doing or 'prioritize' her workload, believing that everything should be done by her with equal thoroughness and commitment.

Ultimately she found she could not resolve the conflict and decided to make a career change.

Discrimination and harassment

Discrimination and harassment because of ethnicity, gender, disability or sexual orientation can be a very significant source of stress for the person concerned. Increasingly employees have been turning to the legal system to get some redress for the adverse consequences of exposure to such stressors. In their study of women police officers, Brown et al. (1995) found that women suffered more general detrimental discrimination than male officers. The factor that best predicted psychological symptoms in women officers was the degree to which they had experienced sexual harassment.

10.3.3 Situational Factors that Influence Stress

Although people respond differently to the same stressful situation, certain characteristics of the stressor have been found to influence the severity of the stress. These are its predictability and controllability, its suddenness and duration.

In general, events over which the person has little or no control, which occur suddenly and unpredictably and which confront a person over a long period of time seem to take the greatest toll on physical and psychological well-being (Lazarus and Folkman, 1984; Taylor, 1991).

10.4 STRESS REACTIONS

As we saw when we looked at emotion (Chapter 3), cognitive and physiological events are integrally linked. How we appraise a situation affects how our bodies respond to it. Emotional arousal plays an extremely important part in our survival.

10.4.1 Physiological Reactions

A mild level of arousal tends to produce alertness and interest in the current situation, and we undoubtedly need a certain amount of arousal to perform any sort of task, whether it be sitting an examination, giving a speech or playing tennis. At very low levels of arousal (for example at the point of waking up or when very relaxed) we will not be attending to sensory information and performance will be relatively poor. If arousal is very high, however, whether the experience is pleasant or unpleasant, performance will be disrupted.

In many situations the relationship between arousal and performance seems to take the shape of an upside-down curve or 'U' curve (Yerkes and Dodson, 1908; Smith and Smoll, 1990).

As physiological arousal increases up to some optimum level, performance improves. But beyond that optimum level, further increases in arousal impair performance.

If we perceive a particular situation as an interesting challenge, then we are more likely to produce the appropriate level of emotional arousal needed to deal with it successfully. If, however, we perceive something as a threat, whatever kind of threat, our bodies react as they have evolved to do by preparing for **fight or flight**. We need quick energy, so extra sugar is released by the liver, and hormones are secreted that convert fat into sugar. Muscles tense and heart rate, blood pressure and breathing rate increase in preparation for expending energy. Saliva and mucus dry up, thereby increasing the size of the airways to the lungs, and non-essential functions such as digestion are decreased. In preparation for injury, surface blood vessels constrict to reduce bleeding, bone marrow produces more white corpuscles to fight infection and endorphins are released.

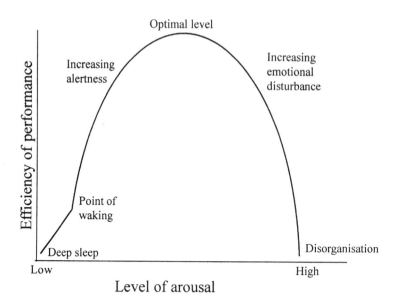

Figure 10.1   Emotional arousal and performance (adapted from Hebb, 1972)

Most of these physiological changes result from the activation of the **sympathetic nervous system** (see Section 3.3). The sympathetic nervous system also stimulates the secretion of **catecholamine**, or stress hormones which increase the general level of physiological arousal. Meanwhile, the adrenal cortex secretes a second group of stress hormones, notably **cortisol**.

Whereas catecholamine secretion (except when secreted at high levels over a long period) can enhance immune system activity, cortisol suppresses it. It does this as part of its function in controlling inflammation. The problem with this is that it does so regardless of whether there is any need (Calabrese et al., 1987). Cortisol's effects generally last much longer than those of the catecholamines and its effects seem to be more damaging; for example, in being responsible (more so than the catecholamines) for fatty deposits in the arteries that lead to heart disease. We shall see in Section 10.6 how the way in which we view situations can affect the secretion of these two hormones.

Increased levels of arousal also involve the release of the hormones **adrenaline** (epinephrine) and **noradrenaline** (norepinephrine) into the tissues and the bloodstream. These hormones are believed also to have an effect on the functioning of the immune system. However, the exact nature of the relationships are still being investigated and it is thought that a number of psychological factors can mediate the relationship between stressors, the autonomic nervous system and the immune system. Such psychological factors include mood, personality, and beliefs about one's personal degree of control.

Although it is possible to demonstrate a variety of somatic consequences following exposure to aversive or noxious stimulations in the laboratory, we cannot assume that such stimulation is equivalent to 'life stress'. Also merely observing that short-term physiological changes can be brought about by stress does not allow us to conclude that such reactions are the necessary and sufficient conditions for bringing about long-term undesirable health effects. There is therefore need for considerable caution in extrapolating from experimental laboratory-based studies of the effects of artificial stress to real-life stress and actual ill health.

10.4.2 Cognitive Impairment

As we have seen, performance on tasks tends to deteriorate at high levels of emotional arousal. At times of stress we find it difficult to concentrate and organize our thoughts. Examination anxiety is a classic case in point. Students or candidates suffering from this type of anxiety are often so beset by negative or other distracting thoughts that they frequently fail to follow instructions and may misread or misinterpret the questions. The intrusion of extraneous thoughts that usually accompany anxiety may also interfere with the retrieval of information necessary for answering the question. (See Section 4.6 on Forgetting.)

But this type of cognitive impairment is not restricted to the examination rooms; it can be a feature of everyday life in times of stress when even the most routine task, such as going to the supermarket, cleaning the house or arranging to have the television set mended can require more effort and concentration than the person can muster.

10.4.3 Behavioural Reactions

Often the last person to realize they are reacting adversely to stressors and stress is the very person who is affected by it. Colleagues, family and friends may be the first to notice some of the behavioural signs that might indicate when a person is 'under stress'. The common non-specific manifestations in people's behaviour include increased irritability, indecisiveness, changes in sleeping and eating patterns, excessive use of alcohol and an increase in smoking.

Thus as well as the possibility of stress having a direct effect on physiological functioning and increasing the risk of disease process it may also have an indirect effect via changes in behaviour. The individual under stress may indulge in behaviours which directly contribute to their risk of disease, e.g. by smoking or by drinking alcohol. Also the person at such times may be more likely to engage in risk-taking behaviours or expose themselves to situations where they might be accidentally injured. Thus behavioural reactions to stress may themselves create more stress by making it more likely that some adverse events will occur.

10.4.4 Emotional Responses

Our emotional responses to stressful situations can range from exhilaration and excitement (when we see the event in question as demanding and manageable) to anger, anxiety and despair (when we are overwhelmed and feel we cannot cope). So the rider may feel a thrill of excitement at the start of a competition; particularly if she knows she is on a good horse and the jumps look manageable. However, if her horse fell at his last outing and the jumps look enormous, she may experience not excitement, but feelings of trepidation and dread, at which point she may wish she'd taken up patchwork or breeding budgerigars for a hobby instead of riding.

Anxiety

As the above example demonstrates anxiety is often related to perceived control over a situation and the extent to which we feel able to cope. Distinctions have been made between normal or **objective anxiety**, which is adaptive and motivates the person to deal with the harmful situation, and **neurotic anxiety**, which is out of proportion to the actual danger posed. But as we can see from the above example, the distinction is not always clear-cut.

Nevertheless, when a person reacts with intense anxiety to a situation which others would see as only mildly stressful, it may be reasonable to suppose that the source of danger is related more to internal feelings than any external source. Different theorists have viewed this sort of internally derived anxiety somewhat differently; Freud attributed it to unconscious conflicts whilst behaviourists focus on ways in which anxiety may have become associated with certain situations through learning. Clearly the way in which counsellors or therapists conceptualize anxiety will have a considerable bearing on the way in which they help their clients to work through, manage or resolve these unpleasant feelings.

Anger

Another common reaction to stressful situations is anger, which may lead to aggression. The **frustration–aggression hypothesis** assumes that when a person's efforts to reach a goal are blocked, an aggressive drive is induced that motivates behaviour to injure the object causing the frustration. Although aggression in not an inevitable response, research has shown it is certainly one of them.

Sometimes, of course, it is extremely unwise to express anger directly to the object or person causing it and sometimes the source of frustration is vague and intangible. This may lead to the displacement of anger onto another object, animal (the proverbial 'kicking the cat') or person, possibly the counsellor. In a therapeutic context this would be seen as transference.

Another way of dealing with anger resulting from a frustrating situation is to express it by talking about it to a third person; a friend, partner or counsellor. One difficulty that clients sometimes report, however, is that the friend or partner then tries to help the client resolve the 'problem', when all the client had wanted to do was vent some of the feelings. Counsellors also need to avoid falling into the trap of inappropriate problem-solving. They also may need to make decisions about whether to encourage the expression of frustration or to contain or deflect it.

Finally we should not forget (as we discussed in Section 3.7 on Emotional Expression and Counselling) that the anger may be telling us something about a situation which needs changing or managing in a different way. If we take some action in this respect, then we may no longer experience the anger.

Withdrawal and apathy

Although some people respond to frustration with aggression, others respond with what seems to be the opposite, withdrawal and apathy. If the stressful situation continues, this may lead to depression.

Depression

Quite why one person reacts to frustration with aggression and another with apathy and depression is unclear, although it is thought that learning plays a part. Frustrated children who strike out angrily and then find their needs met are more likely to respond that way again when encountering subsequent frustrations. But children whose aggressive outbursts are never 'successful' and whose needs continue to be unmet, may give up and become apathetic and withdrawn.

10.5 COPING WITH STRESS

Adverse life events and circumstances are not randomly distributed occurrences throughout the population. We know from sociological and psychological research that social class, gender and ethnicity are linked with one's chances of exposure to negative events and chronic ongoing difficulties. We also know that coping resources, such as money or knowledge, are unequally distributed in our society. In understanding any individual's coping strategies, it is therefore necessary to place that individual in a socio-political context in order to appreciate what their range of coping resources and strategies might be.

Psychological coping responses are sometimes divided into **problem-focused coping** and **emotion-focused coping**. Problem-focused coping involves the individual evaluating the stressful situation and doing something about it. Emotion-focused coping, on the other hand, focuses on the emotional response to the problem; the individual tries to reduce their anxiety about the problem without actually dealing with the situation (Lazarus and Folkman, 1984). People are more likely to use problem-focused coping strategies when they perceive they can gain some control over the situation and emotion-focused coping when the problem cannot be solved, such as when facing terminal illness or coping with bereavement.

10.5.1 Problem-focused Coping Strategies

Problem-focused coping strategies are attempts to confront and directly deal with the demands of the situation itself. It may involve problem-solving strategies such as those discussed in Chapter 5; defining the problem, generating alternative solutions, weighing up alternatives and choosing and implementing the selected response.

Other strategies employed for mastering the situation might be

- **changing our goals or aspirations**—so we may decide we will be satisfied with having completed the Open University's Foundation Course and do not want the stress of completing the degree course;
- **working out how to manage time more effectively**—such as making a detailed revision timetable;
- **confronting the difficulty directly**—for example by trying to resolve an issue or misunderstanding with a neighbour or colleague;
- **changing the situation itself**—such as by postponing taking the driving test.

10.5.2 Emotion-focused Coping Strategies

In general, we tend to employ emotion-focused coping if we believe there is nothing we can do to manage or to change the situation. Such strategies are aimed at managing the physiological components of the response, which usually means our anxiety. They include behavioural strategies such as venting anger, having a drink, taking exercise, seeking emotional support and reappraising the situation in a way which minimizes its emotional impact. A good example of this last strategy was provided by a client whose presenting issues had been social anxiety and low self-esteem.

> She had been out with a group of colleagues for Christmas lunch. One of the party was her new supervisor, a lady whom she liked and respected but who had always appeared somewhat reserved and a little distant. On leaving the restaurant she helped this lady into her jacket, but jokingly put it on her back to front. The supervisor got quite irritated by this and told her to behave herself and that she had had too much to drink. The client was left feeling very embarrassed and worried that she had 'overstepped the mark' and had deeply offended her boss who now must be thinking what a stupid person she was. The situation was made worse by the fact that she developed a virus and was off work for a few days and this was followed by the Christmas break. She began to dread going back to work and facing her supervisor.
>
> Although this incident may not sound particularly stressful in itself, in the context of the client's history it was quite significant. In therapy she had been exploring the ways in which she tended to interpret other people's behaviour and on this occasion she was eventually able to change her appraisal of this situation herself. Her thinking, she reported, went something like this: 'What I did was not offensive, it was all part of the fun. She should lighten up a bit. Maybe she is thinking that, and is really embarrassed she couldn't join in.' The stress almost immediately lessened. When she did return to work the supervisor greeted her in a warm and friendly way and the client accordingly felt she might have been right in her reappraisal of the incident.

In this instance, the reappraisal of the problem seems fairly realistic and evidence for this is provided by the supervisor's response when she returned to work. This is not always the case. Sometimes when we appraise situations we deceive ourselves and distort the reality as a way of attempting to reduce anxiety. Freud used the term **defence mechanisms** to refer to this process. Defence mechanisms are thought to be largely unconscious in their operation but are not necessarily maladaptive or unhelpful. Because they function to moderate the degree of anxiety that the individual experiences, they can perform an essential function in helping the person to cope with the demands made upon them. The main defence mechanisms are:

- **repression**—when memories or impulses that are too frightening or painful are excluded from conscious memory;
- **rationalization**—assigning seemingly logical or socially desirable motives to what we do, so it appears that we have acted rationally;
- **projection**—ascribing our own undesirable traits or qualities to others;
- **reaction formation**—concealing a motive from ourselves by giving strong expression to the opposite motive;
- **displacement**—whereby a motive that cannot be gratified in one form is channelled in some other way;
- **denial**—the denial of external reality when it is too unpleasant to face.

Everyone is thought to use such defence mechanisms. Their use is only thought to become problematic when they prevent the person from employing appropriate problem focused coping strategies to deal with life's demands (or possibly when life's demands are too great).

10.6 PROTECTIVE AND VULNERABILITY FACTORS

We have noted above that there are certain characteristics of the situations which may make them more stressful. But what about the characteristics of the particular individual in influencing the severity of their response to stress. We know that the same stressful life event or situation may have very different effects on different people, and indeed, it may affect the same individual in different ways at different times in their life. Psychologists have identified a number of factors which may influence the person's response to stressful events either by increasing their susceptibility to such events (vulnerability factors) or by helping them to cope more effectively (protective factors). These include coping skills, social support, self-efficacy and psychological hardiness.

10.6.1 The Effectiveness of Coping Strategies

We have discussed above two different styles of coping, but what does the research tell us about which is the most effective method? As we have pointed out, different strategies may be appropriate for different types of problem, and a key factor in the effectiveness of coping strategies is the amount of control that people have over stressful situations.

On the whole, the research suggests that problem-focused coping is associated with stable emotional adjustment and emotion focused strategies, particularly those that involve avoidance, denial and wishful thinking seem to be related to depression and less effective adaptation (Folkman and Lazarus, 1988; Revenson and Felton, 1989; Soloman et al., 1988). However, results such as these must be treated with caution. If people are confronted with stressful or traumatic situations over which they have little or no control, it may be this lack of control that determines their responses, rather than the coping strategies they employ.

10.6.2 Social Support

One important factor that has consistently been shown to make stress more bearable is the emotional support and concern of others. Conversely at times of stress, loneliness and social isolation can have devastating effects on physical and mental well-being (House et al., 1988). One study of Israeli parents who had lost a son either through accidents or war, found that those who were widowed or divorced paid more heavily for their bereavement. Their mortality rate in the ten years following the loss was higher than that for parents who could share their grief with each other (Leval et al., 1988).

There is even experimental evidence that suggests that social support enhances immune system functioning (Baron et al., 1990), affects recovery from medical interventions (Kulik and Mahler, 1989) and that people who are under stress are more disease-resistant if they have high levels of social support.

Although parents, friends and partners can undoubtedly be a considerable source of support, we cannot necessarily assume that this will be he case. Sometimes these people act in overprotective ways that may reduce a person's confidence and ability to cope. Alternatively they may minimize the problem or give vacuous assurances that all will be well, possibly as a means of protecting themselves from the impact of vicarious stress. So the parents who assure their son that he will pass his exams may be defending themselves against worry. Counsellors and therapists must also, of course, be wary of, and avoid giving, reassurance for similar reasons. It may make the helper feel better but it probably will not help the client.

In some situations, the cause of the stress may be shared by others or indeed, as in the case of disasters such as earthquakes, floods etc., by many. These sorts of community disasters often seem to bring out the best in people. Sometimes, however, individuals scarred by the same event, or in a similar way, can be so enmeshed in their own distress that they may not have sufficient resources themselves to support the other 'victim' or 'victims', as the examples below highlight.

A husband and wife sought the help of a counsellor after the 'cot death' of their four-month-old child. What had added to the distress was the fact that both were suffering individually so acutely that neither had been able to support the other in their agonizing grief. This had led to considerable anger and resentment in both husband and wife, and it seemed that the marriage, which had previously appeared to have been robust and good to both partners, was deteriorating to the point of breakdown.

Another husband and wife, both professional people, had both received minor head injuries (in a road traffic accident) which resulted in a similar degree of cognitive impairment. The husband had been driving although he was not at fault. Both their careers were affected and again, both were so individually distressed that neither could support the other.

In both of the above cases, the counsellor was able to give temporary emotional support to each partner individually and they were encouraged to seek social support appropriately outside their relationships. As they became less distressed, they were able to turn to their respective partners and both give and receive the support they felt they had lost.

It may also be the case that when we need support the most, we behave in ways that are least likely to elicit it. Indeed it may be difficult to offer support to someone who is constantly 'moaning on' about being on their own or someone who whines, gets 'clingy' or who resorts to excessive drinking.

One client who used alcohol to deal with her loneliness and distress after the death of her husband from Alzheimer's disease was becoming increasingly socially isolated in the small village in which she lived. Although she had a few acquaintances in the village, over the past few years when she had been nursing her husband she had cut herself off from village life and had neglected her appearance as well as her house. Although it seemed from information gained from other sources that her neighbours were sympathetic to her plight, her visits to their houses of an evening when she appeared quite drunk were becoming a source of embarrassment.

In counselling, the client developed problem-focused coping strategies to develop her social relationships and seek appropriate social support. This involved enrolling for evening classes, including GCSE sociology (when asked why she had chosen this subject, she replied 'because it's on a Thursday'!), buying new clothes and attending to her appearance generally, sorting out her house so she could invite people in, joining in village activities etc. Gradually she became fully integrated into community life; she went on holiday with a new-found friend, and, after a thirty-year break, returned to full-time employment, more for reasons associated with companionship and self-esteem than for financial necessity. She subsequently went on to study for an Open University degree in the social sciences. So as it turned out, it was quite fortuitous that sociology took place on Thursday evenings.

10.6.3 Self-efficacy

It has been noted above how our responses to stressful situations are affected by the extent to which we perceive the situation as controllable. Situations which are perceived as being beyond our control are often more stressful than those in which we feel we can do something, to take some hopefully successful action to achieve a satisfactory outcome. The term self-efficacy refers to the *belief* that we can do just this; the belief, as Bandura (1989) puts it, that one is capable of performing the behaviours that are required in order to attain specific goals. People whose self-efficacy is high have confidence that they are capable of overcoming obstacles and meeting their needs. They take the 'I'm sure I can do it' approach.

But what makes us believe that we *can* do it (whatever 'it' may be)? A considerable amount of research effort has gone into identifying the factors that affect self-efficacy. From this research it would seem that the most important determinant is previous success in similar situations. Other important factors are observing others in similar situations, what others tell us about out capabilities and what we tell ourselves, and finally our level of arousal; high emotional arousal that is interpreted as anxiety decreases self-efficacy.

Self-efficacy has been found to be very significant in protecting us from, or making us vulnerable to, stress and clearly the concepts involved are of relevance to many counselling contexts. But what about clients who believes that 'they can do it' in spite of evidence to the contrary? Clearly the counsellor has to assess carefully the status and function of this possibly erroneous belief.

Take, for example, the case of the client from a different culture who seems to be a permanent student. He starts and fails one course after another but he still believes that he can make it. He may be failing for a number of reasons but if it is because he does not have the intellectual capability whilst asserting that he can succeed, he may be employing a form of pseudo self-efficacy as an inappropriate emotionally focused coping strategy. Careful assessment in this case revealed that the function of this defence was to protect him from facing up to his parents' disappointment which he believed would result from his not completing his studies.

The therapist decided that it was appropriate to confront this defence, and after working through some of his feelings of anger and disappointment, the client expressed an overwhelming sense of relief that he no longer had to 'pretend' to his parents, and even more importantly, to pretend to himself.

10.6.4 Stress Resistance and Psychological Hardiness

It is undoubtedly the case that some individuals seem to be more stress-resistant than others; they can experience one stressful event after another and do not seem to fall apart, whilst others become seriously upset by what might appear to be fairly low-level stressors.

Several investigators have tried to identify what makes some people more resistant to stress than others. Most of this work appears to have been conducted with business executives, funded, no doubt by organizations that have a vested interest in employing or maintaining a work-force as stress-free as possible. The relevance of these findings to other populations is, however, debatable.

What these studies have found is that men under stress who responded positively to change and who were rated high on involvement, commitment and feelings of control were healthier than those who scored low on these dimensions (Kobasa, 1979). It could, of course be argued that this was because those who were healthier scored higher precisely because they were healthier, not the other way round. The researchers therefore conducted a second, longitudinal study with similar results (Kobasa et al., 1982).

The most important factor in 'psychological hardiness' appears to be attitude towards change. If change is viewed as a challenge rather than a threat then less stress is likely to be experienced and the situation turned to the individual's advantage. Examples of this would be seeing redundancy as an opportunity to start a new life and an exciting change of direction or a serious medical condition as a chance to work out priorities, to reassess values.

Support for this concept of psychological hardiness comes from research on physiological responses to stress. As noted earlier, two different hormones are secreted, catecholamine and corticosteroids (such as cortisol), as part of the body's response to stress. Both of these hormones mobilize the body to action but the extent to which each of these two systems is activated depends on how a situation is appraised. Catecholamine tends to be secreted if a situation is viewed as positive or a challenge, and cortisol if it is perceived as a threat. Cortisol stays in the system longer, and seems to have more damaging effects than catecholamine.

Nevertheless, it may not be altogether advisable to ask a friend who is about to go in to a stressful interview whether he is secreting catecholamines or cortisol. However, if you are working with clients on changing the way in which they conceptualize stressful situations, they may be interested and possibly find it helpful to understand the physiological rationale behind your interventions.

The notion of psychological hardiness is interrelated with the other factors discussed above that influence the severity or the stress. So 'high involvement' and 'commitment' to others may give a feeling of social support; feelings of control may reflect self-efficacy which also is likely to affect the way in which a situation is appraised, either as a challenge or as a threat.

The work on protective and vulnerability factors has considerable implications for counsellors and therapists working with individuals suffering from stress and stress-related conditions. Summarizing this literature, it would seem that the most powerful factors that can help to protect us from, or leave us vulnerable to, the effects of stress are the way in which we conceptualize, or cognitively construe situations, and our level of social and emotional support.

10.7 STRESS, HEALTH AND ILLNESS

As noted earlier, there is a common belief that 'stress' is responsible for bringing about, or at least contributing to, the onset and maintenance of a wide variety of physical illnesses and disorders. In this section we will discuss this idea at a general level before concentrating on two of the main areas of interest in this respect: heart disease and 'burnout'.

10.7.1 Psychosomatic Disorders

The terms stress-related disorders, psychosomatic disorders and psychophysiological disorders are all used to refer to those physical conditions which could be caused, at least in part, by adverse events, emotions or ways of thinking.

One of the exponents of the view that emotional conflicts could contribute to, and be manifested in, particular physical health problems was the psychoanalyst Franz Alexander (1950). In his view there was a specific type of emotional conflict associated with each of the different physical disorders. Hypertension was thought to be caused by chronic but repressed hostility, and ulcers by unconscious, frustrated needs for love. The particular organ system that would be affected was also thought to depend on constitutional factors; that is, 'vulnerable' systems would be more likely to show disorders.

Although the idea of specific, unconscious conflicts as contributors to physical ill-health has gone out of fashion somewhat, research in the area of stress-related disorders has continued apace. One example is the research which has examined whether recently bereaved spouses have a higher risk of fatal heart disease than those who have not suffered such a bereavement. In an early study Parkes et al. (1969) found a high mortality rate from heart-related problems among widowers in the first few months after their bereavement. However, later studies did not entirely support those findings (e.g. Clayton, 1979).

The difficulty with establishing simple links between one-off events such as bereavements and subsequent ill-health resides in the fact that one type of event (e.g. a bereavement) may well lead to other stressful events (e.g. having to sell the family house) or chronic financial difficulties.

Although such life event research poses a number of methodological problems, evidence is mounting that stress, such as academic pressures and marital difficulties, affects the ability of the immune system to defend the body (Jemmott et al., 1985; Glaser et al., 1986; Kiecolt-Glaser et al., 1988). There is now a considerable body of findings which supports the idea of psychosomatic links, and the growing field of **psychoimmunology** is beginning to discover more about the mechanisms by which stress may be implicated in the aetiology, course and management of physical illness of various kinds (Pitts and Phillips, 1991). Researchers have been interested in, amongst other things, stress as a possible risk factor in essential hypertension, the role of stress in the control of diabetes, whether stress precipitates asthma attacks, the relationship between stress and cancer and one of the most widely researched areas, stress and heart disease.

10.7.2 Heart Disease

Heart disease in general continues to be seen as one of the examples of a stress-related disorder. In studies of animals in 'high stress' conditions it has been found that they show a thickening of the coronary artery wall not seen in 'low stress' conditions. In humans it has been suggested that a particular personality type is more prone to coronary heart disease: the 'Type A' person. The role of Type A personality as a risk factor for coronary heart disease has been extensively studied. Such individuals are overcommitted to work, impatient, easily irritated and competitive. They are time pressured and hard driven. In contrast the Type B person is less pressurized and more easy going. It is also thought that the Type A person shows a greater physiological reactivity. That is, they show much greater changes in heart rate, blood pressure and stress-related hormones than others.

Recent writers on this topic have suggested that it is the negative emotional aspects of Type A behaviour, especially interpersonal hostility, that might be most strongly implicated in the link between Type A and the risk of coronary heart disease. However, despite the considerable research efforts that have gone into exploring these issues, it is not possible to conclude simply that Type A behaviour causes coronary heart disease. It is possible that some underlying genetic or constitutional factors produce both physiological overactivity and Type A personality styles. Such a personality style might, in turn, generate more stressors for that particular individual because of the habitual ways in which they interact with the world.

10.7.3 Burnout

Burnout is a term used for a severe reaction to stress that affects physical and psychological well-being and that leaves the person in a state of chronic fatigue and feeling emotionally drained. People suffering from burnout may feel exhausted during the day, but sleep badly at night. They often report feelings of depression, helplessness, loss of confidence, resentment, disillusionment and anger. They can become irritable and difficult to deal with and may appear rigid and inflexible, possibly as a way of coping with the increasing demands made upon them.

Burnout is a feature particularly, although by no means exclusively, of the 'helping' and public service professions. It often affects the most dedicated and idealistic members (Pines and Aronson, 1981). In the current economic and political climate seemingly ever-increasing demands are made on personnel in most areas of work. These external demands, coupled with personal features and qualities often (or once) valued highly, such as commitment to high standards, conscientiousness and feelings of responsibility, can result in burnout. As with all forms of stress, the result is an interaction, and sometimes a conflict, between situational and personal demands. The ultimate impact on the person, however, will depend, in part, on how he or she copes with these demands.

10.8 STRESS MANAGEMENT PROGRAMMES

Psychologists have devised a number of cognitive–behavioural methods for helping people to cope with stress. These are both emotion-focused and problem-focused. Emotion-focused methods are aimed at controlling arousal by, for example, relaxation training and biofeedback of physiological responses and by cognitive restructuring. Here, people are taught to modify aspects of their cognitive appraisals that lead to inappropriate emotional responses.

Problem-focused methods include teaching problem-solving techniques, activity scheduling and time management. Also individuals may be helped to improve their social skills or level of assertiveness in order to prevent problems arising in the first instance.

Sometimes these methods may take the form of standardized or semi-standardized 'programmes', usually referred to as 'stress management' treatments or programmes. Similar approaches are adopted in the numerous self-help books that exist to help people with self-management of stress and have also been used with some success in the treatment of essential hypertension (Johnson, 1989).

10.9 CONCLUDING COMMENTS

Although we have broken down the concept of stress into an number of separate areas, it is clear that it is a very broad term involving a transaction between the person and the environment. The psychological research on stress can tell us about the some of the processes which might take place within the person suffering from stress and also highlight a number of issues that it may be important for the counsellor to take into account when working with clients suffering from stress. General stress management programmes can also be useful in helping people identify and manage more 'normal' levels of stress, particularly when the stress comes from external sources.

The literature, however, can tell us little about the individual client, and what counsellors would recognize as the 'internal' sources of stress such as the pressure to succeed brought about by never having had the desired or necessary parental approval; or the strain of constantly ensuring one's actions are 'beyond reproach' and above criticism as a result of past failures and childhood humiliations.

Often the problems counsellors see are of this sort, and taking a standard 'stress-management approach' are unlikely to be successful without the counsellor first gaining a thorough understanding of the interaction between the person and the environment, as the following example demonstrates.

Holes in the net through which red herrings can slip (or 'Floaters that became red herrings')

The client is a 20-year-old man who had withdrawn from his university course after one year. He sought help because he was getting increasingly distressed about 'floaters'—black spots which floated in front of his eyes—which had first appeared a year ago after bungee jumping in Australia (although it had never been established that this was the cause). When he saw the counsellor, he was particularly worried because he was about to take up a job in a Mediterranean resort driving a speed boat for water-skiers. He was concerned that his vision would be impaired by the floaters and this would lead to an accident. He had been 'checked-out' in every possible way—by neurologists, ophthalmologists etc., and had been assured that he had no visual impairment and that he was medically fit to do the job in question.

Although the client described himself as extrovert, the 'life and soul of the party' always in the forefront of everything, further exploration revealed that he had always been a 'worrier'. He worried about the impression he made on people, how he would manage in new situations and he worried about his health. Indeed, after breaking his leg as a young teenager, he became acutely self-conscious and was convinced that he was walking in a peculiar way noticeable to others, in spite of evidence to the contrary. Initially, however, he denied being worried about going into this new situation abroad.

The counsellor then returned to the subject of the floaters and discovered that although they were fairly constant, the way in which they affected the client was not. Most of the time he had learned to ignore them and they did not bother him. By checking in his diary to see when he had consulted his GP because they were particularly troublesome, he discovered that these occasions coincided with times when he was about to enter new interpersonal situations, e.g. joining a new tutorial group at college.

It turned out that his way of managing the social aspects of new situations was to make as big a 'splash' as possible, fearing that unless he made this initial impression he would be ignored and get left behind. He admitted that this put him under considerable stress and he would frequently feel exhausted by it. The therapist at this stage formulated the hypothesis that the client was engaging in denial as an inappropriate emotion-focused way of coping with new situations and projecting the anxiety onto his 'floater' problem.

Therapy accordingly centred on appropriate emotion-focused methods of coping in new situations. This involved a reappraisal of his cognitions about new situations as well as systematic relaxation to help him manage his arousal. A problem-focused approach was also taken to helping him develop appropriate social skills for dealing with new group situations.

It can thus be seen that a stress-management approach which did not take into account the background factors would probably have concentrated on the floaters as the source of stress and might have been less effective. The floaters, whilst mildly troublesome, became something of a red herring.

It is clear from reviewing the literature that there is no single concept of stress that unites the overall field of stress. The sections presented in this chapter therefore reflect the diversities of models, methods and disciplines that have been used in this area. This can make it difficult to get an overview of the area, but it also reflects the reality of investigating and theorizing about a multifaceted and complex phenomenon.

11

Psychological Disorders

CONTENTS

11.1 INTRODUCTION

It is probably the case that most counsellors do not generally conceptualize their clients' experiences in terms of symptomatology or diagnostic labels. However, a knowledge of the symptoms, an understanding of the different perspectives on psychological disorder and an awareness of the range of possible treatments may be of relevance, particularly to those working with more distressed clients. Such information can be important in communicating with health care professionals from different disciplines and will also help the counsellor who may be facing decisions about referring a client elsewhere or recommending a different therapeutic approach.

This chapter begins with a discussion on some of the issues surrounding diagnosis before concentrating on some of the specific psychological disorders which counsellors are most likely to come across in their client work. After a brief introduction and description or definition of the disorder there follows an outline of some of the assessment instruments used mostly by psychiatrists and psychologists for both research and clinical purposes. On the whole, these fall into two categories: those used to assist diagnosis, and those used to assess the severity or the consequences of the disorder. Although in the therapeutic situation such questionnaires and rating scales are not a substitute for a detailed and thorough assessment interview, they can be useful in identifying and assessing the severity of symptoms and also for measuring change.

We then go on to discuss different perspectives on the disorders; biological, psychodynamic, behavioural and cognitive. Because humanistic theory has tended to focus on personal growth and development, its contribution to psychopathology has been rather more limited. This approach does, however, have some intrapsychic features in common with psychodynamic theory.

These perspectives all lead to different ideas about the causes and the treatment of psychological disorders. Some are complementary, others somewhat contradictory. All perspectives, however, as we shall see, have been useful in identifying the multiple and complex factors that may be involved in such disorders.

11.2 CONCEPTS OF NORMALITY AND ABNORMALITY

Often when people choose to see a counsellor it is because they realize, or have pointed out to them, that something is 'wrong'. People sometimes talk about not being their 'usual selves'. When we notice this about our own feelings, thoughts or behaviour, we are often making an implicit comparison between what is 'normal' for us and what is out of the ordinary. However, sometimes the individual does not recognize what is out of the ordinary for him or herself. This might be because the changes that have taken place have been subtle and gradual. Family, friends and colleagues may therefore notice adverse changes before we do ourselves. This may occur for example when an individual becomes more and more depressed and withdrawn over a period of several months. What the person might assume is simply wanting to spend more time by themselves might be seen by others as social avoidance and loss of interest.

In cases where a person has a severe disorder such as a psychosis, this disjunction between the person's understanding of what is happening to them and how others view them can be even more pronounced. This is because one of the characteristics of a psychotic disorder is that the individual concerned may lose 'insight' into themselves and their behaviour. Whereas they themselves may consider their actions to be perfectly appropriate and normal, to the external observer their behaviour can appear bizarre and abnormal.

This difficulty in achieving agreement between people about what is normal and what is abnormal or disordered is not confined to the non-professional. Indeed, the degree of disagreement between experts or practitioners in the field of mental health is often very great and perhaps surprising to the lay public.

Psychiatry has tended to apply what is often termed the 'medical' or categorical model to behaviour in order to classify it as normal or abnormal. This implies that disorders, psychological as well as medical, can be thought about in terms of symptoms, syndromes, diagnosis and treatment. The American Psychiatric Association has published a manual which describes all the various categories of mental disorders. The current version of the manual is called the *Diagnostic and Statistical Manual of Mental Disorders (DSM-IV), (*American Psychiatric Association (APA) 1994).

This manual was first published in the early 1950s and has undergone a series of revisions since that time. DSM IV is known as a *multi-axial* classification scheme because it is concerned not just with the symptoms a person may be experiencing but, in an attempt to take a wider perspective on the person in question, it provides five different 'axes' on which the individual can be assessed. These are listed in Table 11.1.

Table 11.1   DSM-IV Axes

Axis I	Clinical disorders that are associated with mental health problems
Axis II	Personality disorders and also problems that arise from intellectual functioning that is significantly below average
Axis III	Physical medical conditions which might be relevant to any mental health disorder
Axis IV	Psychological or situational problems which might be relevant to any mental health problem
Axis V	Overall assessment of the individual's 'global functioning' or general adaptation in the form of a score

So if we take a particular client, a twenty-eight-year-old woman, and assess her in terms of the DSM-IV criteria, we may find the following:

- **Axis I**   That she suffers from a generalized anxiety disorder (see section 11.3.2 below).
- **Axis II**   That she has a somewhat obsessive compulsive personality (although this does not fulfil the criteria for a personality disorder).
- **Axis III**   She suffers from irritable bowel syndrome.
- **Axis IV**   She lives with her parents, has difficulty making friends and feels trapped in a fairly low grade job, in spite of having a mathematics degree.
- **Axis V**   This yields a score on the Global Assessment of Functioning Scale of 57–58.

DSM-IV covers a very wide range of mental health problems. Examples of the kinds of problems that are included are: disorders of infancy and childhood, substance-related disorders, eating disorders and dementia. However, the use of such a categorical, diagnostic system for understanding normality and abnormality is problematic for a number of reasons. Some critics have suggested that the definition of what constitutes a disorder is often the product of political and practical pressures rather than being firmly based in theory and research. Also, psychologists have pointed out that a categorical approach assumes the inherent distinctiveness of psychological problems from psychological 'normality'. This is, of course, an artificial cut-off since most problems are better thought of in 'dimensional' terms, i.e. being more or less on a particular dimension.

The World Health Organization also produces a classificatory system for both physical and psychiatric disorders: **The International Classification of Diseases (ICD-10)**. Each disorder in this system has a numerical code. These codes are often used alongside the DSM diagnoses. Thus in DSM '300.3 Obsessive compulsive disorder', the 300.3 code is the ICD reference number.

Categorical systems for classifying 'abnormal' behaviour have also been criticized for focusing on the negative or problematic aspects of mental health rather than offering a positive definition of what would constitute good mental health. This is partly because the medical model as exemplified in these classificatory systems tends to be rather atheoretical. Instead, it frequently uses criteria related to subjective distress or discomfort. However, it does not confine itself simply to that criterion because there are often instances, e.g. people with psychotic problems, where the person does not report any great distress yet other people would regard them as in need of help.

An attempt at a more objective criterion for distinguishing normality and abnormality has been made by introducing the notion of 'maladaptiveness'. Such attempts usually focus on how well an individual is managing to function in relation to the various demands of their life. Assessment would therefore be made of the impact of the person's behaviour on their family and school life, their employment and their general environment. Critics of this approach draw attention to the implication that satisfactory adjustment to one's environment is necessarily a good outcome or a desirable situation. Since some environments may be oppressive or harmful to the individual, such as an abusive marital relationship, then it does not make much sense to define good mental health as successful adjustment to such a situation. Indeed, coping with such a situation might be indicative of a rather unhealthy adaptation.

Despite the above-mentioned limitations and cautions about the use of psychiatric diagnosis, there are some advantages to having such a system for classifying abnormal behaviour. Communication between professionals can be facilitated by the use of diagnostic terms which can sum up in a couple of words a whole spectrum of symptoms. Also, diagnosis can give us an immediate sense of the severity, likely course and future prognosis of a particular condition.

Adopting a pragmatic approach to diagnosis does not preclude a full understanding of the person. It would be possible to have both an overall understanding of the person in their context and to apply the relevant diagnostic labels to them for specific purposes of inter-professional communication. There are also some contexts in which it is necessary for the counsellor or therapist to have a good working knowledge of diagnostic categories; for example, when writing court reports or when working in an acute psychiatric setting or in a GP surgery.

In some instances, diagnosis is helpful in deciding upon appropriate treatment or therapy. For example, it might be the case that a client is being seen in therapy for a psychological or counselling approach to their problems as well as taking medication prescribed by their GP or a psychiatrist. Sometimes the prescription of appropriate medication can remove distressing symptoms, thereby giving the client the 'space' and energy to tackle their difficulties within a psychological framework.

11.3 ASSESSMENT OF PSYCHOLOGICAL DISORDERS

There are a number of structured clinical interviews available which are designed to collect information in a reliable and systematic manner in order to arrive at a diagnosis based on the DSM-IV criteria. These include the Diagnostic Interview Schedule (Robins et al., 1981) and the Structured Clinical Interview (Spitzer and Williams, 1986).

Psychologists sometimes use self report questionnaires or rating scales to assess the presence and severity of symptoms. These scales are referred to as 'psychometric' assessments because they have been carefully devised according to rigorous methods to accurately assess the person's psychological state. Such scales must be both *reliable* and *valid*.

If a scale is reliable this means that the scale will give consistent results across time and situations. A valid instrument is something that measures what it claims to measure. For example a depression questionnaire should assess depressive symptoms but not anxiety symptoms. There are various different types of validity that psychologists refer to for different purposes.

Examples of some of the most commonly used psychometric instruments for the assessment of psychological symptoms are given in Table 11.2.

Table 11.2   Examples of scales developed for the assessment of psychological disorders

Type of disorder	Examples of scales
Anxiety	Beck Anxiety Inventory (Beck et al., 1988)
	State-trait Anxiety Inventory (Spielberger et al., 1987)
	Fear Survey Schedule (Wolpe and Lange, 1987)
Depression	Beck Depression Inventory (Beck et al., 1961)
	Montgomery–Asberg Depression Scale (Montgomery and Asberg, 1979)
Post-traumatic symptoms	Revised Impact of Events Scale (Horowitz et al., 1979)
	Penn Inventory (Hammarberg, 1992)
Schizophrenic symptoms	Inventory of Schizotypal Cognitions (Rust, 1988)
	Scale for the Assessment of Negative Symptoms (Walker et al., 1988)
Personality disorders	Millon Clinical Multiaxial Inventory (Millon, 1983)
	Personality Diagnostic Questionnaire (Hyler et al., 1988)

11.4 ANXIETY

The two most common types of neurotic problems that present to GPs, psychologists and counsellors are anxiety and depression. Very often a distressed person will show symptoms of both. The presenting symptoms in these disorders can be 'non-specific' i.e. difficulties in sleeping, worry, loss of appetite, muscle tension or tiredness. Anxiety can also coexist with other pathological conditions such as a somataform disorder where the person presents with some physical or somatic complaint which has no organic basis. Panic and anxiety can also be associated with substance abuse, particularly intoxication and withdrawal states.

The relevance to therapeutic intervention of making a 'correct' diagnosis will depend entirely on the approach adopted. From an existential or a humanistic point of view any such diagnoses would usually be considered irrelevant. However, from a cognitive–behavioural perspective, different diagnoses have different implications for psychological intervention and also for pharmacological treatment.

11.4.1 Signs and Symptoms of Anxiety

The American Psychiatric Association (1994) defines anxiety as apprehension, tension, or uneasiness which stems from the anticipation of danger, the source of which is largely unknown or unrecognized. Although we have all experienced anxiety at some time, anxiety is only considered to be a disorder when the amount or duration of anxiety is out of proportion to the situation or subject that triggers it. Anxiety is not only thought to underlie the various anxiety disorders, but also to contribute to the onset and course of disease and be a factor in post-operative recovery.

Table 11.3 Common signs and symptoms of anxiety

Cognitive/emotional	Somatic
Excessive worry	Palpitations
Feelings of apprehension	Sweating
or dread	Pains in arms or chest
Pre-occupation	Tension headaches
Distractibility	Stomach upsets
	Difficulty swallowing
	Easily startled

11.4.2 Types of Anxiety Disorders

Five types of anxiety disorders are identified in DSM-IV. These are panic disorder, generalized anxiety disorder, phobic disorder, obsessive–compulsive disorder and post-traumatic stress disorder (which we will be discussing separately in Section 11.6).

Panic disorder

A panic attack is an intense but relatively short-lived episode of anxiety in which the person experiences a variety of symptoms which might include shortness of breath, dizziness, nausea, palpitations etc. The person often feels that they might faint, collapse or even die. They may experience 'derealization', that is the feeling that the world is unreal, or 'depersonalization', the feeling that they are unreal.

Panic attacks can happen either entirely 'out of the blue' or may be triggered by certain situations such as being in a queue at the supermarket checkout. In some instances, the person becomes fearful to leave the house unaccompanied because of their fear of having a panic attack. This then constitutes an agoraphobic condition accompanied by panic attacks.

Generalized anxiety disorder

This is a condition with more diffuse and non-specific symptoms characterized by feelings of apprehension, worry and tension. This is often associated with a variety of somatic symptoms which are not related to any particular situations or objects. This type of anxiety is sometimes called 'free floating anxiety'. The absence of any sort of trigger is what distinguishes this type of anxiety from phobias.

Phobias

In phobias, there is an intense fear and avoidance of a particular object (e.g. dogs) or of a particular situation (e.g. heights). Phobic anxiety is generally out of proportion to any real or possible danger posed by the phobic object. The phobias are sometimes subdivided into social phobias (for example, fear of a public situation such as public speaking) and simple phobias (such as a fear of spiders), the latter most commonly being animal phobias.

Obsessive–compulsive disorder

DSM-IV defines obsessive–compulsive disorder as 'recurrent obsessions or compulsions sufficiently severe to cause marked distress, be time-consuming, or significantly interfere with the person's routine, occupational functioning, or with usual social activities or relationship with others. Obsessions are defined as persistent ideas, thoughts, impulses or images that are experienced, at least initially, as intrusive and senseless, while compulsions are defined as repetitive, purposeful and intentional behaviours that are performed in response to an obsession, according to certain rules or in a stereotyped fashion.

The Diagnosis of Anxiety Disorder

As we have suggested above, diagnosis is not always clear-cut. The following client study illustrates this point.

The client is 25 years old and a mother of two children. Her husband is a supervisor with a tyre fitting company and works long hours. She presents with the following complaints:

- *a nervous cough;*
- *pains in her upper arms and in the back of her neck;*
- *intermittent stomach aches;*
- *feelings of dizziness or giddiness especially in crowded places.*

She describes herself as always having been something of a worrier.

Her father left the family when she was six years old, leaving her mother to struggle to bring up her and her three younger siblings. She left school at 16 with few qualifications and took a job in a garage where she met her husband. They got married when she became pregnant, at 19.

She describes her husband as a 'good provider' for herself and the children, now aged six and four. However, he takes little responsibility at home and often spends time with his friends in the pub after work. Although she has sometimes suspected him of having affairs, her husband has always denied this when she has confronted him.

Her mother has recently been diagnosed as having carcinoma of the breast and has undergone a mastectomy.

Although the client suffered with a variety of somatic symptoms, including stomach pains, throughout her adolescence, she never sought any medical help for them. In the last year, her symptoms have intensified and she has also developed some new ones. She has decided to seek help at this time because she sees her physical state as interfering with her ability to look after her children properly. On a number of occasions she has kept her eldest child home from school because she could not face going out in the morning.

Although this client's problems appear at first sight to be very 'physical', in fact it is very common for clients with anxiety problems to describe a range of somatic symptoms as their initial concerns. While the counsellor will obviously be conscious of the need to have any possible organic causes investigated, it should not be too surprising that a psychological state such as anxiety can have such pronounced somatic manifestations. Chapter 10 deals with the physiology of stress in more detail.

The counsellor or therapist would clearly attempt to make sense of these symptoms in terms of the client's past history and current situation. Another approach would be to see how her problems would fit into the diagnostic categories provided by DSM-IV.

There are a number of possible diagnostic categories that such difficulties might match up with. These are:

- agoraphobia, either with or without panic disorder;
- generalized anxiety disorder;
- somatization disorder.

We have already discussed the symptoms of panic disorder, phobias and generalized anxiety disorder. **Somatization disorder** occurs when a person has a number of persistent physical symptoms and problems which have no known organic basis. The full blown condition is relatively rare but it is by no means unusual to see clients with somatic preoccupations or concerns. Somatization is not the same as hypochondriasis. In hypochondriasis, the person believes, or fears, that they have a specific disease. Both hypochondriasis and somatization disorder fall into the Somatoform Disorders group in DSM-IV.

Because of the overlap in symptoms between these various diagnostic categories outlined above, the counsellor might find it useful to conduct a more thorough assessment of the client's difficulties and anxieties. In the case of this client, as we have noted, her initial presentation could potentially fall into several diagnostic categories. This is not necessarily a problem. It might indeed be the case that she has a range and severity of symptoms which would meet the diagnostic criteria for agoraphobia, panic disorder, generalized anxiety disorder and somatization disorder. Alternatively it could be the case that her emphasis on the somatic symptoms she experiences is a result of a belief that she needs to have a 'medical' problem in order to be taken seriously.

11.4.3 Models of Anxiety and Implications for Treatment

Treatment approaches to anxiety will depend very much on the theoretical perspective of the therapist. From a **biological perspective** theories of anxiety focus on the interaction of a number of neurotransmitters that regulate feelings of anxiety. Biochemical abnormalities have been found for panic attacks (Bradwejn et al., 1989) and obsessive-compulsive disorder (Baxter et al., 1988), although environmental experiences undoubtedly play an important role.

The somatic symptoms of anxiety are often treated by GPs via the prescription of anti-anxiolytic (i.e. anti-anxiety) medication. The most common pharmacological treatment of anxiety is the benzodiazepines, such as diazepam (Valium) or lorezepam (Ativan). In some cases, antidepressants, which have been found to be helpful in the treatment of panic attacks (Black et al., 1993) are prescribed. We also know that many individuals use alcohol as a means of dampening down anxiety or helping them to relax or get off to sleep.

Like alcohol, benzodiazepines depress the action of the central nervous system, reducing tension and causing drowsiness. They also suffer from some of the same drawbacks as the use of alcohol does. They can lead to dependence, withdrawal and rebound effects. They can, however, be very useful for short-term or emergency treatment.

Beta blockers, such as popranolol (Inderal) which are more commonly used in the treatment of hypertension, are also prescribed for people suffering from anxiety. Although they do not seem to affect psychological symptoms such as worry, tension and fear, they do reduce autonomic symptoms such as palpitations, sweating and tremor.

In addition psychologists have often used physically focused strategies such as teaching progressive muscular relaxation as a way of helping the person feel more in control of their physical symptoms or allowing them to stay and face a feared object rather than simply avoiding it.

From a **psychodynamic perspective**, sources of anxiety are assumed to be internal and unconscious. Anxiety, according to this view, results when unconscious impulses (such as sex or aggression) threaten to burst into consciousness.

Generalized anxiety and panic attacks are thought to occur when our defences are not strong enough to control or contain the anxiety. Phobias, on the other hand, are seen to be ways of coping with these unacceptable impulses by displacing the anxiety onto an object or situation which can then be avoided. Obsessions and compulsions are similarly seen to be ways of handling anxiety with the obsession being less threatening than the underlying impulse. In this way they protect the individual from the 'true' source of the anxiety.

The emphasis in psychodynamic approaches to the treatment of anxiety is on fostering insight into the unconscious motives and conflicts which are believed to lie at the heart of the patient's symptoms.

Behavioural understandings of anxiety problems have emphasized the role of learned responses and how these are maintained by particular reinforcers in the person's environment. In general terms, anxiety is seen as a normal and adaptive feature of human experience. However, anxiety can become maladaptive if it becomes associated with a particular object and then leads the person to arrange their life in order to avoid that object. Through the process of avoidance, the person finds that their anxiety is reduced and thus avoidance becomes a reinforcing behaviour. These behavioural explanations of anxiety are sometimes called **operant models** of anxiety.

It is easy to see how this theory works by looking at the case of someone who has a simple phobia such as a dog phobia. If a child has been frightened by a large dog unexpectedly jumping up to lick their face, they may come to associate that feeling of fear with all dogs. The sight of a dog may arouse within the child the feelings of anxiety and fear. The child then avoids dogs by refusing to go to the park, by crossing to the opposite side of the road from any dogs and by insisting on friends confining their dogs to the garden when they are visiting. Because avoidance of dogs brings relief from the anxiety, the child will continue to avoid dogs and may never have a chance to learn that the fear of dogs is not realistic.

This model of understanding how anxiety develops and is maintained has led to specific behavioural treatments including:

- systematic desensitization;
- *in vivo* desensitization;
- modelling;
- positive reinforcement.

These elements of behavioural treatments are often used in combination. For example, the therapist might start by having the client construct a 'hierarchy' of their fears from the least anxiety provoking (looking at a picture of a dog in a book) to the most anxiety provoking (being alone with a large, barking dog in an enclosed space). The client is then taught to relax deeply and while in this state, to imagine a situation from the 'easy' end of the hierarchy (e.g. hearing a dog barking in a nearby house) and to remain relaxed while thinking of this situation. This is sometimes called imaginal exposure.

This systematic desensitization procedure may then merge into an *in vivo* approach where the client is gradually exposed to real dogs in situations of increasing fearfulness for the client. The important point about such exposure is that it is carried out at a pace with which the client feels comfortable and while maintaining the client's sense of control over their autonomic anxiety by the use of relaxation techniques. The therapist can also use *in vivo* techniques to model appropriate behavioural or cognitive coping strategies and to use positive reinforcement such as praise or encouragement. A helpful description of some of these behavioural techniques is provided by Goldfried and Davison (1994).

Obviously not all anxieties are as specific or easily identified as those experienced by dog phobics. For example, in panic attacks the person may be fearful of their own internal bodily feelings which they misinterpret as a sign of an imminent collapse (Agras 1993). These diversities in the types of anxieties experienced and some conceptual limitations of the behavioural model have led therapists to look at the role of cognitive processes in the development and maintenance of anxiety disorders. The most influential writer in this area is Beck (Beck et al., 1979; Beck and Emery, 1985).

One of the main problems that anxious clients experience is worrying or anxious thoughts. However, thoughts are obviously more difficult to observe and assess than behaviours such as avoidance. **Cognitive theories** of anxiety maintain that negative, anxious thoughts are themselves produced by a set of maladaptive beliefs that are held by the anxious person. Examples of some of the kinds of beliefs that anxious clients report are given below.

- 'The world is unpredictable and unsafe.'
- 'I am likely to face difficulties that I cannot cope with in the future.'
- 'If something goes wrong, I won't know what to do.'
- 'When I am with other people, I won't know what to say and I'll be embarrassed.'
- 'If I don't do anything, then no-one can criticize me.'
- 'It is better to avoid difficulties than to face up to them.'

Panic attacks, from a cognitive perspective, would be seen as arising from an oversensitivity to and cognitive catastrophizing about physical signs such as an increased heart rate or sweaty palms.

Cognitive approaches to the treatment of anxiety problems therefore focus on challenging and modifying those beliefs that are believed to underlie the person's problems.

11.5 DEPRESSION

While clients often describe symptoms of both anxiety and depression, depression can be a separate condition in its own right. The classification of the depressive disorders has been the subject of considerable debate and controversy. Depression is sometimes called a **mood disorder** or an **affective disorder**.

11.5.1 Descriptions and Definitions of Depression

Because the term depression is used in everyday language to describe a mood state that everyone experiences from time to time, it can be difficult when the term is also used to mean an extreme state in which the person may feel entirely hopeless and even suicidal. The chief differences between 'normal' depression and that which may be regarded as 'clinical' depression are that clinical depression persists for weeks or months and affects the person in many different ways. Although we usually think of depression as a disorder of mood, it also manifests itself in cognitive, motivational and physical symptoms.

Mood symptoms

Depression is often characterized by feelings of hopelessness, isolation sadness and dejection. But equally pervasive, is a loss of gratification and pleasure in life. Activities that used to bring pleasure seem dull and joyless, to have lost their meaning.

Cognitive symptoms

The most pronounced cognitive symptoms are negative thoughts. Depressed people often feel hopeless about their situation and future and feel pessimistic about improving things. They tend to feel inadequate, suffer from low self-esteem and are full of self-blame, and sometimes self-loathing.

Motivational symptoms

Depression affects the ability to 'get going' and even to do the things which used to give pleasure. Everything seems too much effort and in extreme cases even movements and speech may be slowed down.

Physical symptoms

Physical symptoms of depression include sleep disturbance, loss of appetite and libido, weight loss (in moderate to severe depression), tiredness and fatigue.

An individual need not have all these symptoms to be diagnosed depressed but such symptoms will be familiar to most counsellors and therapists. The following is a fairly typical example of a client referred for counselling by his GP.

The client says that he cannot remember when he was last his 'usual' self. Over the last 6 months or so, he has become increasingly bored at work and irritable at home. He has withdrawn from his friends and stopped pursuing his interests in fishing and DIY. At work his motivation and drive have gone and he is procrastinating about several important tasks. Trivial decision making has become a problem, as has prolonged concentration. The client says that he has 'no idea' what is wrong with him.

11.5.2 Types of Depressive Disorders

DSM-IV distinguishes between a number of different kinds of clinical depressions. These include:

- **major depression**—a severe episodic depressive disorder with symptoms for at least two weeks;
- **dysthymic disorder**—less severe than major depression with insidious onset;
- **major depression—seasonal pattern (seasonal affective disorder)**—depression that comes with shortened daylight in winter and autumn and disappears during spring and summer;
- **bipolar disorder (manic depression)**—the individual alternates between depression and normal mood and between extreme, sometimes wild, elation and normal mood;
- **cyclothymia**—a less severe chronic and non-psychotic form of bipolar disorder.

11.5.3 Models of Depression and Implications for Treatment

Biological factors undoubtedly play an influential role in regulating mood, and mood disorders involve biochemical changes in the nervous system. The neurotransmitter systems involved in regulating mood are extremely complex but a widely held view is that depression is associated with a deficiency of one or both of the neurotransmitters serotonin and norepinephrine. The question that has yet to be resolved, however, is whether the physiological changes are the cause or the result of psychological changes.

Various studies also suggest that **genetic factors** are somehow involved and that inherited predispositions make people more vulnerable to depression when under stress.

The most commonly used pharmacological treatments for depression are the tricyclic antidepressants such as imipramine and amitriptyline, monoamine oxidase inhibitors (MAOIs), the newer serotonin re-uptake inhibitors (SSRIs) such as fluoxetine (Prozac) and lithium carbonate (which is used mostly in the treatment of bipolar disorder). **Seasonal affective disorders**, those depressions that seem to occur mostly in the winter, are treated with exposure to full spectrum light but the efficacy of these treatments remains in question. The controversial question of the use of electroconvulsive treatment is beyond the scope of this chapter but an overview can be found in Weiner (1989).

Counsellors and therapists sometimes find it frustrating when the client, with whom they have been working hard on addressing 'underlying issues', decides not to continue with counselling because their symptoms, for which they had originally sought help, have been alleviated by anti-depressant medication. Sometimes, however, the fact that the client is no longer experiencing the distressing mood, cognitive, motivational or physical symptoms of depression can be enough for them to address the difficulties themselves. Alternatively, they may return to counselling at a later stage.

Psychoanalytic models of depression have emphasized the role of early loss, self-esteem and dependency. According to this view, for some reason the individual's needs for care, approval and affection would not have been satisfied in childhood and a loss in later life re-stimulates this early distress and causes the person to regress to the original helpless, dependent state. The picture is further complicated by angry feelings towards the deserting person. Psychodynamic therapy would probably focus on the issues of overdependence, on external approval and internalization of anger.

Behavioural approaches in the early 1970s drew attention to the way in which depressed persons seemed to be lacking in reinforcement for positive behaviours, particularly social reinforcement, and in contrast how their negative behaviours (e.g. crying) seemed to be reinforced by attention from others. It was suggested that people, when depressed, seemed to be on 'extinction schedules' for antidepressive behaviours.

Cognitive models have built on the behavioural models but switched attention from the person's behaviour in their social environment to the person's internal world. Beck (1967, 1976) described how when people became depressed they manifested a negative cognitive triad: a negative view of self, world and future. The depressed person sees their world through a series of negative filters or cognitive schemas. The schemas are underlying beliefs which influence the way in which a person perceives and interprets what happens to them. Such a person habitually makes a number of cognitive errors in their understanding of their world which then maintains their depressive view of self, world and future.

Usually a combination of behavioural and cognitive models are adopted by clinical psychologists when treating depression. Cognitive behaviour therapy for depression is fully described in a number of texts (e.g. Beck et al., 1979; Blackburn and Davidson, 1990). Example of the techniques that are integrated into cognitive behaviour therapy include the following:

- monitoring and scheduling of activities;
- distraction;
- graded tasks and homework tasks;
- Socratic questioning;
- identifying and answering negative thoughts or assumptions.

Cognitive behaviour therapy is marked by a structured and systematic approach which stresses the need for the client to generalize the insights gained in therapy to their real life setting by the use of 'homework' exercises and 'experiments'.

11.6 POST-TRAUMATIC STRESS DISORDER

While it has long been observed that various stressors can bring about a variety of psychological disorders, the role of traumatic stress and any resulting disorder has been a matter of considerable debate. The general role of stress in relation to distress has previously been examined in Chapter 10. Traumatic stressors can range from natural disasters, such as earthquakes and floods, to being in a life-threatening car accident. Traumatic stressors can also be long-term, such as physical, sexual or emotional abuse in childhood or living in a prison camp as a prisoner of war.

11.6.1 Description and Definition

Reactions to such traumatic stressors can include anxiety and depression. However, more recently it has been suggested that there is a specific syndrome—post-traumatic stress disorder (PTSD) which is associated with exposure to a traumatic stressor or event. The symptoms which are included in PTSD are:

- **persistent re-experiencing of the event**—e.g. through dreams, images, thoughts;
- **avoidance of any reminders of the event**—e.g. inability to recall important aspects of trauma;
- **numbing of responsiveness**—e.g. feelings of detachment;
- **increased arousal**—e.g. difficulty concentrating, exaggerated startle response.

In order to meet the full diagnostic criteria, as described in DSM-IV (American Psychiatric Association, 1995), these symptoms need to have been present for at least a month. PTSD is classified as an anxiety disorder in DSM-IV.

11.6.2 Models of PTSD

Models of PTSD range from the biological and psychodynamic to cognitive and behavioural. **Biological models** draw attention to the extreme hyperarousal and aggression experienced in PTSD and suggest that this may be attributable to neurotransmitter activity in the brain. People suffering from PTSD may be prescribed appropriate antianxiolytic or anti-depressant medication and also taught progressive relaxation techniques to reduce arousal.

Psychodynamic understandings of the effects of trauma have centred on the failure of the ego to cope with overwhelming threat. This, it is suggested, leads to attempts to defend the ego against the assault.

The process of conditioning is emphasized in **behavioural models** of PTSD. Here, the person is believed to learn to associate fear and anxiety with a range of stimuli that might be connected to the original trauma (Keane et al., 1985).

Cognitive models suggest that trauma either overwhelms the person's information processing capacities or else that the experience of trauma may shatter some of the person's fundamental beliefs about the world being a safe and predictable place (Foa et al., 1989).

Horowitz (1993) proposes a model of PTSD which combines both cognitive and psychodynamic elements.

11.6.3 Treatment of PTSD

Although each of the above models has specific implications for treatment, in reality, most counsellors and therapists would draw on understandings gained from more than one approach. Psychotherapists in the field (e.g. Scurfield, 1985) have suggested that the following components are important in the treatment of PTSD:

- establishing a trusting therapeutic relationship;
- education about coping with trauma;
- stress-management training;
- re-experiencing the trauma;
- integration of traumatic event into client's experience.

As we have discussed in Section 3.7 on Emotional Expression and Counselling, re-experiencing the trauma is usually considered to be the most important element of therapy for PTSD. The precise techniques employed for this will depend on the orientation of the therapist. One way is through **trauma desensitization**, a variation on systematic desensitization. Here the client is taught basic relaxation and is gradually encouraged to relive the trauma, through discussion, description, fantasy and visualization of the event whilst maintaining a state of low arousal.

Any individual's response to trauma, however will be coloured by their past experiences, as the following example demonstrates.

A client sought counselling some three months after a serious car crash. He had been a passenger in a vehicle which hit a tree late at night. Trapped in the car for some time before the emergency services arrived, he could smell petrol and was very fearful that the car was going to explode. He reported that he had never felt so helpless and trapped before.

Despite the nature of the crash, the client only suffered minor physical injuries but had a range of adverse psychological symptoms. He often dreamt about situations in which he was trapped and awoke from these dreams crying and very frightened. He could no longer see very far ahead and had a feeling of anxious foreboding that he was not going to live much longer. Bangs, loud noises or even the telephone ringing made him feel very startled and anxious. He had become very irritable at home and at work and felt considerable rage and resentment towards the driver of the car, who had escaped without injury.

The client recounted how he had lost his trust in the world as a safe place and now looked for dangers wherever he went. This meant a constant scanning of the environment for any dangers or threats. Avoidance of anything that reminded him of

the accident became habitual and he would only travel by car if absolutely neces-
sary. This anxiety generalized to any confined spaces such as lifts or underground
trains and the client had restricted his activities because of these fears.

Over the course of time, through exploring his feelings with the counsellor, the
client came to recognize that the feelings of being trapped and helpless were very
similar to the feelings that he had when sent to boarding school at the age of ten fol-
lowing the death of his mother. He had hated the boarding school and been unable
to understand why his father had not responded to his pleas to be taken away from
the school.

The client came to realize that his fears of being abandoned in a dangerous situ-
ation were something that had predated the accident but had been reawakened and
strengthened by the crash. He also became aware that he had considerable unre-
solved grief and anger about his childhood losses which he had not dealt with pre-
viously.

This example of someone who has suffered a post traumatic reaction reminds us that
pre-existing vulnerabilities can exacerbate or prolong psychological problems that
might arise after trauma. We know that people who have had experience of trauma or
severe psychological problems in the past are likely to suffer more if they have a subsequent trauma.

11.7 SCHIZOPHRENIA AND RELATED DISORDERS

Schizophrenia is one of the most complex and devastating of human conditions. Many
approaches have been taken to its study and the literature is extensive and diverse.
Considerable discussion and controversy surrounds the concept and definition of schizophrenia

Most workers in the field agree that it is a disorder or condition that is characterized
by psychotic symptoms and which involves disturbances in feeling, thinking and
behaviour which impair to some significant degree the person's ability to function.
Although there are problems with defining schizophrenia, it is possible to estimate the
prevalence at around one per cent (Sartorius et al., 1986) which makes schizophrenia
the most common of the major psychiatric disorders.

There are also a number of related psychotic disorders. these include:

- **brief reactive psychosis**—where the symptoms are less than one month's duration
  and are secondary to identifiable psycho-social stress;
- **schizoaffective disorder**—where symptoms of schizophrenia partially overlap
  with symptoms of mood disorder—mania or depression;
- **delusional disorder**—where the main symptom is a fixed and unshakable delusion
  (previously known as paranoid disorder);
- **schizophreniform disorder**—where symptoms may be identical to schizophrenia
  but of less than six months' duration.

Some individual psychotic symptoms can be seen within other types of disorder. For example, someone with very severe depression may have a delusional belief that they have a terminal illness. Also in some organic conditions, such as dementia, psychotic symptoms may be present.

11.7.1 Description and Definition of Schizophrenia

The complexity of the various possible symptom pictures, and the rather slow and insidious onset in some cases, means that there can be some difficulty and also disagreement about diagnosis in this area. There are also cultural and ethnic differences which impact on the diagnosis and have generated considerable research. Because of these conceptual and practical difficulties, it has sometimes been suggested that the diagnosis of schizophrenia should be revised or even abandoned altogether (e.g. Bentall 1990).

With the above reservations in mind, the following can provide a guide to the signs and symptoms of schizophrenia.

- **impaired overall functioning**—below the expected level to achieve or highest previous level;
- **abnormal content of thought**—e.g. delusions, poverty of content, ideas of reference;
- **illogical form of thought (thought disorder)**—e.g. loosening of associations, tangentiality, over-inclusiveness, neologisms;
- **distorted perception**—e.g. auditory, visual, tactile or olfactory hallucinations;
- **changed affect**—e.g. flat, blunted, silly, inappropriate or labile;
- **impaired sense of self**—e.g. gender confusion, loss of ego boundaries;
- **altered volition**—e.g. inadequate motivation, marked ambivalence;
- **impaired interpersonal functioning**—e.g. social withdrawal, inappropriate sexual behaviour;
- **change in psychomotor behaviour**—e.g. agitation, withdrawal, catatonia, grimacing, posturing.

In DSM-IV, five subtypes of schizophrenia are described: catatonic, paranoid, disorganized, undifferentiated and residual. These different types are distinguished by the particular symptom patterns.

A more recently suggested system proposes a distinction between 'positive symptoms' and 'negative symptoms'. **Positive symptoms** are those symptoms that are obvious because of their presence: delusions, hallucinations, bizarre behaviours, disorganized speech, whereas **negative symptoms** refers to the deficits that are found in schizophrenia: social withdrawal, lack of affect or emotional responsiveness, loss of initiative and energy.

Given that psychotic disorders such as schizophrenia can have an insidious onset and that delusional beliefs can appear to have some element of truth in them, it can be difficult for the counsellor to know when they should suspect that their client might be suffering from a psychotic disorder and refer them for a psychiatric opinion.

> *A client has referred himself for counselling because of feelings of loneliness and isolation. He has been seen on four occasions and the counsellor has found him to be somewhat rambling and circumstantial in his speech and to be a little eccentric and dishevelled in appearance. The counsellor has a feeling that something isn't quite right but cannot quite identify what is causing concern. In the next session the client confides that he is being courted by a member of the Royal family who regularly sends him coded messages through the 'For Sale' column of the local newspaper. Although they have never met, the client describes how they have a strong spiritual bond which unites them. The client also admits that the reason he does not seek other people's company is because no other relationship could ever match his royal affair.*

11.7.2 Course and Outcome in Schizophrenia

The onset of schizophrenia, which may be acute or insidious, is often preceded by symptoms of anxiety, perplexity, terror or depression. Although traditionally schizophrenia has been considered to be a severe and progressive disorder, recent evidence suggests that this is unnecessarily pessimistic (Harding et al., 1992). The evidence from several studies indicates that about a third of all schizophrenic patients recover fairly well after their initial serious episode; another third continue to experience intermittent episodes that may require hospitalization (or, if it exists, care in the community); the remaining third tend to follow a deteriorating course (Cutting, 1986).

Research has shown that prognosis in schizophrenia is related to a number of factors. The prognosis seems to be better when the onset is acute and related to obvious precipitating stress factors, where there is a good pre-morbid level of social and work functioning, a predominance of positive symptoms and where there are mood symptoms (depression and a family history of mood disorder). Those who fare less well tend to be those for whom the onset is insidious, who have poor pre-morbid social and work functioning, who are withdrawn and socially unskilled, with a predominance of negative symptoms and a family history of schizophrenia.

11.7.3 Aetiological Factors in Schizophrenia

Biological factors

The causes of schizophrenia are still something of a mystery, despite years of research and theoretical speculation. Biological researchers have concentrated their efforts on attempting to track down particular genes or in looking for abnormalities in brain structure or chemistry.

The search for a particular brain abnormality in schizophrenia has until recently been hampered by the fact that evidence could only be gathered from post mortem examinations of the brains of patients. It was therefore very problematic to interpret any observed differences between schizophrenic and normal brains since they might have been due to the effects of antipsychotic medication or physical health problems. However, advances in medical technology have now allowed researchers to look at live people's brains, via magnetic resonance imaging (MRI) and CT scans. These studies (e.g. Andreasen et al., 1990, 1992) have found that some people with schizophrenia have enlarged ventricles in the brain and some also have reduced blood flow in the frontal regions of the brain. However, the significance of these findings and their implications for the understanding and treatment of schizophrenia remains unclear. There are similar problems with those studies which have sought evidence for the role of particular brain chemicals, such as the neurotransmitter dopamine (cf. Davis et al., 1991).

Other researchers have explored the genetic factors in schizophrenia, and epidemiological studies of family patterns in schizophrenia have examined the relative risk of the disorder in family members. Such studies have often looked at identical and non-identical twins (e.g. Torrey, 1992) or at children of a schizophrenic parent who are adopted into 'normal' families (e.g. Tienari et al., 1987). Overall this research has suggested that there is a genetic contribution to risk of developing schizophrenia but it has also highlighted the important role that environmental factors play.

Family interaction

It has been suggested by a number of writers and researchers in the 1960s and 1970s that family styles of interaction and communication are implicated in the onset of schizophrenia (Singer and Wynne, 1963; Liem, 1980). However, although some differences in communication style were found between the families of schizophrenics and 'normal' controls, the evidence did not support the idea that 'faulty' family communication patterns caused schizophrenia. Nevertheless there has since been a body of research which has found that family relationships as manifested in patterns of *expressed emotion* (*defined as hostile, critical* or *emotionally over-involved*) can contribute to risk of relapse in schizophrenia (e.g. Brewin et al., 1991).

Stressful life events

Brown and Birley (1968) found in their study that there was an increase in stressful events in the three week period before the onset of a schizophrenic episode. Their findings have been confirmed in a number of studies since that time. A helpful review can be found in Day (1989).

Needless to say, the search for a single causal agent for a complex phenomenon such as schizophrenia is not likely to succeed unless the investigators are able to provide a model for the causation of schizophrenia which can account for the various risk factors and the different manifestations of the disorder. Because at the present time this seems unlikely to be achieved, some of the more recent workers in the field have abandoned the notion of studying schizophrenia as a discrete diagnostic entity altogether. Instead, some have concentrated on examining the individual symptoms of the disorder such as hallucinations and delusions and others on exploring the idea of schizophrenia existing at the extreme end of a continuum of normal functioning in the same way in which depression can be seen to be at one end of a dimension of mood.

11.7.4 Treatment of Schizophrenia

The nature of the symptoms in schizophrenia means that hospitalization is often necessary as well as treatment with antipsychotic medication. Antipsychotic drugs are sometimes referred to as **neuroleptics** or **major tranquillizers**. Specific medications that are used to treat schizophrenia include chlorpromazine (Largactil), haloperidol (Serenace) and trifluoperazine (Stelazine) and the newer risperidone (Risperdal). Drug therapy in schizophrenia usually helps to reduce the positive symptoms such as delusions and disordered thinking but is generally less effective in treating the negative symptoms. Some schizophrenic sufferers require long-term maintenance therapy which should be provided via community psychiatric services, but there are often difficulties in achieving compliance with a medication regime due, in part, to a range of adverse side effects.

Psychosocial treatments for schizophrenia are often used alongside drug therapy. These approaches aim both to reduce the likelihood of relapse and to re-build social, occupational and self-care skills. The two most widely used psychosocial treatment approaches are **family therapy**, developed from the theory and research on expressed emotion, and **social skills training**, which builds upon information-processing models of skill (e.g. Wilkinson and Canter, 1984; Halford and Hayes, 1991).

Although there have been occasional references in the past to a cognitive approach to schizophrenia (Beck, 1952; Hole et al., 1979) it has only been relatively recently that a systematic cognitive behavioural treatment has been elaborated. **Cognitive behavioural techniques** have now been applied to some psychotic features, such as delusional beliefs, with claimed efficacy (Kingdon and Turkington, 1994).

11.7.5 Schizophrenia and Counselling

The therapies mentioned above and generally discussed in the research literature are designed to target quite specific behaviours or symptoms associated with schizophrenia. But when we work therapeutically with clients with schizophrenia we are working with individuals, not merely a set of symptoms.

These clients, as well as experiencing difficulties which result directly from the disorder itself, such as distressing auditory hallucinations, may have problems which are secondary to the condition, such as the effects of loss: loss possibly of job and career, maybe of old friends and relationships, loss of self-esteem and perhaps loss of the sense of continuity of their lives. In addition, they may, of course, suffer from the sorts of difficulties and troubles that anyone might experience which have nothing to do with the disorder itself. There are, therefore, many ways in which the experienced counsellor working in a psychiatric setting can help such clients.

11.8 PERSONALITY DISORDERS

Personality traits, as we discussed in Chapter 2, are those relatively permanent qualities and consistent aspects of the person which influence how we perceive, understand and interact with our environment. We talk about **personality disorders** when these long-standing patterns or traits become maladaptive and lead to subjective distress or significant impairment of social or occupational functioning.

11.8.1 Classification of Personality Disorders

Considerable controversy surrounds the categories and diagnoses of personality disorder: they are difficult to identify reliably, their aetiology is poorly understood and there is little evidence to indicate that they can be treated successfully (Oltmanns and Emery, 1995). There are also important discrepancies between DSM-IV and ICD-10. The categories, therefore, should not be accepted uncritically.

As noted in Section 11.1 above, the personality disorders are grouped together on Axis II of DSM-IV. The ten specific types of personality disorder are organized into three clusters (see Table 11.4 below). The first cluster includes **asocial** people—those who tend to be odd or eccentric; the second includes **flamboyant** people—those who appear to be excessively dramatic, emotional or erratic; and the third cluster **anxious** people, who appear to be excessively fearful.

11.8.2 Aetiology and Models of Personality Disorders

The personality disorders are relatively new to DSM and less is known about what factors cause them than many other disorders. There is thought to be a genetic component particularly in paranoid, schizoid, schizotypal and antisocial personality disorders. Some form of organic brain injury may also play a part in schizotypal and borderline disorders.

Disturbed early relationships, loss and possibly abuse are believed to contribute to paranoid, schizoid, schizotypal, narcissistic and dependent personality disorders. Other disorders are seen to result from, or be associated with, rather more specific parental (or carer) behaviours such as excessive overt parental deprecation in dependent personality disorder and harsh discipline in the case of obsessive–compulsive personality disorder.

Psychodynamic approaches to personality disorders have stressed the role of early experience and view such disorders as resulting from fixation at certain developmental stages or from faulty relationships with parents.

Table 11.4 Personality disorders listed in DSM-IV

	Charactersistic features
Cluster A	
• Paranoid	Distrust and suspiciousness of others
• Schizoid	Detachment from social relationships and restricted range of expression of emotions
• Schizotypal	Discomfort with close relationships, cognitive and perceptual distortions, eccentricities of behaviour
Cluster B	
• Antisocial	(Previously called psychopathic) Disregard for, and frequent violation of, rights of others
• Borderline	Instability of interpersonal relationships, self-image, emotions and control over impulses
• Histrionic	Excessive emotionality and attention seeking.
• Narcissistic	Grandiosity, need for admiration and lack of empathy
Cluster C	
• Avoidant	Extreme social discomfort and timidity
• Dependent	Excessive need to be taken care of, submissive and clinging behaviour
• Obsessive–compulsive	Preoccupation with orderliness and perfectionism at the expense of flexibility

Beck (Beck et al., 1990), one of the founders of cognitive therapy, sees core beliefs and schemas formed by critical incidents in childhood as significant in the development of personality disorder. He has described how the various types of personality disorders may be differentiated by these beliefs or schemas. For example, someone with a dependent personality disorder may hold the belief 'I cannot do anything by myself' while a person with an obsessive compulsive personality disorder may have as a characteristic belief 'I must be completely in control of my environment'.

11.8.3 Treatment of Personality Disorders

Personality disorders have traditionally been considered to be extremely difficult to treat psychologically. This is hardly surprising in view of the fact that psychological therapy involves, some would say relies on, a close personal relationship between client and therapist and difficulty in making and maintaining relationships is a central feature of most personality disorders. Working with people who can be manipulative, emotionally labile, overly dependent, suspicious or alternate between over-idealization and devaluation can be extremely challenging for the therapist. As might be expected, there is not a great deal of evidence for the effectiveness of therapy with this client population. Kelly et al. (1992), for example, found that between one half and two thirds of all patients with borderline personality disorder discontinue therapy within the first few weeks of treatment.

While there has been a considerable amount written about the treatment of personality disorders, most approaches are based on theory and speculation rather than on evidence from research. However, a number of texts have been published in the last few years about cognitive behavioural treatments for personality disorders (Beck et al., 1990; Layden et al., 1993; Young, 1990), which hopefully will prove to be rather more promising.

Where does this leave the counsellor or therapist in relation to working with clients with personality disorders? This is difficult to answer and will, of course, depend on the background and experience of the counsellor and the context of the therapy. Most of the research looking at the effectiveness of therapeutic intervention has been conducted with clients with severe borderline, schizotypal and antisocial disorders. But in a therapeutic context, mental health professionals often use these terms rather more loosely. It is not unusual to hear, or read in the case-notes, that Mrs X, it is suspected, may be a bit 'borderline'. What is probably meant is that Mrs X shows some of the characteristics of borderline personality disorder, that the problems may be deep-rooted and that she may not be amenable to therapeutic change. The counsellor may not necessarily agree.

Counselling with clients with severe personality disorders would, as a rule, be carried out in a mental health or similar facility. Clearly any counsellor coming across such clients in whatever setting would need to be aware of the difficulties, the limitations and in some cases the dangers of working with such clients.

11.9 CONCLUDING COMMENTS

This chapter has examined some of the conditions usually termed 'psychological disorders'. There has been much criticism, some of it justified, of the use of diagnostic labels. Such labelling can stigmatize the person, devalue their experience, place the individual in a 'patient' role and separate them from the rest of the world. Whilst this undoubtedly does happen, a diagnostic label can, in some cases, be reassuring to the individual, possibly giving them 'permission' to stop and take time out to reassess their life situation.

It is also important to bear in mind that when we talk about mental states such as anxiety and depression, we are referring to a dimension of severity from normal to very severe rather than some qualitatively different condition, although undoubtedly somewhere along the dimension there comes a point at which the person could be described as having a 'disorder'. There is good evidence that this is also the case with schizophrenia (Claridge, 1990).

So when the symptoms which an individual is experiencing become sufficiently pronounced that a diagnosis is made, the label can tell us something about the severity and the range of symptoms a person might be experiencing. If, for example, we hear or suspect from a person's mood that they are depressed, we can expect (although not assume) that they may be experiencing a number of different symptoms—cognitive, motivational and physical—in addition to their depressed mood.

As well as telling us something about which symptoms co-vary or 'hang together', a diagnosis should ideally tell us something about the aetiology, course, treatment and prognosis of a disorder. This is not always the case, and the diagnosis of schizophrenia has been brought into question partly for this reason. We come a little closer to this ideal in the case of depression. Here, the diagnosis can tell us something in a general way about the vulnerability factors, genetic and environmental, about the possible progress of depression, about appropriate treatments, pharmacological and psychological and about expected prognosis.

The diagnosis, however, tells us nothing about the person. For that we need to make a psychological formulation. This is a psychological explanation of how (and possibly why) this person is experiencing these difficulties/symptoms in this way at this particular point in time. Such an explanation will take into account background factors, precipitating factors, vulnerability factors, aspects such as social support, cognitive and emotional style, pre-morbid personality and functioning.

On the whole, diagnosis is the province of the psychiatrist and formulation that of the psychological therapist. Most psychiatrists, however, make use of psychological formulations and many psychological therapists use diagnostic categories. An awareness and some knowledge of this system can add to the counsellor's understanding of the client and the client's experience; it can assist them in their choice of therapeutic approach, possibly indicate the need for other forms of therapy, such as pharmacological therapy, and facilitate communication with other professionals or workers in the field.

References

Abelson R P (1976) 'Script processing in attitude formation and decision making' in J S Carroll and J W Payne (Eds) *Cognitive and Social Behaviour* Hillsdale, N J: Erlbaum

Adams J A (1989) *Human Factors Engineering* New York: Macmillan

Adams C (1991) 'Qualitative age differences in memory for text: A life-span developmental perspective' *Psychology and Aging* **6**, 323–336

Adelmann P K and Zajonc R B (1989) 'Facial efference and the experience of emotion' *Annual Review of Psychology* **40**, 249–280

Agras W S (1993) 'The diagnosis and treatment of panic disorder' *Annual Review of Medicine* **44**, 39–51

Ainsworth M D (1989) 'Attachments beyond infancy' *American Psychologist*, **44**, 709–716.

Ainsworth M D, Blehar M C, Waters E and Wall S (1978) *Patterns of Attachment*, Hillsdale, N J: Erlbaum.

Aldrich E K (1963) 'The dying patient's grief' *Journal of the American Medical Association* **184**, 329–331

Alexander F (1950) *Psychosomatic Medicine: Its Principles and Applications* New York: Norton

Alexander J F, Holtzworth-Monroe A and Jameson P (1994) 'The process and outcome of marital and family therapy: Research review and evaluation' in A E Bergin and S L Garfield (Eds) *Handbook of Psychotherapy and Behavior Change* (4th edn) New York: Wiley

Allison P and Faustenberg F F (1989) 'How marital dissolution affects children: variations by age and sex' *Child Development* **25**, 540–549

Allport G W (1937) *Personality: A Psychological Interpretation* New York: Henry Holt

Altman I and Taylor D A (1973) *Social Penetration: The Development of Interpersonal Relationships* New York: Holt, Rinehart and Winston

Amabile T M (1983) *The Social Psychology of Creativity* New York: Springer-Verlag

Ambady N and Rosenthal R (1992) 'Thin slices of expressive behaviour as predictors of interpersonal consequences: A meta-analysis', *Psychological Bulletin* **111**, 256–274

American Psychiatric Association (1994) *Diagnostic and Statistical Manual of Mental Disorders* (4th edn), Washington, DC: American Psychiatric Association

Andreasen N C, Swayze V W, Flaum M, Yates W R, Arndt S and McChesney C (1990) 'Ventricular enlargement in schizophrenia evaluated with computed tomographic scanning: Effects of gender, age and stage of illness' *Archives of General Psychiatry* **47**, 1008–1015

Andreasen N C, Rezai K, Alliger R, Swayze V W, Flaum M, Kirchner P, Cohen G and O'Leary D S (1992) 'Hypofrontality in neuroleptic-naive patients and in patients with chronic schizophrenia: Assessment with Xenon 133 single photon emission computed tomography and the Tower of London' *Archives of General Psychiatry* **49**, 943–958

Argyle M (1988) 'Social relationships' in M Hewstone, W Stroebe, J Codol and G M Stephenson (Eds) *Introduction to Social Psychology: A European perspective* Oxford: Blackwell

Argyle M and Henderson M (1984) 'The rules of friendship' *Journal of Personal and Social Relationships* **1**, 211–237

Argyle M and Henderson M (1985) *The Anatomy of Relationships* London: Heinemann; Harmondsworth: Penguin

Argyle M and Kendon A (1967) 'The experimental analysis of social performance' *Advances in Experimental Social Psychology* **3**, 55–98

Arieti S and Bemporad J (1978) *Severe and Mild Depression* New York: Basic Books

Arizmendi T G, Beutler L E, Shanfield S, Crago M and Hagman R (1985) 'Client–therapist value similarity and psychotherapy outcome; A microscopic approach' *Psychotherapy; Theory, Research and Practice* **22**, 16–21

Asher S R, Erdley C A and Gabriel S W (1993) 'Peer relations' in M Rutter and D Hay (Eds) *Development Through Life: A Handbook for Clinicians* London: Blackwell

Atkinson D and Schein S (1986) 'Similarity in Counseling' *The Counseling Psychologist* **14**, 319–354

Atkinson R L, Atkinson R C, Smith E E, Bern D S and Hilgard E R (1990) *Introduction to Psychology*, 10th edition, San Diego, CA: Harcourt Brace Jovanovich

Baddeley A (1990) *Human Memory* Needham Heights, MA: Allyn and Bacon

Baddeley A (1993) *Your Memory: A User's Guide* Harmondsworth: Penguin

Baddeley A and Logie R (1992) 'Auditory imagery and working memory' in D Reisberg (Ed) *Auditory Imagery* Hillsdale NJ: Erlbaum

Baker R A (1990) *They Call it Hypnosis* Buffalo, NY: Prometheus

Bandura A (1977) *Social Learning Theory* Englewood Cliffs, NJ: Prentice Hall.

Bandura A (1982) 'Self efficacy mechanisms in human agency' *American Psychologist* **37** 122–147

Bandura A (1986) *Social Foundations of Thought and Action: A Social–Cognitive Theory* Englewood Cliffs, NJ: Prentice Hall

Bandura A (1989) 'Self-efficacy mechanism in physiological activation and health promoting behaviour' in J Madden IV, S Mattysse and J Barchas (Eds) *Adaptation, Learning and Affect* New York: Raven Press

Baron R A and Byrne D (1991) *Social Psychology: Understanding Human Interaction* (6th edn) Boston: Allyn and Bacon

Baron R S, Cutrona C E, Hicklin D W and Lubaroff D M (1990) 'Social support and immune responses among spouses of cancer patients' *Journal of Personality and Social Psychology* **59**, 344–352

Barrett M S and Berman J S (1991) 'Is psychotherapy more effective when therapists disclose information about themselves?', Paper presented at the North American Society for Psychotherapy Research, Panama City, FL

Barry R (1993) 'Bereavement care as a preventative health measure in older adults' in D R Trent and C Reed (Eds) *Promotion of Mental Health, Volume 2* Aldershot: Avebury.

Bartlett F C (1932) *Remembering: A Study in Experimental and Social Psychology* New York: Cambridge

Bass E and Davis L (1988) *The Courage to Heal* New York: Harper and Row

Baxter L R Jr, Schwartz J M, Mazziota J C, Phelps M E, Phal J J, Guze M D and Fairbanks L (1988) 'Cerebral glucose metabolic rates in nondepressed patients with obsessive–compulsive disorder' *American Journal of Psychiatry* **1455**, 1560–1563

Beck A T (1952) 'Successful outpatient psychotherapy of a chronic schizophrenic with a delusion based on borrowed guilt' *Psychiatry* **15**, 305–312

Beck A T (1967) *Depression: Clinical, Experimental and Theoretical Aspects* New York: Harper and Row

Beck A T (1976) *Cognitive Theory and the Emotional Disorders* New York: International Universities Press

Beck A T and Emery G (1985) *Anxiety Disorders and Phobias: A Cognitive Perspective* New York: Basic Books

Beck A T, Brown G, Steer R A, Eidelson J I and Riskind J H (1987) 'Differentiating anxiety and depression: A test of the cognitive-content-specificity hypothesis' *Journal of Abnormal Psychology* **96**, 179–183

Beck A T, Ward C H, Mendelson N, Mock J and Erbaugh J (1961) 'An inventory for measuring depression' *Archives of General Psychiatry* **4**, 561–585

Beck A T, Rush A J, Shaw B F and Emery G (1979) *Cognitive Therapy of Depression* New York: Guilford Press

Beck A T, Epstein N, Brown G and Steer R A (1988) 'An inventory for measuring clinical anxiety' *Journal of Consulting and Clinical Psychology* **56**, 893–897

Beck A T, Freeman A and Associates (1990) *Cognitive Therapy of Personality Disorders* New York: Guilford Press

Beck D F (1988) *Counselor Characteristics: How They Affect Outcomes* Milwaukee, WI: Family Services of America

Bee H (1994) *Lifespan development* New York: HarperCollins

Bentall R P (1990) *Reconstructing Schizophrenia* London: Routledge

Berscheid E (1984) *The Problem of Emotion in Close Relationships* New York: Plenum

Berzins J I (1977) 'Therapist–patient matching' in A S Gurman and A M Razin (Eds) *Effective psychotherapy: A handbook of research* Elmsford, NY: Pergamon

Beutler L E and Clarkin J (1990) *Systematic Treatment Selection: Towards Targeted Therapeutic Interventions* New York: Brunner/Mazel

Beutler L E, Machado P P P and Neufeldt S A (1994) 'Therapist Variables' in A E Bergin and S L Garfield (Eds) *Handbook of Psychotherapy and Behavior Change* (4th edn) New York: Wiley

Bixler E O, Kales A, Soldatos C R, Kales J D and Healey S (1979) 'Prevalence of sleep disorders in the Los Angeles metropolitan area' *American Journal of Psychiatry* **136**, 1257–1262

Black D W, Wesner R, Bowers W and Gabel J (1993) 'A comparison of fluoxamine, cognitive therapy and placebo in the treatment of panic disorder' *Archives of General Psychiatry* **50**, 44–50

Blackburn I M and Davidson K M (1990) *Cognitive Therapy for Depression and Anxiety: A Practitioner's Guide* Oxford: Blackwell Science Publishers

Blaye A, Light P, Joiner R and Sheldon S (1991) 'Collaboration as a facilitator of planning and problem solving on a computer-based task' *British Journal of Developmental Psychology* **9**, 471–484

Block J H, Block J and Gjerde P F (1986) 'The personality of children prior to divorce: a prospective study' *Child Development* **57**, 827–840

Bloom B L, White S W and Asher S J (1979) 'Marital disruption as a stressful event' in C Levinger and O C Moles (Eds) *Divorce and Separation: Context, Causes, and Consequences* New York: Basic Books

Blumstein P and Schwartz P (1983) *American Couples: Money, Work, Sex* New York: William Morrow

Bohannon N J (1988) 'Flashbulb memories and the space shuttle disaster: A tale of two theories' *Cognition* **29**, 179–196

Boldero J and Moore S (1990) 'An evaluation of de Jong–Giervald's loneliness model with Australian adolescents' *Journal of Youth and Adolescence* **10**, 133–147

Bootzin R R (1972) 'A stimulus control technique for insomnia' *Proceedings of the American Psychological Association* pp. 395–396

Bootzin R R and Nicassio P M (1978) 'Behavioral treatments for insomnia' *Progress in Behaviour Modification*, **6**, 1–45

Bouchard T J, Henston L, Eckert E, Keyes M and Resnick S (1981) 'The Minnesota study of twins reared apart: Project description and sample results in the developmental domain' *Twin Research 3: Intelligence, Personality and Development* New York: Alan R Liss

Bower G H (1981) 'Mood and memory' *American Psychologist* **36**, 129–148

Bowlby J (1953) *Child Care and the Growth of Love* Harmondsworth: Penguin

Bowlby J (1980) *Attachment and Loss,* Vol. 3: *Loss, Sadness and Depression* London: Hogarth

Bowlby J (1988) *A Secure Base: Clinical Applications of Attachment Theory* London: Routledge

Bradwejn J, Koszycki D and Meterissian G (1989) 'Cholecystokinin tetrapeptide induces panic attacks identical to spontaneous panic attacks in patients suffering from panic disorder' *Canadian Journal of Psychiatry* **35**, 83–85

Brannen J and Moss P (1987) 'Fathers in dual-earner households: through mothers' eyes' In C Lewis and M O'Brien (Eds) *Reassessing Fatherhood: New Observations on Fathers and the Modern Family* London: Sage

Breakwell G M (1986) *Coping with Threatened Identities* London: Methuen

Brehm J W and Self E A (1989) 'The intensity of motivation' *Annual Review of Psychology* **40**, 109–131

Brewer M B (1988) 'A dual process model of impression formation' in T K Scrull and R S Wyer (Eds) *Advances in Social Cognition,* Vol. 1: *A Dual Process Model of Impression Formation* Hillsdale, NJ: Lawrence Erlbaum Associates

Brewin C R, MacCarthy B, Duda K and Vaughn C E (1991) 'Attribution and expressed emotion in the relatives of patients with schizophrenia' *Journal of Abnormal Psychology* **100**, 545–554

British Psychological Society (1995) *Recovered Memories* Leicester: British Psychological Society

Brown G W and Birley J (1968) 'Crises and life changes in the onset of schizophrenia' *Journal of Health and Social Behaviour* **9**, 217–244

Brown G W and Harris T O (1978) *Social Origins of Depression* London: Tavistock

Brown G W and Harris T O (1989) (Eds) *Life Events and Illness* London: Unwin Hyman

Brown J, Campbell E and Fife-Schaw C (1995) 'Adverse impacts experienced by police officers following exposure to sexual discrimination and sexual harassment' *Stress Medicine* **11**, 221–228

Bryant P E (1972) *Perception and Understanding in Young Children* London: Methuen

Buck R, Miller R E and Caul W F (1974) 'Sex, personality and physiological variables in the communication of affect via facial expression' *Journal of Personality and Social Psychology*, **30**, 587–596

Bushnell I W R, Sai F and Mullen J T (1989) 'Neonatal recognition of the mother's face' *British Journal of Developmental Psychology* **7**, 3–15

Butler R (1963) 'The life review: An interpretation of reminiscence in the aged' *Psychiatry* **26**, 65–76

Buyer L S (1988) 'Creative problem solving; A comparison of performance under different instructions' *Journal of Creative Behaviour* **22**, 55–61

Byrne D, Clore G L and Smeaton G (1986) 'The attraction hypothesis: Do similar attitudes affect anything?' *Journal of Personality and Social Psychology* **51**, 1167–1170

Calabrese R J, Kling M A and Gold P W (1987) 'Alterations in immunocompetence during stress, bereavement and depression: Focus on neuroendocrine regulation' *American Journal of Psychiatry* **144**, 1123–1134

Carskadon M A, Mitler M M and Dement W C (1974) 'A comparison of insomniacs and normals: Total sleep time and sleep latency' *Sleep Research* **3**, 130

Cartwright R D (1974) 'The influence of a conscious wish on dreams: A methodological study of dream meaning and function' *Journal of Abnormal Psychology* **83**, 387–393

Caspi A and Herbener E S (1990) 'Continuity and change: Assortative marriage and the consistency of personality in adulthood' *Journal of Personality and Social Psychology* **58**, 250–258

Cattell R B (1965) *The Scientific Analysis of Personality* Baltimore, MD: Penguin Books

Cattell R B (1986) *Handbook for the Sixteen Personality Factor Questionnaire* Champaign, Ill: Institute for Personality and Ability Testing

Cattell R B and Nesselrode J R (1967) 'Likeness and completeness theories examined by 16 personality factor measures in stable and unstable married couples' *Journal of Personality and Social Psychology* **7**, 351–361

Champion L A and Goodall G (1993) 'Social support: Positive and negative aspects' in D Tantam and M Birchwood (Eds) *Seminars in Psychology and the Social Sciences* London: Gaskell Press

Charone J K (1981) 'Patient and therapist treatment goals related to psychotherapy outcome' *Dissertation Abstracts International* **42**, 365B

Chi M T (1978) 'Knowledge structures and memory development' in R S Siegler (Ed) *Children's Thinking: What Develops?* Hillsdale, NJ: Erlbaum

Chwalisz K, Diener E and Gallagher D (1988) 'Autonomic arousal feedback and emotional experience: Evidence from the spinal cord injured' *Journal of Personality and Social Psychology* **54**, 820–828

Claridge G (1990) 'Can a disease model of schizophrenia survive?' in R P Bentall (Ed) *Reconstructing schizophrenia* London: Routledge

Clarke-Stewart, A (1989) 'Infant day care: Maligned or malignant?' *American Psychologist* **44**, 266–273

Clayton P J (1979) 'The sequelae and nonsequelae of conjugal bereavement' *American Journal of Psychiatry* **136**, 1530–1534

Collinson D R (1980) 'Hypnosis and respiratory disease' in G D Burrows and L Dennerstein (Eds) *Hypnosis and Psychosomatic Medicine* Amsterdam: Elsevier/North-Holland Biomedical Press

Costello C G and Selby M M (1965) 'The relationship between sleep patterns and reactive and endogenous depression' *British Journal of Psychiatry* **111**, 497–501

Craik F I M and Lockhart R S (1972) 'Levels of processing: A framework for memory research' *Journal of Verbal Learning and Verbal Behaviour* **11**, 671–684

Crasilneck H B and Hall J A (1985) *Clinical hypnosis: Principles and applications* Orlando, FL: Harcourt Brace Jovanovich

Crick F and Michison D (1983) 'The function of dream sleep' *Nature* **304**, 111–114

Crick F and Michison D (1986) 'Sleep and neural nets' *Journal of Mind and Behaviour* **7**, 229–250

Crisp A H and Stonehill E (1977) *Sleep, Nutrition and Mood* London: Wiley

Cushway D and Sewell R (1992) *Counselling with dreams and nightmares* London: Sage

Cutting J (1986) *The Psychology of Schizophrenia* London: Churchill Livingstone

Daniels M and Coyle A (1993) ' "Health dividends": The use of co-operative inquiry as a health promotion intervention with a group of unemployed women' in D R Trent and C Reed (Eds) *Promotion of Mental Health:* Vol. 2, Aldershot: Avebury

Darwin C (1872) *The Expression of Emotion in Man and Animals* New York: Philosophical Library

Davies P M, Hickson F C I, Weatherburn P and Hunt A J (1993) *Sex, Gay Men and AIDS* London: The Falmer Press

Davis K L, Kahn R S, Ko G and Davidson M (1991) 'Dopamine in schizophrenia: A revised and reconceptualization' *American Journal of Psychiatry* **148**, 1474–1486

Day R (1989) 'Schizophrenia' in G W Brown and T Harris (Eds) *Life Events and Illness* London: Unwin Hyman

DeLongis A, Coyne J C, Dakof G, Folkman S and Lazarus R S (1982) 'Relationship of daily hassles, uplifts and major life events to health status' *Health Psychology* **1**, 119–136

Dement W C and Wolpert E (1958) 'The relation of eye movements, bodily motility and external stimuli to dream activity: An objective method to the study of dreaming' *Journal of Experimental Psychology* **55**, 543–553

Dent H and Flin R (1992) *Children as Witnesses* Chichester: Wiley

Dick P K (1972) *Do Androids Dream of Electric Sheep?* London: Granada

Doise W and Mugny G (1984) *The Social Development of Intellect* Oxford: Pergamon

Donaldson M (1978) *Children's Minds* London: Fontana

Dorsey C M (1993) 'Failing to sleep: Psychological and behavioral underpinnings of insomnia' in T H Monk (Ed) *Sleep, Sleepiness and Performance* Chichester: Wiley

Dufault K and Martocchio B C (1985) *Nursing Clinics of North America*, Vol. 20, No. 2

Dunleavy D L F and Oswald I (1973) 'Phenalzine, mood response and sleep' *Archives of General Psychiatry* **28**, 353–356

Dunn J (1988) *The Beginnings of Social Understanding* Oxford: Blackwell

Dunn J and Kendrick C (1982) *Siblings* Cambridge, MA: Harvard University Press

Dunn J and Munn P (1985) 'Becoming a family member: Family conflict and the development of social understanding in the second year' *Child Development* **56**, 480–492

Dywan J and Bowers K S (1983) 'The use of hypnosis to enhance recall' *Science* **222**, 184–185

Ebbesen E, Duncan B and Konecni V (1975) 'Effects of content of verbal aggression on future verbal aggression: A field experiment', in *Journal of Experimental Psychology* **11**, 192–204

Ebbinghaus H (1885, 1913) *Memory* Translation by H Ruyer and C E Bussenius, New York: Teachers College, Columbia University

Edwards W (1987) 'Decision making' in G Salvendy (Ed) *Handbook of Human Factors* New York: Wiley

Egon G (1986) *The Skilled Helper; A Systematic Approach to Effective Helping* Pacific Grove, CA: Brooks/Cole

Eibl-Eibesfeldt I (1973) 'The expressive behavior of the deaf- and-blind born' in M von Cranach and I Vine (Eds) *Social Communication and Movement* New York: Academic Press

Eich J E (1989) 'Theoretical issues in state dependent memory' in H L Roediger and F I Craik (Eds) *Varieties of Memory and Consciousness* Hillsdale, NJ: Lawrence Erlbaum Associates

Eich J E, Weingartner H, Stillman R C and Gillin J C (1975) 'State dependent accessibility of retrieval cues in the retention of a categorized list' *Journal of Verbal Learning and Verbal Behaviour* **14**, 408–417

Eisenberg N and Fabes R A (1992) *Emotion and its Regulation in Early Development: New Directions for Child Development*, San Francisco: Jossey-Bass

Ekman P (1982) 'Methods of measuring facial action' in K R Scherer and P Ekman (Eds) *Handbook of Methods in Nonverbal Behaviour Research* Cambridge: Cambridge University Press

Ekman P, Levenson R W and Friesen W V (1983) 'Autonomic nervous system distinguishes amongst emotions' *Science* **221**, 1208–1210

Ellman S J and Antrobus J S (1991) *The Mind in Sleep: Psychology and Psychophysiology* (2nd edn) New York: Wiley

Empson J (1993) *Sleep and Dreaming* New York: Harvester Wheatsheaf

Erdelyi M H (1985) *Psychoanalysis: Freud's Cognitive Psychology* New York: Freeman

Erikson E H (1956) 'The problem of ego identity' *Journal of the American Psychoanalytic Association* **4**, 56–121

Erikson E H (1959) 'Identity and the life cycle' *Psychological Issues 1* (Monograph no. 1)

Erikson E H (1968) *Identity: Youth and Crisis* New York: Norton

Evans C (1984) *Landscapes of the Night: How and Why we Dream* New York: Viking

Eysenck H J and Eysenck S B G (1969) *Personality Structure and Measurement* San Diego: RR Knapp

Faraday A (1974) *The Dream Game* New York: Harper and Row

Feinberg I, Koresko R L and Heller N (1967) 'EEG sleep patterns as a function of normal and pathological aging in man' *Journal of Psychiatric Research* **5**, 107

Festinger L, Schachter S and Back K (1950) *Social Pressures in Informal Groups: A Study of Human Factors in Housing* Stanford, California: Stanford University Press

Fischoff B and MacGregor D (1982) 'Subjective confidence in forecasts' *Journal of Forecasting* **1**, 155–172

Fischoff B, Slovic P and Lichenstein S (1977) 'Knowing with certainty: The appropriateness of extreme confidence' *Journal of Experimental Psychology: Human Perception and Performance* **3**, 552–564

Fiske S T and Ruscher J B (1989) 'On-line processes in category based and individuating impressions: Some basic principles and methodological reflections' in J N Bassili (Ed) *On-line Cognition in Person Perception* Hillsdale, NJ: Lawrence Erlbaum Associates

Fiske S T and Taylor S E (1991) *Social Cognition* (2nd edn) New York: McGraw-Hill

Fleming I, O'Keeffe M K and Baum A (1991) 'Chronic stress and toxic waste: The role of uncertainty and helplessness' *Journal of Applied Social Psychology* **21**, 1889–1907

Foa E B, Steketee G and Rothbaum B O (1989) 'Behavioural/cognitive conceptualisations of post-traumatic stress disorder' *Behaviour Therapy* **20**, 155–176

Foenander G and Burrows G D (1980) 'Phenomena of hypnosis: 1. Age regression' in G D Burrows and L Dennerstein (Eds) *Hypnosis and psychosomatic medicine* Amsterdam: Elsevier/North-Holland Biomedical Press

Folkman S and Lazarus R S (1988) 'Coping as a mediator of emotion' *Journal of Personality and Social Psychology* **54**, 466–475

Fonte R J and Stevenson J M (1985) 'The use of propranolol in the treatment of anxiety disorders' *Hillside Journal of Clinical Psychiatry* **7**, 54–62

Freud S (1905/1948) *Three Contributions to the Theory of Sex* (4th edn) New York: Nervous and Mental Disease Monograph

Friedman M and Rosenman R H (1974) *Type A Behavior* New York: Knopf

Frodi A M, Lamb M E, Leavitt L A and Donovan W L (1978) 'Fathers' and mothers' responses to infant smiles and cries' *Infant Behaviour and Development* **1**, 187–189

Gaillard J M, Nicholson A N and Pascoe P A (1989) 'Neuro-transmitter systems' in M H Kryger, T Roth and W C Dement (Eds) *Principles and Practice of Sleep Medicine* Philadelphia: W B Saunders

Gelman R and Gallistel R (1978) *The Child's Understanding of Number* Cambridge, MA: Harvard University Press

Gergen K J (1968) 'Personal consistency and presentation' in C Gordon and K J Gergen (Eds) *The Self in Social Interaction* Reading, MA: Addison-Wesley

Gerson L W, Jarjoura D and McCord G (1987) 'Factors related to impaired mental health in urban elderly' *Research on Aging* **9**, 356–371

Glaser R, Rice J, Speicher C E, Stout J C and Kiecolt-Glaser J K (1986) 'Stress depresses interferon production by leucocytes concomitant with a decrease in natural killer-cell activity' *Behavioral Neuroscience* **100**, 675–678

Glucksberg S (1962) 'The influence of strength of drive on functional fixedness and perceptual recognition' *Journal of Experimental Psychology* **63**, 36–41

Goldfarb W (1945) 'Effects of psychological deprivation in infancy and subsequent stimulation' *American Journal of Psychiatry* **102**, 18–33

Goldfried M R and Davison G C (1994) *Clinical Behaviour Therapy* New York: Wiley

Goldman-Rakic P S (1992) 'Working memory and the mind' *Scientific American* **267**, 110–117

Goldsmith H H (1983) 'Generic influences on personality from infancy to adulthood' *Child Development* **54**, 331–355.

Gottman J M (1979) *Marital Interaction: Experimental Investigation* New York: Academic Press

Gould R L (1978) *Transformations: Growth and Change in Adult Life* New York: Simon & Schuster

Green C (1968) *Lucid Dreams* Oxford: Institute for Psychophysical Research

Greene R L (1992) *Human Memory: Paradigms and Paradoxes* Hillsdale, NJ: Erlbaum

Haefele J W (1962) *Creativity and Innovation* New York: Reinhold

Haider I and Oswald I (1971) 'Effects of amylobarbitone and nitrazepam in the electrodermogram and other features of sleep' *British Journal of Psychiatry* **118**, 519–522

Halford W K and Hayes R (1991) 'Psychosocial rehabilitation of chronic schizophrenic patients: Recent findings on social skills training and family psychoeducation' *Clinical Psychology Review* **11**, 23–44

Halikas J A, Goodwin D W and Guze S B (1971) 'Marijuana effects: A survey of regular users' *Journal of American Medical Association* **217**, 692–694

Hamilton D L (1988) 'Understanding Impression formation: What has memory research contributed?' in P Soloman, G R Goethals, C M Kelly and B Stephens (Eds) *Memory: An interdisciplinary approach* New York: Springer-Verlag

Hammarberg M (1992) 'Penn Inventory for Post-Traumatic Stress Disorder: Psychometric properties' *Psychological Assessment* **4**, 67–76

Harber K D and Pennebaker J W (1992) 'Overcoming traumatic memories' in S-A Christianson (Ed) *The handbook of emotion and memory* Hillsdale, NJ: Lawrence Erlbaum Associates

Harding C M, Zubin J and Strauss J S (1992) 'Chronicity in schizophrenia: revisited' *British Journal of Psychiatry* **161**, 27–37

Harlow H F and Zimmerman R R (1959) 'Affectional responses in the infant monkey' *Science* **130**, 421–432

Hartman E (1976) 'Long-term administration of psychotropic drugs: effects on human sleep' in R L Williams and I Karacan (Eds) *Pharmacology of human sleep* New York: Wiley

Hartman E (1978) *The Sleeping Pill* New Haven: Yale University Press

Hartmann H (1939) *Ego Psychology and the Problem of Adaptation* New York: International Universities Press

Hatfield E (1988) 'Passionate and companionate love' in R J Sternberg and M L Barnes (Eds) *The Psychology of Love* New Haven, CT: Yale University Press

Hathaway S and McKinley J C (1943) *Minnesota Multiphasic Personality Inventory: Manual* New York: Psychological Corporation

Hathaway S and McKinley J C (1989) *Manual for Administration and Scoring MMPI-2* Minneapolis: University of Minnesota Press

Havighurst R J (1972) *Developmental Tasks and Education:* (3rd edn) New York: David McKay

Hayslip B and Panek P E (1993) *Adult Development and Aging* (2nd edn) New York: HarperCollins

Hearne K (1990) *The Dream Machine* Wellingborough: Aquarian Press

Hebb D O (1972) *Textbook of Psychology* (3rd edn) Philadelphia: Saunders

Heider F (1958) *The Psychology of Interpersonal Relations* New York: Wiley

Herzog A R, House J S and Morgan J N (1991) 'Relation of work and retirement to health and well-being in older age' *Psychology and Aging* **6**, 202–211

Hetherington E M (1989) 'Coping with family transitions: winners, losers and survivors' *Child Development* **60**, 1–14

Hilgard E R (1965) *Hypnotic Susceptibility* New York: Harcourt, Brace and World

Hilgard E R (1977) *Divided Consciousness* New York: Wiley

Hilgard E R (1980) 'Hypnosis and the treatment of pain' in G D Burrows and L Dennerstein (Eds) *Hypnosis and Psychosomatic Medicine* Amsterdam: Elsevier/North-Holland Biomedical Press

Hohmann G W (1962) 'Some effects of spinal cord lesions on experienced emotional feelings' *Psychophysiology* **3**, 143–156

Hole R W, Rush A J and Beck A T (1979) 'A cognitive investigation of schizophrenic delusions' *Psychiatry* **42**, 312–319

Holmes D S (1974) 'Investigations of repression: Differential recall of material experimentally or naturally associated with ego threat' *Psychological Bulletin* **81**, 632–653

Holmes D S (1984) 'Meditation and somatic arousal reduction: A review of the experimental evidence' *American Psychologist* **39**, 1–10

Holmes T H and Rahe R H (1967) 'The social readjustment rating scale' *Journal of Psychosomatic Research* **11**, 213–218

Hopson B (1981) 'Response to the papers by Schlossberg, Brammer and Abrego' *Counseling Psychologist* **9**, 36–39

Horne J (1981) 'The effects of exercise on sleep: A critical review' *Biological Psychology* **12**, 241–290

Horne J (1988) *Why We Sleep: The Functions of Sleep in Humans and Other Animals* New York: Oxford

Horner K W, Rushton J P and Vernon P A (1986) 'Relation between aging and research productivity of academic psychologists' *Psychology and Aging* **1**, 319–324

Horowitz M J (1993) 'Stress response syndromes: a review of post-traumatic stress and adjustment disorders' in J P Wilson and B Raphael (Eds) *International Handbook of Traumatic Stress Syndromes* New York: Plenum Press

Horowitz M, Wilmer N and Alvorez W (1979) 'The Impact of Events Scale: A measure of subjective distress' *Psychosomatic Medicine* **41**, 209–218

House J S, Landris K R and Umberson D (1988) 'Social relationships and health' *Science* **241**, 540–545

Hunt R and Rouse W B (1981) 'Problem solving skills of maintenance trainees in diagnosing faults in simulated power plants' *Human Factors* **23**, 317–328

Hyler S E, Reider R O, Williams J B W, Spitzer R L, Hendler J and Lyons M (1988) 'The Personality Diagnostic Questionnaire: development and preliminary results' *Journal of Personality Disorders* **2**, 229–237

Izard C E (1971) *The Face of Emotion* New York: Appleton-Century-Crofts

Izard C E (1977) *Human Emotions* New York: Plenum

Izard C E (1989) 'The structure and functions of emotions: Implications for cognition, motivation and personality' in I S Cohen (Ed) *The G Stanley Hall lecture series* (Vol 9) Washington, DC: American Psychological Association

Izard C E (1990) 'Facial expressions and the regulation of emotion' *Journal of Personality and Social Psychology* **58**, 487–498

Jacobi J (1968) *The Psychology of C G Jung* London: Routledge and Kegan Paul

James W (1890) *The Principles of Psychology* New York: Dover

Janis I L and Mann L (1977) *Decision Making: A Psychological Analysis of Conflict* New York: Free Press

Janis I L and Mann L (1982) 'A theoretical framework for decision counselling' in I L Janis (Ed) *Counselling on Personal Decisions; Theory and Research on Short-term Helping Relationships* New Haven, CT: Yale University Press

Jemmott J B III, Borysenko M R, McClelland D C, Chapman R, Meyer D and Benson H (1985) 'Academic stress, power motivation and decrease in salivary secretory immunoglobulin: A secretion rate' *Lancet* **1**, 1400–1402

Johnson D W (1989) 'Will stress management prevent coronary heart disease?' *The Psychologist: Bulletin of the British Psychological Society* **2**, 275–278

Jourard S M (1971) *The Transparent Self* Princeton, NJ: Van Nostrand Reinhold

Kagan J (1989) *Unstable Ideas: Temperament, Cognition and Self* Cambridge, MA: Harvard University Press

Kahneman D and Tversky A (1979) 'Prospect theory: an analysis of decisions under risk' *Econometrica* **47**, 263–291

Keane T M, Zimmerling R T and Caddell J M (1985) 'A behavioural formulation of post-traumatic stress disorder in Vietnam veterans' *The Behaviour Therapist* **8**, 9–12

Kelly G (1955) *The Psychology of Personal Constructs*, Vols 1 and 2 New York: Norton

Kelly H H (1973) 'The process of causal attribution' *American Psychologist* **28**, 107–128

Kelly H (1979) *Personal Relationships: Their Structures and Processes* Hillsdale, NJ: Lawrence Erlbaum Associates

Kelly T, Soloff P H, Cornelius J, George A, Lis J A and Ulrich R (1992) 'Can we study (treat) borderline patients? Attrition from research and open treatment' *Journal of Personality Disorders* **6**, 417–433

Kiecolt-Glaser J K, Kennedy S, Malkoff S, Fisher L, Speicher C E and Glaser R (1988) 'Marital discord and immunity in males' *Psychosomatic Medicine* **50**, 213–229

Kihlstrom J F (1985) 'Hypnosis' *Annual Review of Psychology* **36**, 385–418

Kihlstrom J F (1987) 'The cognitive unconscious' *Science* **237**, 1445–1452

Kingdon D G and Turkington D (1994) *Cognitive–Behavioural Therapy of Schizophrenia* Hove, UK: Lawrence Erlbaum Associates

Kitzinger C and Coyle A (1995) 'Lesbian and gay couples: Speaking of difference' *The Psychologist* **8**, 64–69

Kobasa C S (1979) 'Stressful life events, personality and health: An inquiry into hardiness' *Journal of Personality and Social Psychology* **37**, 1–11

Kobasa C S, Hilker R J and Maddi S (1979) 'Psychological hardiness' *Journal of Occupational Medicine* **21**, 595–598

Kobasa C S, Maddi S R and Kahn S (1982) 'Hardiness and Health: A prospective study' *Journal of Personality and Social Psychology* **42**, 168–177

Kroger J (1989) *Identity in Adolescence: The Balance Between Self and Other* London: Routledge

Kubler-Ross E (1969) *On Death and Dying* London: Tavistock

Kulik J A and Mahler H I M (1989) 'Social support and recovery from surgery' *Health Psychology* **8**, 221–238

Kurdek L A (1994) 'The nature and correlates of relationship quality in gay, lesbian, and heterosexual cohabiting couples: A test of the individual difference, interdependence, and discrepancy models' In B Greene and G M Herek (Eds) *Lesbian and Gay Psychology: Theory, Research, and Clinical Applications* Thousand Oaks, CA: Sage

Kurdek L A and Schmitt J P (1987) 'Perceived emotional support from family and friends in members of homosexual, married, and heterosexual cohabiting couples' *Journal of Homosexuality* **14**, 57–68

La Berge S (1985) *Lucid Dreaming* New York: Ballantyne Books

Labouvie-Vief G (1980) 'Beyond formal operations: Uses and limits of pure logic in life-span development' *Human Development* **23**, 141–161

Labouvie-Vief G (1990) 'Modes of knowledge and the organization of development' in M L Commons, C Armon, L Kohlberg, F A Richards, T A Grotzer and J D Sinnott (Eds) *Adult Development, Vol. 2, Models and Methods in the Study of Adolescent and Adult Thought* New York: Praeger

LaFrance M and Banaji M (1992) 'The gender–emotion relationship' in M S Clark (Ed) *Emotion and Social Behaviour* Newbury Park, CA: Sage

Laird J D (1974) 'Self-attribution of emotion: The effects of expressive behaviour on the quality of emotional experience' *Journal of Personality and Social Psychology* **33**, 475–486

Laird J D and Bresler C (1992) 'The process of emotional experience: A self-perception theory' in M S Clark (Ed) *Emotion*, Newbury Park, CA: Sage

Langer E J (1975) 'The illusion of control' *Journal of Personality and Social Psychology* **32**, 311–328

Langer E J (1989) *Mindlessness* Reading, MA: Addison-Wesley

Laurence J and Perry C (1983) 'Hypnotically created memory among highly hypnotizable subjects' *Science* **222**, 523–524

Layden M A, Newman C F, Freeman A and Morse S B (1993) *Cognitive Therapy of Borderline Personality Disorder* Boston, MA: Allyn and Bacon

Lazarus R S (1991a) 'Progress on a cognitive-motivational-rational theory of emotion' *American Psychologist* **46**, 819–834

Lazarus R S (1991b) 'Cognition and motivation in emotion' *American Psychologist* **46**, 352–367

Lazarus R S and Folkman S (1984) *Stress, Appraisal and Coping* New York: Springer

Lehman D R, Ellard J E and Wortman C B (1986) 'Social support for the bereaved: Recipients' and providers' perspectives on what is helpful' *Journal of Counselling and Clinical Psychology* **54**, 438–446

Leval I, Friedlander Y, Kark J D and Periz E (1988) 'An epidemiological study of mortality among bereaved parents' *New England Journal of Medicine*, **319**, 457–461

Levinson D J, Darrow D N, Klein E B, Levinson M H and McKee B (1978) *The Seasons of a Man's Life* New York: A A Knopf

Lewinsohn P M and Rosenbaum M (1987) 'Recall of parental behaviour by acute depressives, remitted depressives and nondepressives' *Journal of Personality and Social Psychology* **52**, 611–619

Liem J H (1980) 'Family studies of schizophrenia: An update and commentary, *Schizophrenia Bulletin* **6**, 429–455

Lindsay D S and Read J D (1994) 'Incest resolution psychotherapy and memories of childhood sexual abuse' *Applied Cognitive Psychology* **8**, 281–338

Loftus E F (1980) *Memory* Reading, MA: Addison-Wesley

Loftus E F and Loftus G R (1980) 'On the permanence of stored information in the human brain' *American Psychologist* **35**, 409–420

Loftus E F and Palmer J C (1974) 'Reconstruction of automobile destruction: An example of interaction between language and memory' *Journal of Verbal Learning and Verbal Behaviour* **13**, 585–589

Loftus E F, Miller D G and Burns H J (1978) 'Semantic integration of verbal information into visual memory' *Journal of Experimental Psychology: Human Learning and Memory* **4**, 19–31

Lynn S J and Rhue W J (1988) 'Fantasy proneness' *American Psychologist* **43**, 35–44

Major B, Carrington P I and Carnevale P J D (1984) 'Physical attractiveness and self-esteem; Attributions for praise from an other-sex evaluator' *Personality and Social Psychology Bulletin* **10**, 43–50

Malmquist C P (1986) 'Children who witness parental murder: Post traumatic aspects' *Journal of American Academy of Child Psychiatry* **25**, 320–325

Marcia J E (1980) 'Identity in adolescence' in J Adelson (Ed) *Handbook of Adolescent Psychology* New York: Wiley

Markus H R (1977) 'Self schema and processing information about the self' *Journal of Personality and Social Psychology* **35**, 63–78

Markus H R and Nurius P (1986) 'Possible selves' *American Psychologist* **41**, 954–969

Marshall V (1975) 'Age and awareness of finitude in developmental gerontology' *Omega* **6**, 113–129

Maslow A H (1954) *Motivation and personality* New York: Harper and Row

Maslow A (1968) *Towards a new psychology of being* New York: Van Nostrand-Reinhold

Maslow A (1970) *Motivation and Personality* (2nd edition) New York: Harper and Row

Mauro R, Sato K and Tucker J (1992) The role of appraisal in human emotions: A cross-cultural study, *Journal of Personality and Social Psychology* **62**, 301–317

McCloskey M and Zaragoza M (1985) 'Misleading post-event information and memory for events: Arguments and evidence against memory impairment hypotheses' *Journal of Experimental Psychology; General* **114**, 1–16

McCrae R R and Costa P T (1988) 'Psychological resilience among widowed men and women: A 10-year follow-up of a national sample' *Journal of Social Issues* **44**, 129–142

Meier-Ewart K, Matsubayashi K and Benter L (1985) 'Propranolol: Long-term treatment in narcolepsy–cataplexy' *Sleep* **8**, 95–104

Meltzoff A N and Moore M K (1983) 'Newborn infants imitate adult facial gestures' *Child Development* **54**, 702–709

Metts S, Cupach W R and Bejlovec (1989) ' "I love you too much to ever start liking you": Redefining romantic relationships' *Journal of Social and Personal Relationships* **6**, 259–274

Miller G (1956) 'The magical number seven, plus or minus two: Some limits on our capacity for processing information' *Psychological Review* **63**, 81–87

Millon T (1983) *Millon Clinical Multianxial Inventory Manual* (3rd edn) Minneapolis: National Computer

Mischel W (1968) *Personality and Assessment* New York: Wiley

Mischel W (1986) *Introduction to Personality: A New Look* (4th edn) New York: Holt, Rinehart and Winston

Montgomery S and Asberg M (1979) 'A new depression scale designed to be sensitive to change' *British Journal of Psychiatry* **134**, 382–389

Morgan C D and Murray H A (1935) 'A method for investigating fantasy: the thematic apperception test' *Archives of General Psychiatry* **34**, 289–386

Negrete J C and Kwan M W (1972) 'Relative value of various etiological factors in short-lasting, adverse psychological reactions to cannabis smoking' *International Pharmacopsychiatry* **7**, 249–259

Neimeyer R A and Mitchell K A (1988) 'Similarity and attraction; A longitudinal study' *Journal of Social and Personal Relationships* **5**, 131–148

Nicholson A N and Pasco P A (1988) 'Studies on the modulation of sleep and wakefulness in man by fluoxetine, a 5-HT uptake inhibitor' *Neuropharmacology* **27**, 597–602

Norris F H (1990) 'Screening for traumatic stress: A scale for use in the general population' *Journal of Applied Social Psychology* **20**, 1704–1718

Oltmanns T F and Emery R E (1995) *Abnormal Psychology* Englewood Cliffs, NJ: Prentice Hall

Orne M T, Sheehan P W and Evans F J (1968) 'Occurrence of posthypnotic behaviour outside the experimental setting' *Journal of Personality and Social Psychology* **9**, 189–196

Osgood C E, Suci G J and Tannenbaum P H (1957) *The Measurement of Meaning* New York: Viking

Overton D A (1984) 'State dependent learning and drug discriminations' in L L Iverson, S H Iverson and S H Snyder (Eds) *Handbook of Psychopharmacology*, Vol. 18 New York: Plenum Press

Papousek H (1967) 'Experimental studies of appetitional behaviour in human newborns and infants' in H W Stevenson (Ed) *Early Behavior* New York: Wiley

Park B (1989) 'Trait attributions as on-line organizers in person impressions' in J N Bassili (Ed) *On-line Cognition in Person Perception* Hillsdale, NJ: Lawrence Erlbaum Associates

Parkes C M (1980) 'Bereavement counselling: Does it work?' *British Medical Journal* **281**, 3–6

Parkes M C, Benjamin B and Fitzgerald R G (1969) 'Broken heart: a statistical study of increased mortality among widowers', *British Medical Journal* **1**, 740–743

Pasnau, R O, Naitoh R, Stier S and Kollar E J (1968) 'The psychological effects of 205 hours of sleep deprivation' *Archives of General Psychiatry* **18**, 496–505

Pennebaker J W and Beall S K (1986) 'Confronting a traumatic event: Towards an understanding of inhibition and disease' *Journal of Abnormal Psychology* **95**, 274–281

Pennebaker J W, Hughes C and O'Heeron R (1987) 'The psychophysiology of confession: Linking inhibitory and psychosomatic processes' *Journal of Personality and Social Psychology* **52**, 781–793

Pennebaker J W, Kielcolt-Glaser J and Glaser R (1988) 'Disclosure of traumas and immune function: Health implications for psychotherapy' *Journal of Consulting and Clinical Psychology* **56**, 239–245

Pennebaker J W, Barger S and Tiebout J (1989) 'Disclosures of traumas and health amongst Holocaust survivors' *Psychosomatic Medicine* **51**, 577–589

Peplau L A (1991) 'Lesbian and gay relationships' in J C Gonsiorek and J D Weinrich (Eds) *Homosexuality: Research Implications for Public Policy* Newbury Park, CA: Sage

Peplau L A and Cochran S D (1990) 'A relationship perspective on homosexuality' in D P McWhirter, S A Sanders and J M Reinisch (Eds) *Homosexuality/ Heterosexuality: The Kinsey Scale and Current Research* New York: Oxford University Press

Perls F S (1947) *Ego, Hunger and Aggression: The Beginning of Gestalt Therapy* New York: Random House

Perls F S (1973) *The Gestalt Approach and Eyewitness to Therapy* Palo Alto, CA: Science and Behaviour Books

Perls F S, Hifferine R F and Goodman R (1951) *Gestalt therapy: Excitement and growth in personality* New York: Julian Press.

Pfohl B, Stangl D and Zimmerman M (1982) *Structured interview for DMS-III Personality Disorders (SIDP)* Iowa: University of Iowa Hospitals and Clinics

Phinney J S and Rosenthal D S (1992) 'Ethnic identity in adolescence: Process, context and outcome' In G R Adams (Ed) *Adolescent Identity Formation* Newbury Park, CA: Sage

Piccione C, Hilgard E R and Zimbardo P G (1989) 'On the degree of measured hypnotizability over a 25 year period' *Journal of Personality and Social Psychology* **56**, 289–295

Pillemer D B, Goldsmith L R, Panter A T and White S H (1988) 'Very long-term memories of first year in college' *Journal of Experimental Psychology: Learning, Memory and Cognition* **14**, 709–715

Pines A and Aronson E (1981) *Burnout: From Tedium to Personal Growth* New York: Free Press

Pitts M and Phillips K (1991) *The Psychology of Health* London: Routledge

Plomin R and Thompson L (1987) 'Life-span developmental behavioral genetics' in P B Baltes *et al.* (Eds) *Life-Span Development and Behavior* Vol. 7, Hillsdale, NJ: Erlbaum

Polya G (1957) *How to Solve It* New York: Anchor

Popper K R (1959) *The Logic of Scientific Discovery* London: Hutchinson

Powers S I, Hauser S T and Kilner L A (1989) 'Adolescent mental health' *American Psychologist* **44**, 200–208

Priest R (1983) 'Sleep and its disorders' in R N Gaine and B L Hudson (Eds) *Current Themes in Psychiatry* London: Macmillan

Prochaska J O and Norcross J C (1994) *Systems of Psychotherapy: a Transtheoretical Analysis* (3rd edn) Pacific Grove, CA: Brookes/Cole

Raphael B (1984) *The Anatomy of Bereavement* London: Hutchinson

Reizenzein R (1983) 'The Schaachter theory of emotion: Two decades later' *Psychological Bulletin* **94**, 239–264

Repetti P L (1989) 'Effects of daily workload on subsequent behaviour during marital interaction: The roles of social withdrawal and spouse support' *Journal of Personality and Social Psychology* **57**, 651–659

Revenson T A and Felton B J (1989) 'Disability and coping as predictors of psychological adjustment to rheumatoid arthritis' *Journal of Consulting and Clinical Psychology* **57**, 344–348

Richards M P M (1988) 'Developmental psychology and family law: A discussion paper' *British Journal of Developmental Psychology* **6**, 169–182

Robins L N, Herlzer J E, Croghan J and Ratcliff K S (1981) 'National Institute of Mental Health: Diagnostic interview schedule' *Archives of General Psychiatry* **38**, 381–389

Rogers C R (1951) *Client-centred Therapy: Its Current Practice, Implications and Theory* Boston, MA: Houghton Mifflin

Rogers C R (1961) *On Becoming a Person: A Therapist's View of Psychotherapy* Boston, MA: Houghton Mifflin

Rorschach H (1942) *Psychodiagnostics: A Diagnostic Test Based on Perception* New York: Grune & Stratton

Rosa R R, Bonnet M H and Kramer M (1983) 'The relationship between sleep and anxiety in anxious subjects' *Biological Psychology* **16**, 119–126

Rotter J B (1972) *Applications of a Social Learning Theory of Personality* New York: Holt, Rinehart and Winston

Ruch J C, Morgan A H and Hilgard E R (1973) 'Behavioral predictions from hypnotic responsiveness when obtained with and without prior induction procedures' *Journal of Abnormal Psychology* **82**, 543–546

Rust J (1988) 'The Rust Inventory of Schizotypal Cognitions (RISC)' *Schizophrenia Bulletin* **14**, 317–322

Rutter M (1981) *Maternal Deprivation Reassessed* (2nd edn) Harmondsworth: Penguin

Rutter M and Madge N (1976) *Cycles of Disadvantage* London: Heinemann

Ryan W (1977) *Blaming the Victim* New York: Vintage Books

Sachs J D S (1967) 'Recognition memory for syntactical and semantic aspects of connected discourse' *Perception and Psychophysics* **2**, 237–442

Sai F and Bushnell I W R (1988) 'The perception of faces in different poses by 1 month olds' *British Journal of Developmental Psychology* **6**, 35–42

Salamy J (1970) 'Instrumental responding to internal cues associated with REM sleep' *Psychomotor Science* **18**, 342–343

Salthouse T A (1982) *Adult Cognition: An Experimental Psychology of Human Aging* New York: Springer-Verlag

Sanders C M (1989) *Grief: The Mourning After* New York: Wiley-Interscience

Sanders G S and Simmons W L (1983) 'Use of hypnosis to enhance eye witness accuracy: Does it work?' *Journal of Applied Psychology* **68**, 70–77

Sargent W (1967) *The Unquiet Mind* London: Heinemann

Sarnoff I and Zimbardo P G (1961) 'Anxiety, fear and social affiliation' *Journal of Abnormal and Social Psychology* **62**, 356–363

Sartorius N, Jablensky A, Korten A, Ernberg G, Anker M, Cooper J E and Day R (1986) 'Early manifestations and first-contact incidence of schizophrenia in different cultures: A preliminary report on the initial evaluation phase of the WHO Collaborative Study on Determinants of Outcome of Severe Mental Disorders' *Psychological Medicine* **16**, 909–928

Schaachter S and Singer J E (1962) 'Cognitive, social and physiological determinants of emotional state' *Psychological Review* **69**, 379–399

Schactel E G (1947) 'On memory and child amnesia' *Psychiatry* **10**, 1–26

Schaeffer H R and Emerson P E (1964) 'The development of social attachments in infancy' *Monographs of the Society for Research in Child Development* **29**, 94

Scurfield R M (1985) 'Posttrauma stress assessment and treatment: Overview and formulations' in C R Figley (Ed) *Trauma and its Wake* New York: Brunner/Mazel

Selye H (1956) *The Stress of Life* New York: McGraw-Hill

Selye H (1982) 'Stress: Eustress, distress and human perspectives' in S B Day (Ed) *Lifestress* New York: Van Nostrand Reinhold

Shapiro D H and Giber D (1978) *Meditation: Self-regulation Strategy and Altered States of Consciousness* New York: Aldine

Shaver P, Hazan C and Bradshaw D (1988) 'Love and attachment; The integration of three behavioral systems' in R J Sternberg and M L Barnes (Eds) *The Psychology of Love* New Haven, CT: Yale University Press

Sheehan P W and Statham D (1989) 'Hypnosis, the timing of its introduction, and acceptance of misleading information' *Journal of Abnormal Psychology* **98**, 170–176

Siddique C M and D'Arcy C (1984) 'Adolescence, stress and psychological well-being' *Journal of Youth and Adolescence* **13**, 459–474

Simonton D K (1988) 'Age and outstanding achievement: What do we know after a century of research?' *Psychological Bulletin* **104**, 251–267

Singer M and Wynne L C (1963) 'Differentiating characteristics of the parents of childhood schizophrenics' *American Journal of Psychiatry* **120**, 476–487

Skuse D (1984) 'Extreme deprivation in early childhood II: Theoretical issues and a comparative review' *Journal of Child Psychology and Psychiatry* **25**(4), 543–572

Smith C A and Ellsworth P C (1987) 'Patterns of appraisal and emotion related to taking an exam' *Journal of Personality and Social Psychology* **52**, 475–488

Smith R E and Smoll F L (1990) 'Sport performance anxiety' in H Leitenberg (Ed) *Handbook of social and evaluation anxiety* New York: Plenum

Smith S M, Glenberg A M and Bjork R A (1978) 'Environmental context and human memory' *Memory and Cognition* **6**, 342–355

Snyder M (1984) 'When belief creates reality' in L Berkowitz (Ed) *Advances in Experimental Social Psychology*, Vol. 18 New York: Academic Press

Snyder M (1987) *Public Appearances, Private Realities: The Psychology of self-monitoring* New York: Freeman

Solomon Z, Mikulincer M and Autizur E (1988) 'Coping, locus of control, social support and combat related posttraumatic stress disorder: a prospective study' *Journal of Personality and Social Psychology* **55**, 279–285

Spence M J and DeCasper A (1982) 'Human fetuses perceive maternal speech' Paper presented at the Meeting of the International Congress on infant studies, Austin, Texas.

Sperling G (1984) 'A unified theory of attention and signal detection' in R Parasuraman and D R Davies (Eds) *Varieties of Attention* New York: Academic Press

Spielberger C D, Gorsuch R and Lushene R E (1987) *The State-Trait Anxiety Inventory* Windsor, UK: NFER-Nelson

Spitzer R and Williams J D W (1986) *Structured Clinical Interview Schedule for DSM-IIIR* New York State Psychiatric Institute Biometrics Research Division

Sternberg R J (1988) 'Triangulating love' in R J Sternberg and M L Barnes (Eds) *The Psychology of Love* New Haven, CT: Yale University Press

Sternberg R J and Grajek S (1984) 'The nature of love' *Journal of Personality and Social Psychology* **47**, 312–329

Stone B M (1980) 'Sleep and low doses of alcohol' *Electroencephalography and Clinical Neurophysiology* **48**, 706–709

Strack F, Martin L L and Stepper S (1988) 'Inhibiting and facilitating conditions of facial expressions: A non-intrusive test of the facial feedback hypothesis' *Journal of Personality and Social Psychology* **54**, 768–777

Streufert S, Pogash R, Piasecki M and Post G M (1990) 'Age and management team performance' *Psychology and Aging* **5**, 551–559

Stroebe W and Stroebe M S (1986) 'Beyond marriage: The impact of partner loss on health' in R Gilmour and S Duck (Eds) *The Emerging Field of Personal Relationships* Hillsdale, NJ: Lawrence Erlbaum

Sugarman L (1986) *Life-span Development: Concepts, Theories and Interventions* London: Methuen

Suls J and Marco C (1991) 'The self' in R M Baron, W G Graziano and C Stangor (Eds) *Social Psychology* Fort Worth, TX: Holt, Rinehart and Winston

Super C M and Harkness S (1982) 'The development of affect in infancy and child-hood' in D Wagner and H Stevenson (Eds) *Cultural Perspectives on Child Development* San Francisco, CA: W H Freeman

Sutton-Smith B and Rosenberg B (1970) *The Sibling* New York: Holt, Rinehart and Winston

Sweeney P D, Anderson K and Bailey S (1989) 'Attributional style in depression: A meta-analytic review' *Journal of Personality and Social Psychology* **50**, 974–991

Syer J and Connolly C (1984) *Sporting Body, Sporting Mind: An Athlete's Guide to Mental Training* Cambridge, MA: Cambridge University Press

Tamir L M (1982) *Men in Their Forties: The Transition to Middle Age* New York: Springer

Taylor S E (1991) *Health Psychology* (2nd edition) New York: McGraw-Hill

Tesser A and Brodie M (1971) 'A note on the evaluation of a "computer date" *Psychometric Science* **23**, 300

Thibault J W and Kelley H (1967) *The Social Psychology of Groups* New York: Wiley

Thomas A and Chess S (1977) *Temperament and Development* New York: Bruner-Mazel

Thompson A M (1986) 'Adam – a severely deprived Columbian orphan: A case report' *Journal of Child Psychology and Psychiatry* **27**, 689–695

Thompson R A and Lamb M E (1986) 'Infant–mother attachment: New directions for theory and research' in P B Baltes, D L Featherman and R M Lerner (Eds) *Life-span Development and Behaviour, vol. 7* Hillsdale NJ: Lawrence Erlbaum

Thompson R A, Lamb M E and Estes D (1982) 'Stability of infant–mother attachment and its relationship to changing life circumstances in an unselected middle-class sample' *Child Development* **53**, 144–148

Tienari P, Sorri A, Lahti I, Naarala M, Wahlberg K E, Moring J, Pohjola J and Wynne L C (1987) 'Genetic and psychosocial factors in schizophrenia: The Finnish Adoptive Family Study' *Schizophrenia Bulletin* **13**, 477–484

Torrey E F (1992) 'Are we overestimating the genetic contribution to schizophrenia?' *Schizophrenia Bulletin* **18**, 159–170

Trower P, Bryant B and Argyle M (1978) *Social Skill and Mental Health* London: Methuen

Tulving E (1983) *Elements of Episodic Memory* Oxford: Oxford University Press

Tulving E and Thompson D M (1973) 'Encoding specificity and retrieval processes in episodic memory' *Journal of Experimental Psychology* **80**, 352–373

Tversky A and Kahneman D (1973) 'Extensional vs. intuitive reasoning: The conjunction fallacy in probability judgment' *Psychological Review* **90**, 293–315

Tversky A and Kahneman D (1974) 'Judgement under uncertainty: heuristics and biases' *Science* **211**, 453–458

Wagner N E, Schubert H J P and Schubert D S P (1985) 'Family size effects: a revision' *Journal of Genetic Psychology* **146**, 65–78

Walker E F, Harvey P and Perlman D (1988) 'The positive/negative symptom distinction in psychoses: A replication and extension of previous findings' *Journal of Nervous and Mental Disease* **176**, 359–363

Wallbott H and Scherer K (1988) 'How universal and specific is emotional experience? Evidence from 27 countries and five continents' in K Scherer (Ed) *Facets of Emotion: Recent Research* Hillsdale, NJ, Erlbaum

Wallerstein J S, Corbin S B and Lewis J M (1988) 'Children of divorce: a ten year study' in E M Hetherington and J A Rasteh (Eds) *Impact of Divorce, Single-parenting and Step-parenting on Children* Hillsdale, NJ: Erlbaum

Walters W J and Lader M H (1970) 'Hangover effects of hypnotics in man' *Nature* **229**, 637–638

Warr P, Jackson P and Banks M (1988) 'Unemployment and mental health: Some British studies' *Journal of Social Issues* **44**, 47–68

Watkins J G (1989) 'Hypnotic hypermnesia and forensic hypnosis: A cross-examination' *American Journal of Clinical Hypnosis* **32**, 71–83

Webb W B (1974) 'Sleep as an adaptive response' *Perceptual and Motor Skills* **38**, 1023–1027

Webb W B (1975) *Sleep the gentle tyrant* Englewood Cliffs, NJ: Prentice Hall

Weber A L, Harvey J H and Stanley M A (1987) 'The nature and motivations of accounts for failed relationships' in R M Burnett, P McGhee and D Clarke (Eds) *Accounting for relationships: Explanation, Representation and Knowledge* London: Methuen

Wegner D, Shortt J W, Blake A W and Page M S (1990) 'The suppression of exciting thoughts' *Journal of Personality and Social Psychology* **58**, 409–418

Weiner B (1992) *Human Motivation: Metaphors, Theories and Research* Newbury Park, CA: Sage

Weiner R D (1989) 'Electroconvulsive therapy' in H I Kaplan and B J Sadock (Eds) *Comprehensive Textbook of Psychiatry* Vol 5 (5th edn) Baltimore, MD: Williams and Wilkins

Wilkinson (1985) The Assessment of Social Skill of Schizophrenics in Remission Unpublished doctoral thesis, University of Surrey, England

Wilkinson J and Canter S (1982) *Social Skills Training: Assessment, Programme Design and Management of Training* Chichester: Wiley

Williams J M G (1992) 'Autobiographical memory and emotional disorders' in S-A Christianson (Ed) *The Handbook of Emotion and Memory* Hillsdale, NJ: Lawrence Erlbaum Associates

Wolfe J and Lange P (1987) *Fear Survey Schedule* Windsor, UK: NFER-Nelson

Wood A J J (1984) 'Pharmacologic differences between beta blockers' *American Heart Journal* **108**, 1070–1077

Wright C M (1993) Experiences of AIDS-related Bereavement among Gay Men Unpublished MSc dissertation: University of Surrey

Yerkes R M and Dodson J D (1908) 'The relation of strength of stimulus to rapidity of habit formation' *Journal of Comparative Neurological Psychology* **18**, 459–482

Young J E (1990) *Cognitive Therapy for Personality Disorders: A Schema Focused Approach* Sarasota, FL: Professional Resource Exchange

Zajonc R B (1984) 'On the primacy of affect' *American Psychologist* **39**, 117–123

Zajonc R B, Murphy S T and Inglehart M (1989) 'Feeling and Facial efference: Implications of a vascular theory of emotion' *Psychological Review* **96**, 395–416

Glossary of Frequently Used Terms

AFFECT A general term used more-or-less interchangeably with emotion, feeling or mood

AFFECTIVE EXPERIENCE An emotional experience

AROUSAL The overall level of excitation, activation or readiness for activity at any given time in a person or animal

ATTACHMENT An emotional tie, secure or insecure, that develops between infants and their care-givers and are theorized to be related to subsequent development

ATTENTION The focusing of perception giving rise to a heightened awareness of a limited range of stimuli

ATTITUDE A reaction, whether positive or negative, to particular classes of people, objects, social issues, abstract ideas or events

ATTRIBUTION The process by which we attempt to explain the causes of behaviour or events

AUTONOMIC NERVOUS SYSTEM A division of the peripheral nervous system that regulates the activity of the glands and internal organs

BEHAVIOUR Activities, responses, reactions, movements or processes that are observable or can be measured

BEHAVIOURAL PERSPECTIVE An approach that focuses only on observable behaviour and tries to explain it in terms of the organism's interaction with the environment

BIOFEEDBACK A technique that allows individuals to monitor their own bodily functions and learn to control them

BIOLOGICAL PERSPECTIVE An approach that tries to explain behaviour in terms of electrical and chemical impulses particularly within the brain and nervous system

BORDERLINE PERSONALITY DISORDER A personality disorder characterized by serious instability in emotional control, relationships and identity

COGNITION An individual's thoughts, understandings, interpretations, knowledge or ideas

COGNITIVE APPRAISAL   The process of interpreting internal or external events or situations

COGNITIVE PERSPECTIVE   An approach that attempts to explain behaviour in terms of mental processes such as perceiving, remembering, reasoning, and problem-solving

COGNITIVE PROCESSES   The mental processes of perception, memory and information processing involved in acquiring information, making plans and solving problems

COGNITIVE SCHEMA   See **schema**

CONCEPT   A mental grouping of a class of objects or events that are related in some way

CONSCIOUSNESS   An individual's experience of mental awareness including thoughts, perceptions, memories and feelings

CONSTRUCT   Generally speaking, a synonym for concept, in that both are concerned with logical and intellectual creations where there is a relationship between several objects or events

COUNTER-TRANSFERENCE   The analyst's (or therapist's) emotional involvement in the therapeutic process which can involve the therapist's displacement of affect

DATA   The information, often expressed in a numerical form, that results from scientific observation

DEDUCTIVE REASONING   Reasoning from general principles to a particular case

DEFENCE MECHANISMS   In psychoanalytic theory, the habitual and often unconscious psychological strategies used by the ego to avoid or reduce anxiety

DELUSION   A false beliefs firmly held in spite of compelling evidence to the contrary

DENIAL   A defence mechanism that protects the person from unacceptable impulses or ideas

DEVELOPMENTAL TASK   A skill which must be mastered or some personal change that must occur at a particular life stage in order for healthy development to take place

DISSOCIATION   The process that allows certain thoughts, feelings and behaviours to lose their relationship to other aspects of consciousness and occur independently of one another

DRIVE   The motivational state that results from either deprivation of a need, such as food or a drug, or from the presence of some noxious stimulus such as excessive heat or cold, or a loud noise

EGO   In psychoanalytic theory, the executive portion of the personality which is charged with directing rational, realistic behaviour

EMOTION   An innate or acquired response (cognitive, psychological and behavioural) to certain internal or external events that relates to important goals or motives and which motivates the person to take some action

EMOTIONAL AROUSAL   See **arousal**

EMPIRICAL METHOD   Involving the collection and evaluation of data in a systematic way on the basis of some conceptual scheme

ENCODING   The process of putting information into a form that the memory system can accept and use

ENDOCRINE SYSTEM   The system of glands that secrete hormones into the bloodstream and thereby affect many bodily functions

ENVIRONMENT   The sum total of all external conditions and influences affecting the life and development of a person or animal

EXISTENTIAL THERAPY   A therapeutic approach that focuses on the problems of existence, such as death, meaning, choice and responsibility

FIXATION   In Freudian theory, arrested development resulting from anxiety or frustration at a particular stage of psychosexual development

GESTALT THEORY   A humanistic approach to therapy which emphasizes the importance of affective awareness, emotional expression and the integration of fragmented experiences

HEURISTIC   A rule-of-thumb approach to solving problems that involves mental shortcuts

HORMONE   A chemical secreted by the glands of the endocrine system into the bloodstream allowing the gland to stimulate remote cells with which it has no connection

HUMANISTIC PERSPECTIVE   An approach in psychology that emphasizes the uniqueness of the personality which is believed to be created out of each individual's way of perceiving and interpreting the world

HYPOTHESIS   A statement of proposition that serves as a tentative explanation of certain facts and which is presented in such a way as to be amenable to empirical test and either supported or rejected by evidence

ID   In psychoanalytic theory, the unconscious part of the personality that contains primitive drives that demand gratification

IDENTITY   The subjective concept of one's own essential and continuous self

IMPLICIT PERSONALITY THEORY   A person's beliefs about how various traits or behaviours are related to one another

INDIVIDUAL DIFFERENCES   Relatively persistent dissimilarities in traits, characteristics or behaviour

INFORMATION PROCESSING   In cognitive psychology, the process of organizing, interpreting and responding to stimuli

INNATE   Inherited or inborn traits or characteristics

INSTINCT   An innate, automatic, unlearned tendency to respond in a particular way when confronted with a specific stimulus

INTELLIGENCE   The ability to acquire knowledge, to think and reason effectively, to learn from experience and to deal adaptively with the environment

INTRAPSYCHIC   Related to internal covert factors or personality processes that influence behaviour

LEARNING   A relatively permanent change in behaviour or mental processes that occurs as a result of practice or past experience

LIMBIC SYSTEM   A group of brain structures that plays an important part in regulating emotion and memory

LONG-TERM MEMORY   The relatively limitless and permanent component of the memory system

LONGITUDINAL STUDY   A research method that studies the individual over time

MEMORY   The mental processes that allows us to record and retain information about stimuli and retrieve it at a later time

MENTAL MODEL   A cluster of propositions that represents people's understanding of how (usually physical) things work

MENTAL SET   The tendency to approach the solution of a problem in a certain way based on past experience, even though it may not be the most efficient method of solving that problem

MODELLING   Learning through observation and imitation

MOTIVATION   An internal state that activates behaviour or directs it towards some goal

MOTIVE   (1) A state of arousal that drives an organism to action. (2) A rationalization that a person gives as a reason for a particular action

NATURE–NURTURE DEBATE   The longstanding controversy concerning the relative importance of biological and environmental determinants of development

NEUROTRANSMITTER   A chemical substance involved in the transmission of nerve impulses across the synapse from one neuron to another

NORM   (1) What is expected or accepted behaviour in specific situations. (2) Statistically, an average or common standard of a particular group which may be used as a basis of comparison for individual cases

PARASYMPATHETIC NERVOUS SYSTEM   The part of the autonomic nervous system that slows down bodily processes and reduces physiological arousal

PATTERN RECOGNITION   The perceptual process of determining what an object is

PERCEPTION   The process by which sensory input is organized and interpreted by the brain using knowledge, experience and understanding of the world so that sensations become meaningful experiences

PERSONALITY   The distinctive pattern of relatively unchanging psychological and behavioural characteristics that makes each person a unique individual

PERSONALITY DISORDER   Longstanding, inflexible and maladaptive patterns of behaviour and functioning that begins by early adulthood and results in social, emotional or occupational distress to the individual or to others

PHYSIOLOGICAL AROUSAL   See **arousal**

PROJECTION   A defence mechanism whereby people attribute their own undesirable traits to others as a means of protecting themselves

PROPOSITION   A statement that relates objects, events or properties to each other and that asserts something about somebody or something else

PSYCHOACTIVE DRUG   A drug that affects consciousness, mood and behaviour

PSYCHOANALYSIS   The method of psychotherapy originally developed by Freud for treating neurosis

PSYCHOANALYTIC THEORY   Freudian theory of personality that emphasizes unconscious forces and internal conflicts in its explanation of behaviour

PSYCHODYNAMIC PERSPECTIVE   A view of behaviour that focuses on inner causes such as unconscious beliefs, fears and motives

PSYCHOMETRICS   Mathematically based methods for designing and evaluating psychological tests

PSYCHOPATHOLOGY   The manifestation of mental disorder and the study of its causes

PSYCHOPHYSIOLOGY   The study of changes in the functioning of body that result from physiological experience

PSYCHOSEXUAL STAGES   The oral, anal, phallic and genital stages during which, according to Freud's theory of personality development, various personality traits are formed

PSYCHOSIS   Severe mental disorder in which the person is out of contact with reality

PSYCHOSOMATIC DISORDERS   A physical disorder caused by, or greatly exacerbated by, psychological factors

QUALITATIVE DATA   Data that is descriptive, such as what people say in interviews

RATING SCALE   A list of various personality traits or aspects of behaviour on which a person is rated

RECONSTRUCTIVE MEMORY   The process whereby a person's previous experiences are retrieved in terms of the person's reconstruction of events, which can be affected by later experiences

REINFORCEMENT   An event that increases the possibility that a particular response will occur, or that brings about learning

RELIABILITY   (1) The degree to which a test can be repeated with the same results. (2) Diagnostic agreement among clinicians

REPRESSION   (1) The most basic Freudian defence mechanism in which a memory or impulse which might arouse anxiety or guilt is excluded from conscious awareness. (2) A theory of forgetting

RETRIEVAL   The process by which information is brought out of long-term memory

REWARD   Anything that produces pleasure or satisfaction; a positive reinforcer

SAMPLE   A designated group of people (subjects) from whom data are collected in order to draw conclusions about the larger population

SCHEMA   A mental structure stored in memory that provides a framework for interpreting experience

SCRIPT   An abstract cognitive representation or 'schema' of social interactions and situations (for example, asking someone out)

SELF-AWARENESS   Consciousness of oneself as a person

SELF-CONCEPT   The way one thinks about oneself

SELF-CONSCIOUSNESS   A state of heightened self-awareness

SELF-EFFICACY   The belief that one is capable of performing the behaviours necessary to achieve specific goals

SELF-ESTEEM   The degree to which one values oneself

SELF-MONITORING   (1) The process of observing and evaluating one's own behaviour. (2) The tendency to regulate behaviour in accordance to the situation (high self-monitoring) or in accordance to internal factors (low self-monitoring)

SELF-PERCEPTION   A person's awareness of himself or herself. It differs from self-consciousness in that it may take the form of an objective self-appraisal

SELF-SCHEMA   An organized collection of feelings and beliefs about oneself

SENSORY CODING   Codes used by the sense organs to transmit information to the brain

SENSORY REGISTER   The part of the memory system that receives incoming information from the senses and briefly retains it so that it can be interpreted

SHORT-TERM MEMORY   The memory system that holds small amounts of information for relatively brief time periods

SOCIAL COMPARISON   A method of evaluating oneself by comparing oneself with others

SOCIAL IDENTITY   The part of one's identity that is based on group memberships

SOCIAL LEARNING THEORY   An approach to the development of the personality that emphasizes the role of learning through observation and imitation

SOCIAL ROLE   A pattern of behaviour that is expected of someone who occupies a particular position in a social group

SOCIAL SKILLS TRAINING   A method of teaching cognitive and behavioural skills involved in effective social interaction

STEREOTYPE   A rigid and oversimplified impression or schema of an entire group of people that involves the false assumption that all members of the group share the same characteristics

STIMULUS   Any thing or event, internal or external, that has some effect on an organism and that evokes a response

STRESS   (1) The physiological and psychological response that occurs when confronted by a challenge or a threat. (2) A stimulus, event or set of circumstances that place excessive demands on the individual (also referred to as the stressor). (3) A transaction between the stressor and the organism that responds to it

STRESSOR   See **stress**

SUBCONSCIOUS PROCESSES   Stimuli that are registered and evaluated and of which we are not consciously aware

SUPEREGO   In Freud's theory of personality, the part that represents the internalization of values and morals of society that controls the impulses of the id

SUPPRESSION   Conscious exclusion of impulses, thoughts and desires that are felt to be unacceptable to the individual

SURVEY METHOD   A method of obtaining information by questioning a large sample of people

SYMPATHETIC NERVOUS SYSTEM   A division of the autonomic nervous system active in emotional excitement and to some extent antagonistic to the parasympathetic division

SYNAPSE   The microscopic space between neurons across which the nerve impulse must pass

TEMPERAMENT   An individual's characteristic patterns of emotionality and reactions to the environment that are visible from early infancy and appear to be genetically based

THEORY   A set of assumptions that can be used to explain existing data and predict new events

THINKING   The ability to imagine or represent objects or events in memory and to operate on these representations in order to reason, solve problems, make decisions, understand situations etc.

TRAIT   A persisting characteristic or dimension of personality

TRANSFERENCE   In psychoanalysis, clients' unconscious tendency to respond to their therapists as if they were important figures in their life history

UNCONSCIOUS   (1) Contents of the mind that are not accessible to consciousness. (2) In psychoanalytic theory, the part of the mind that is beyond consciousness and contains instinctual drives and repressed material

VALIDITY   (1) The degree to which a test measures what it is supposed to measure. (2) The extent to which diagnostic categories capture actual disordered behaviour patterns

VARIABLE   In an experiment, any specific factor or characteristic that changes or can be made to change

Index